Simplified Student's Notes In OBS/GYN Vol. II

OrangeBooks Publication

1st Floor, Rajhans Arcade, Mall Road, Kohka, Bhilai, Chhattisgarh 490020

Website: **www.orangebooks.in**

© Copyright, 2025, Author

All rights reserved. No part of this book may be reproduced, stored in a retrieval system, or transmitted, in any form by any means, electronic, mechanical, magnetic, optical, chemical, manual, photocopying, recording or otherwise, without the prior written consent of its writer.

First Edition, 2025
ISBN: 978-93-6554-028-4

SIMPLIFIED STUDENT'S NOTES
IN OBS/GYN VOL II

Dr. Vvarsha Sachin Patil

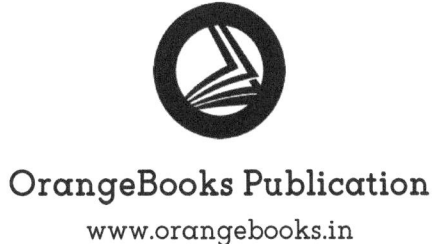

OrangeBooks Publication
www.orangebooks.in

Disclaimer

The author has made every effort to ensure that all information presented in this book is accurate and up-to-date at the time of publication. However, the author does not assume and hereby disclaims any liability to any party for any loss, damage, or disruption caused by errors or omissions, whether such errors or omissions result from negligence, accident, or any other cause.

All images, links, and data included in this book are used for educational and illustrative purposes only. Every attempt has been made to properly credit and cite original sources. If any copyrighted material has been unintentionally included without proper acknowledgment, please contact the author so that the appropriate corrections/ removal can be made in future editions.

External links provided in this book are for the reader's convenience. The author/publisher is not responsible for the content, accuracy, or reliability of any external websites and does not endorse any views expressed therein.

The inclusion of data, case studies, or examples does not imply endorsement of any particular organization, individual, or methodology. Readers are encouraged to critically evaluate the sources and apply their own judgment when interpreting the content.

Index

1	Adolescence	1
2	Amenorrhea	4
3	Basic Terminologies In OBS/GYN	15
4	Benign Tumours Of Overies	28
5	Breast Lump	37
6	Cancer Of Cervix	46
7	Cervical Erosion (Cervical Ectropion)	63
8	Cervical Polyp	71
9	Chemotherapy And Radiotherapy In OB/GYN	78
10	Colposcopy	81
11	Congenital Uterine Anomalies	84
12	Contraception	88
13	Dilatation And Curettage	114
14	Dysfunctional Uterine Bleeding (DUB)	118
15	Dysmenorrhea	124
16	Dyspareunia	130
17	Endometrial Cancer	134
18	Endometrial Polyp	138
19	Endometriosis	144
20	Fibroid Uterus	156
21	Genital Prolapse	174
22	Genital Tuberculosis	185

23	Harmone Replacement Thearapy...	193
24	Hysterectomy	196
25	Infertility	205
26	Leucorrhea	218
27	Malignant Tumours Of Ovary	232
28	Menstrual Cycle	242
29	Menopause & Syndrome	251
30	Menorrhagia	262
31	Metrorrhagia	267
32	New Mechanically Aided Techniques In Male Infertility: Diagnosis & Treatment	272
33	Obstrectric Fistula	279
34	PAP Smear	286
35	Pelvic Inflammatory Disease (PID)	291
36	Pelvic Pains	312
37	Puberity	320
38	Puberity Menorrhagia	329
39	Polycystic Overies	333
40	Retroversion Of Uterus	341
41	Study Methods to Rule Out Ovulation.	347
42	USG In OBS/GYN	359
43	Vaginitis	367
44	Vaginismus	372
45	Various Obstrectric And Gynaecological Procedure	376

Adolescence

Definition of Adolescence

Adolescence is a developmental stage that marks the transition from childhood to adulthood, typically occurring between the ages of 10 and 19. It is characterized by rapid physical, emotional, cognitive, and social changes, as individuals prepare for adulthood.

The World Health Organization (WHO) defines adolescence as the period of life between childhood and maturity, during which individuals experience significant growth and developmental milestones.

Types of Adolescence

Adolescence can be broadly divided into three stages:

1. **Early Adolescence (10-13 years):**
   - Onset of puberty.
   - Development of primary and secondary sexual characteristics.
   - Emergence of abstract thinking begins.

2. **Middle Adolescence (14-17 years):**
   - Heightened emotional and social development.
   - Formation of personal identity.
   - Increased independence from family.

3. **Late Adolescence (18-19 years):**
   - Consolidation of identity and emotional maturity.
   - Preparation for adult roles and responsibilities.
   - Stabilization of physical growth.

Changes Occurring During Adolescence

1. **Physical Changes:**
   - **Puberty:** Hormonal changes triggered by the hypothalamic-pituitary-gonadal axis.
   - Growth spurts in height and weight.
   - Development of sexual organs and secondary sexual characteristics (e.g., breast development, voice deepening).
   - Acne and changes in body composition.

2. **Cognitive Changes:**
   - Development of abstract and logical thinking.
   - Enhanced problem-solving abilities.
   - Increased capacity for planning and decision-making.

3. **Emotional Changes:**
   - Heightened sensitivity to emotions and stress.
   - Mood swings due to hormonal fluctuations.
   - Exploration of self-identity and personal values.

4. **Social Changes:**
   - Peer relationships take precedence over family.
   - Development of intimate and romantic relationships.
   - Increased risk-taking behaviors.

Common Abnormalities in Adolescence

1. **Physical Abnormalities:**
   - **Delayed Puberty:** Failure to start puberty at the expected age.
   - **Precocious Puberty:** Early onset of puberty before the age of 8 in girls and 9 in boys.

2. **Emotional and Behavioral Abnormalities:**
   - Depression and anxiety disorders.
   - Eating disorders (e.g., anorexia nervosa, bulimia nervosa).
   - Substance abuse and addiction.
   - Self-harm or suicidal tendencies.

3. **Cognitive and Learning Abnormalities:**
   - Learning disabilities (e.g., dyslexia, ADHD).
   - Difficulty with executive functioning.

4. **Social and Environmental Issues:**
   - Peer pressure leading to risky behaviors.
   - Social isolation and bullying.

Diagnosis and Management of Adolescent Abnormalities

General Approach:

1. **Assessment:**
   - Comprehensive history-taking (physical, emotional, social, and academic history).
   - Physical examination and growth monitoring.
   - Psychological evaluations using standardized tools.

2. **Investigations:**
   - Hormonal tests for puberty-related issues.
   - Imaging (e.g., X-ray for bone age in delayed puberty).
   - Psychological assessments for mental health conditions.

3. **Management Strategies:**
   - **Medical Management:** Hormonal therapy for puberty abnormalities, medications for mental health disorders.
   - **Psychotherapy:** Cognitive-behavioral therapy (CBT), family therapy, and counseling.
   - **Lifestyle Modifications:** Balanced diet, regular exercise, and stress management techniques.
   - **Educational Support:** Special education plans and accommodations for learning disabilities.

Role of Homoeopathic Remedies in Adolescence

Homeopathy provides a holistic approach to managing various challenges of adolescence by addressing the physical, emotional, and mental aspects of the individual. Key remedies include:

1. **For Physical Complaints:**
   - **Calcarea Phosphorica:** For delayed growth and development, especially during puberty.
   - **Silicea:** For acne and other skin issues.
   - **Pulsatilla:** For hormonal imbalances and irregular menstruation.

2. **For Emotional and Behavioral Issues:**
   - **Ignatia Amara:** For mood swings, grief, and emotional sensitivity.
   - **Natrum Muriaticum:** For depression and social withdrawal.
   - **Stramonium:** For aggressive or violent tendencies.

3. **For Cognitive and Learning Difficulties:**
   - **Lycopodium:** For lack of confidence and poor memory.
   - **Baryta Carbonica:** For delayed mental development and immaturity.
   - **Anacardium Orientale:** For forgetfulness and poor concentration.

4. **For Social and Environmental Stressors:**
   - **Staphysagria:** For issues arising from suppressed emotions or bullying.
   - **Sepia:** For feelings of isolation or disconnection.

Amenorrhea

Definition

Absence of menstruation is amenorrhea.

Factors affecting menstruation cycle-

- **Hypothalamus**: Controls your pituitary gland, which affects ovulation (releasing an egg).
- **Ovaries**: Store and produce the egg for ovulation and the hormones estrogen and progesterone.
- **Uterus**: Responds to the hormones by thickening your uterine lining. This lining sheds as your menstrual period if there's no pregnancy.
- Primary amenorrhea
- Primary amenorrhea is when you haven't gotten your first period by age 15 or within five years of the first signs of puberty .

Types Of Amenorrhea-

Primary amenorrhea

Primary amenorrhea is when you haven't gotten your first period by age 15 or within five years of the first signs of puberty

Common causes are congenital genital and gonadal defects, hormonal disfunctions, chromosomal abnormalities and syndromes.

Secondary amenorrhea

Secondary amenorrhea is when you've been getting regular periods, but you stop getting your period for at least three months

Common Risk factors for amenorrhea include:

- Family history of amenorrhea or early menopause.
- Genetic or chromosomal condition that affects your ovaries or uterus.
- Obesity or being underweight.
- Eating disorder.
- Over-exercising.
- Poor diet.
- Stress.
- Chronic illness.

Aetiology-

Table 1. Major Causes of Amenorrhea

Outflow tract	Pituitary	Hypothalamic	Other endocrine gland disorders
Congenital	Autoimmune disease	Eating disorder	Adrenal disease
Complete androgen resistance	Cocaine	Functional (overall energy deficit)	Adult-onset adrenal hyperplasia
Imperforate hymen	Cushing syndrome		Androgen-secreting tumor
Müllerian agenesis	Empty sella syndrome	Gonadotropin deficiency (e.g., Kallmann syndrome)	Chronic disease
Transverse vaginal septum	Hyperprolactinemia		Constitutional delay of puberty
Acquired	Infiltrative disease (e.g., sarcoidosis)	Infection (e.g., meningitis, tuberculosis, syphilis)	Cushing syndrome
Asherman syndrome (intrauterine synechiae)	Medications	Malabsorption	Ovarian tumors (androgen producing)
Cervical stenosis	Antidepressants	Rapid weight loss (any cause)	Polycystic ovary syndrome (multifactorial)
Primary ovarian insufficiency	Antihistamines		Thyroid disease
Congenital	Antihypertensives	Stress	**Physiologic**
Gonadal dysgenesis (other than Turner syndrome)	Antipsychotics	Traumatic brain injury	Breastfeeding
Turner syndrome or variant	Opiates	Tumor	Contraception
Acquired	Other pituitary or central nervous system tumor		Exogenous androgens
Autoimmune destruction	Prolactinoma		Menopause
Chemotherapy or radiation	Sheehan syndrome		Pregnancy

Information from references 1, 2, and 4 through 11.

Common causes of secondary amenorrhea

Secondary amenorrhea is when you miss your period for three or more months after previously having a normal period. Common causes include:

- Some birth control methods, such as Depo-Provera®, intrauterine devices (IUDs) and certain birth control pills.
- Chemotherapy and radiation therapy for cancer.
- Previous uterine surgery with scarring (for example, if you had a dilation and curettage, often called D&C).
- Stress.
- Poor nutrition.
- Weight changes — extreme weight loss or gain.
- Extreme exercise routines.
- Certain medications-steroids, testesteron derivatives, antipsychiatric drugs, antiepileptic drugs
- Post brain surgery or trauma

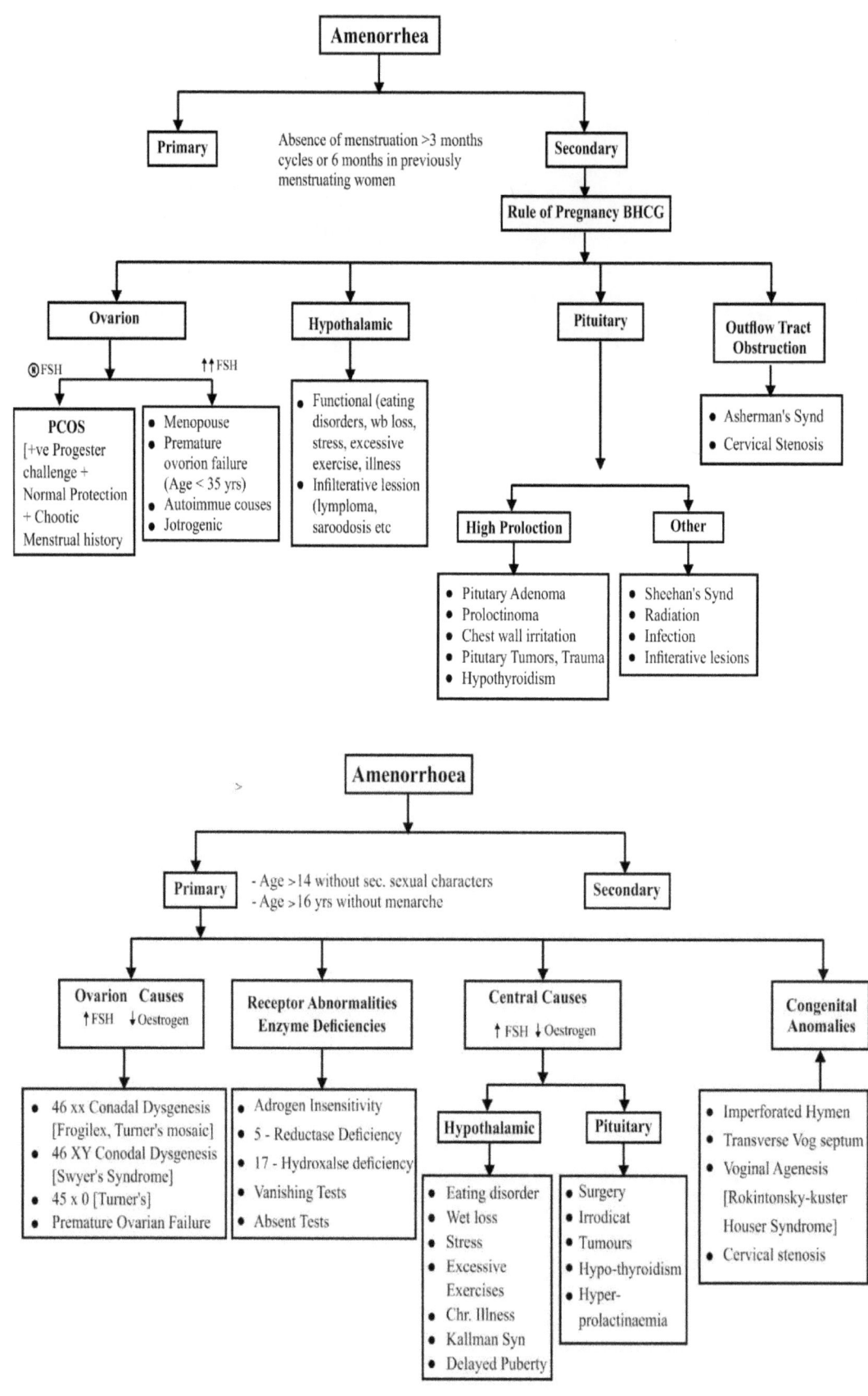

The following medical conditions may also cause secondary amenorrhea:
- Primary ovarian insufficiency (POI), when your ovaries stop working before age 40.
- Hypothalamic amenorrhea, a condition where amenorrhea occurs due to an issue with your hypothalamus.
- Pituitary disorders, such as a benign pituitary tumor or excessive production of prolactin.
- Hormonal imbalances as a result of conditions like polycystic ovary syndrome, adrenal disorders or hypothyroidism.
- Ovarian tumors.
- Obesity.
- Ongoing illness or chronic illness (like kidney disease or inflammatory bowel disease).

Diagnosis / Investigations-

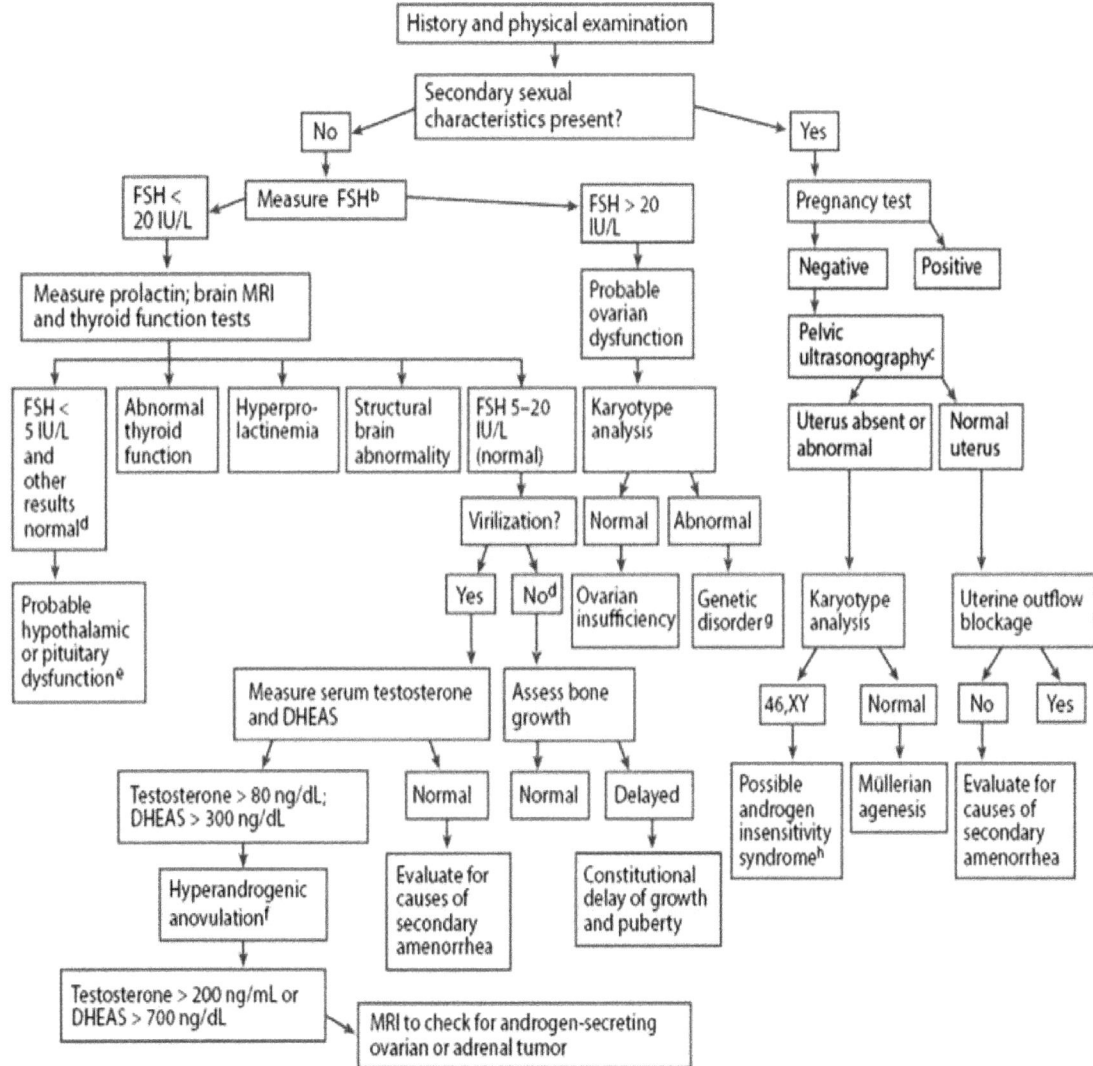

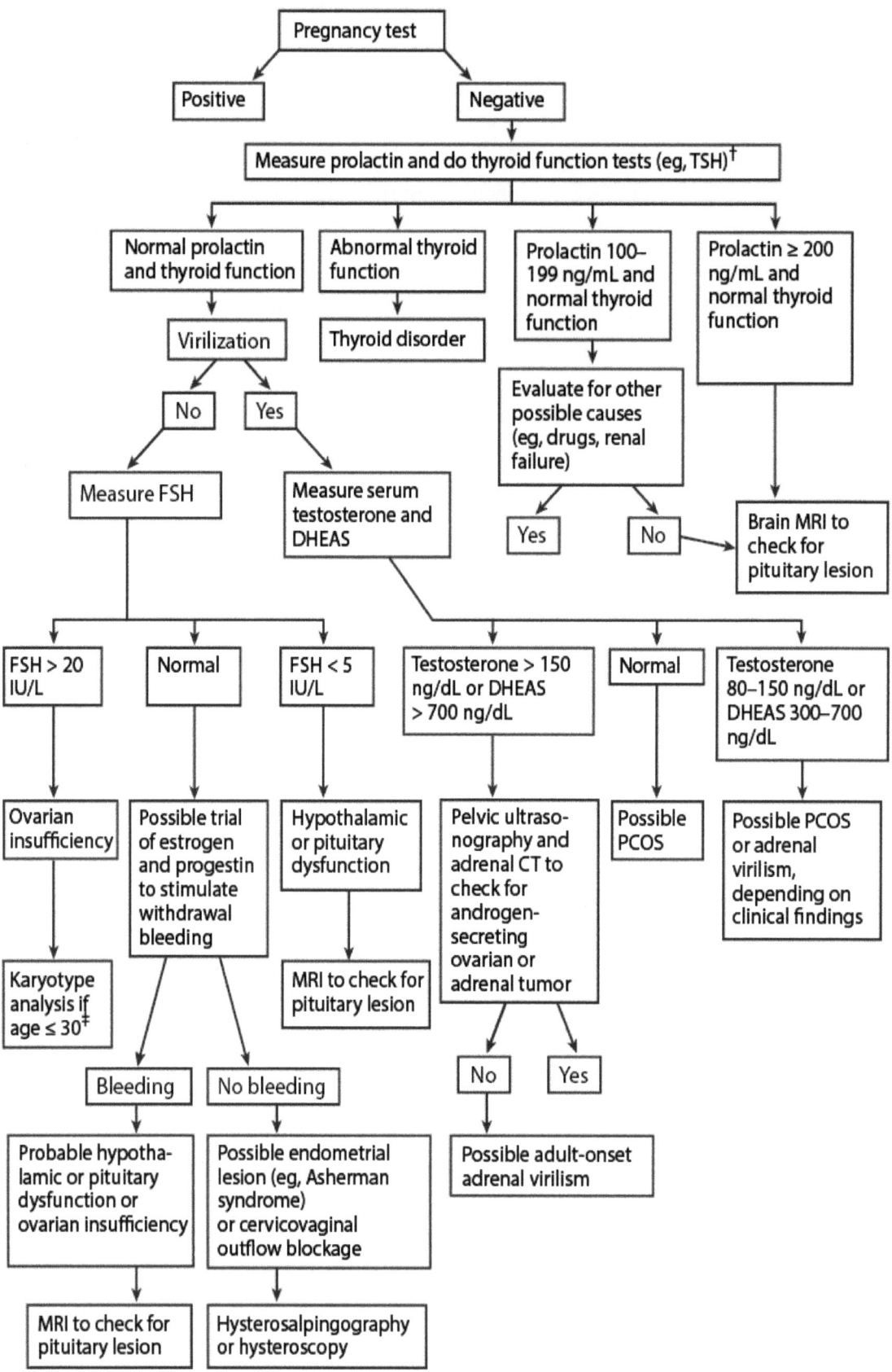

- Clinical history taking to rule out family history, development of sec.sexual characters, mentle stress or trauma or sudden shock.
- BMI
- UPT- For confirmation of pregnancy
- Harmonal assay to find out cause related to thyroid [T3,T4,TSH] harmone disfunctions or LH, FSH, Prolactin imbalance
- AMH level, below normal indicates premature ovarian failure, high than normal indicates PCOD
- USG Abdomen- to rule out structural abnormality of reproductive system e.g, ovarian atropy, small underdeveloped uterus, cryptomenorrhea with transverse uterine septum
- CT /MRI scan to rule out cns causes
- Instrumental investigations like hysteroscopy, laparoscopy to find out congental anomalies regarding reproductive system.
- Karyotyping for genetic abnormality analysis like Turner syndrome

Clinical Features-

Depends on cause of amenorrhea-

e.g, DELAYED PUBERITY- Late appearance of secondary sexual characters, short stature due to absence of hight spert.

POCD- obesity, hirsutism, masculine features like male,pimples over face, moon face,strie marks due to overstretching due to excessiuve fat deposition

PREGNANCY- nausea, vomiting, increased sleep, frequent micturation, mornig sickness, gradual abdominal distention, movement feeling if amenorrhea more than 4 months,

BRAIN TUMOURS- headache, blurred vision, vomiting, vertigo .

HYPOTHYRODISM- Weightgain, cold intolerance, hyperglycemia, oedema, sluggishness in activities, all body metabolism slow, anorexia etc.

MENOPAUSE- Hot flushes, increased perspiration, mood variations, depression, backache, dry vagina, loss of libido, loss of sexual interest.

HYPERPROLACTINEMIA- Milk discharge from nipples

TURNER SYNDROME- short stature, shield thorax, shorten metacarpels, poor breast development which are wide placed, small fingernails, rudimentary or underdeveloped gonads and genitals, brown spots, elbow deformity.

KALLMANN SYNDROME- deficient GnRH and anosmia, bone anomalies, renal anomlies, cleft palate & cleft lip, colour blindness

Management – Treat The Cause

- If cause is physiological like prepubertal, pregnancy, lactation, menopause, no treatment is necessary.

- Obesity management with diet and exercise plan
- Mentle stress management with cauncelling.
- HRT in menopausal syndrome,
- Combined ocpills in hypoestrogenic amenorrhea.
- Only progesterone in eugenic amenorrhea.
- Ocpills, hormonal management according hormonal assay.
- Levothyroxin, Thyronine in hypothyroidism
- Surgical management in CNS tumours, Intact hymen and transverse vaginal septum if cryptomenorrhea.
- Stop overusing of steroids.
- No treatment available for chromosomal anomaly causes.
- If Y chromosome present, gonadectomy

Drug Management of Primary and Secondary Amenorrhea

1. Hormonal Therapy

Drug	Indication	Dosage (Posology)
Estrogen + Progesterone (Oral Combined Hormonal Therapy)	Hypogonadism, Turner Syndrome, Hypothalamic Amenorrhea	Ethinyl Estradiol (20-50 mcg) + Progesterone (Norethindrone 1 mg) daily
Cyclic Progestins	Secondary Amenorrhea (Progesterone Challenge Test)	Medroxyprogesterone Acetate (MPA) 10 mg/day for 10-14 days
Estrogen Replacement Therapy (ERT)	Hypogonadotropic Hypogonadism, Premature Ovarian Insufficiency	Conjugated Estrogens 0.625 mg/day or Estradiol 1-2 mg/day
Progesterone (Micronized)	Secondary Amenorrhea due to PCOS	Micronized Progesterone 200-300 mg/day for 10-14 days per cycle

2. Ovulation Induction Agents (For amenorrhea due to anovulation/PCOS)

Drug	Indication	Dosage
Clomiphene Citrate	PCOS, Ovulation Induction	50 mg/day from Day 2-5 of cycle, max 150 mg/day
Letrozole (Aromatase Inhibitor)	PCOS-related Anovulation	2.5-7.5 mg/day for 5 days starting Day 2 of cycle

Drug	Indication	Dosage
Gonadotropins (FSH, hMG, hCG)	Resistant PCOS, Hypogonadotropic Hypogonadism	FSH 75-150 IU/day SC/IM, followed by hCG 5,000-10,000 IU for ovulation trigger

3. **Dopamine Agonists (For Hyperprolactinemia-Induced Amenorrhea)**

Drug	Indication	Dosage
Cabergoline	Prolactinoma, Hyperprolactinemia	0.25-0.5 mg twice weekly
Bromocriptine	Prolactinoma, Hyperprolactinemia	1.25-2.5 mg/day, max 15 mg/day

4. **Insulin-Sensitizing Agents (For PCOS-related Amenorrhea)**

Drug	Indication	Dosage
Metformin	PCOS with Insulin Resistance	500-2000 mg/day (divided doses)
Myo-Inositol + D-Chiro Inositol	PCOS-related Amenorrhea	2-4 g/day

5. **Surgery (If Indicated)**
   - **Müllerian Agenesis** – Vaginal reconstruction
   - Imperforate Hymen – Hymenotomy
   - **Prolactinoma** – Transsphenoidal surgery if resistant to medical therapy
   - **Asherman's Syndrome** – Hysteroscopic adhesiolysis

Homeopathic Management of Amenorrhea

Remedy	Primary Amenorrhea Indications	Secondary Amenorrhea Indications	Key Symptoms
Pulsatilla Nigricans	Delayed puberty, no menses in young girls, hormonal imbalance	Suppressed menses due to emotions, stress, PCOS	Mild, weeping nature, thirstless, changeable mood
Sepia Officinalis	Late puberty, weak reproductive organs	Secondary amenorrhea from prolapse, hormonal changes, menopause	Indifference to loved ones, bearing-down pains, dislike of company

Remedy	Primary Amenorrhea Indications	Secondary Amenorrhea Indications	Key Symptoms
Cimicifuga Racemosa	Delayed puberty, uterine atony	Amenorrhea from ovarian dysfunction, mental shock	Extreme sadness, headache with menstrual suppression, muscular pain
Graphites	Late menarche in obese girls, delayed puberty	Amenorrhea with obesity, dry skin, sluggish metabolism	Cold, constipated, depressed, tendency to skin eruptions
Kali Carb	No menses in anemic, weak girls	Secondary amenorrhea from exhaustion, anemia, post-delivery	Anxiety, weakness, lower back pain, early waking
Ferrum Metallicum	Delayed puberty with anemia, pale complexion	Amenorrhea due to **severe anemia**, weakness, headaches	Sensitive, palpitations, flushes of heat, intolerance to cold
Lachesis Mutus	Delayed menarche in talkative, overactive girls	Suppressed menses due to hormonal imbalance (PCOS, thyroid issues)	Hot flushes, loquacious, intolerance to tight clothing
Conium Maculatum	Puberty delay due to glandular suppression	Amenorrhea after grief, celibacy, breast lumps	Hard glandular swellings, breast tenderness
Ignatia Amara	Menses absent due to grief, emotional trauma	Secondary amenorrhea due to **shock, stress, bereavement**	Deep sighing, mood swings, lump in throat sensation
Calcarea Carbonica	Late menarche in obese, slow-growing girls	Amenorrhea from thyroid disorders, excessive fatigue	Chilly, sweats on head, craving eggs
Natrum Muriaticum	Absent menses in thin, introverted girls	Suppressed menses due to **grief, sun exposure**	Reserved, weeps alone, headache, craving for salt

Remedy	Primary Amenorrhea Indications	Secondary Amenorrhea Indications	Key Symptoms
Apis Mellifica	No menarche in hot, restless girls	Amenorrhea from ovarian cysts, PCOS	Burning sensation, thirstless, intolerance to heat
Senecio Aureus	Amenorrhea in young girls with underdeveloped uterus	Suppressed periods from stress, overwork	Irritable, urinary complaints, heaviness in pelvis
Thuja Occidentalis	Amenorrhea due to PCOS, vaccine effects	Absent menses in obese, warty skin, cystic conditions	History of vaccination, greasy face, cold extremities
Lilium Tigrinum	Suppressed menses from uterine displacement	Amenorrhea with pelvic congestion, strong sexual desire	Irritable, hurried, bearing down pains
Phosphoric Acid	Delayed puberty in mentally exhausted girls	Amenorrhea after mental shock, loss of fluids, weakness	Apathy, memory loss, premature graying of hair
Ustilago Maydis	No periods with weak ovaries	Amenorrhea from chronic ovarian inflammation, uterine fibroids	Dark, stringy discharge if menses return

Conclusion

- Primary Amenorrhea remedies focus on constitutional support for puberty and glandular development (e.g., Pulsatilla, Graphites, Calcarea Carb).
- Secondary Amenorrhea remedies are chosen based on underlying causes like PCOS (Thuja, Apis, Lachesis), emotional stress (Ignatia, Natrum Mur), or hormonal imbalance (Sepia, Cimicifuga).

Cryptomenorrhea

Defination-

Concealed haemorrhage i.e, menses occurs but remains hidden due to closure of outlet below internal cervical os.

Aetiology-

Primary / Congenital
- Imperforated hymen
- Transverse vaginal septum
- Congenital cervical atresia
- Congenital vagianl aplasia

Secondary / Aquired
- Theurapeutic cervical coniation
- Post radiotherapy
- Cevical cauterization
- Vaginal synachie
- Cervical stenosis

Clinical Features-
- Absence of menstruation.
- Distention of lower abdomen
- Abdominal pains
- pressure symptoms like retention urine, dysurea, constipation, painfull
- Defaecation.
- Uniform globular mass in the abdomen
- Backache
- Bearing down sensation
- O/E-
- P/V; blush membranous bulging of hymen .
- P/A; Severe tenderness

Complications-
- Retrograde menstruation causes hematocolpos, hematometra, Hematosalphinx.

Management-
- Hymenectomy
- Removal of transverse vaginal septum
- F/B Drainage of internal bleed
- Dilatation of cervix in cervical stenosis
- Vaginoplasty in vaginal stenosis or atresia

Basic Terminologies In OBS/GYN

OBSTRETRICS- A branch of science that deals with care of mother and child during pregnancy, labour and post delivery i.e related to pregnancy and products of pregnancy.

GYNAECOLOGY- A branch of science that deals with diseased or pathological conditions of female genital tract.

DECIDUA- Endometrium of pregnant uterus.

PLACENTA / CHORION - A fleshy disc like structure implanted and adherent to maternal uterine wall due to which establishes maternal and faetal connection.

CORD /UMBILICAL CORD- A long tune like structure joining the placenta and umbilicus of baby,containing umbilical vessels for materno.faeto circulation.

FAETUS- A viable conceptive product inside the uterus.i.e, intrauterine baby.

AMNIOTIC SAC- A bag like structure which contains the growing baby during pregnancy.

AMNIOTIC FLUID / LIQUOR- A amino acid rich fluid inside the amniotic sac which surrounds the baby and provides nutritions,protection and space for growing baby.

AFI [AMNIOTIC FLUID INDEX]- The sonografic measurement of amniotic fluid around baby in centimeter.

NORMAL AMNIOTIC FLUID INDEX= 10 TO 15 cm

OLIGOHYDROMNIOS- when AFI is less thsn 10cm

POLYHYDROMNIOS- When AFI is more than 15cm.

AMNIOCENTENSIS- Tapping out of amniotic fluid from amniotic sac.

AMNIOINFUSION- Filling of normal saline in amniotic sac.

PREGNANCY DURATION- 40 TO 42 WKS

ABORTION- Expulsion of product of conception before viability,.

VIABILITY- ability to servive independent with or without life saving supports.

PERIOD OF VIABILITY- After 20 wks.

EARLY ABORTION- When occur in 1st trimaster i.e, in 1st three months of pregnancy.

MIDTERM ABORTION- When it occurs in 2nd trimaster I.e, in middle 3 months of pregnancy.

PRETERM BABY- When viable baby delivered after 28th wk of gestational week but before the completion of 37 wk gestational age.

FULLTERM BABY- When baby delivered between 37th completed wks.G.A . upto 40 wks.G.A.

POST-TERM BABY- When baby delivered after 40WKS. completed wks of G.A.

G.A. [GESTATIONAL AGE]- Age of intrauterine existence of faetus in pregnancy i.e, apporox.duration since the woman's L.M.P.

CERVICAL INCOMPITANCE- Cervical length less than normal i.e, less than 3 cm

CERVICAL STITCH OR LIGATION- A minor cervical procedure in pregnancy of women with cervical incompetence where a circular cervical stitching is done to prevent early delivery.

LABOUR- pains before delivery due to rhythmic contraction and retraction of pregnant uterus.

ANTEPARTUM PERIOD- The duration from conception till starting of true labour pains.

INTRAPARTUM- The duration in between starting of true labour pains till the delivery of baby.

POSTPARTUM- 24HRS. duration following delivery of baby

NEONATE- A newly born baby upto 7th day age.

ASPHYXIA- Inability to breath.

L.M.P.- Last menstrual period..considerating 1st day of menstrual flow.

E.D.D- Expected date of delivery…i.e, 9 months and 7 days counding from L.M.P. i.e, approx.40 wks.

NAGELE'S RULE OF EDD-

Substract 3months from month of L.M.P.and add 7 days in 1st day of L.M.P.

GRAVIDA- It is the number of times ,the mother get conceived ,regardless of whether these pregnancies were carried to term.

NULLIPAROUS OR GRAVIDA '0'- A woman never conceived or never has been pregnant.

PRIMI GRAVIDA OR GRAVIDA '1'- A woman who is pregnant for '1st' time.

MULTIGRAVIDA- A woman has been pregnant for more than one time.

ELDERLY GRAVIDA- When pregnancy occurred in woman above age of 35yrs.

ELDERLY PRIMI GRAVIDA- When pregnancy occurred 1st time in woman with age above 35yrs.

PARITY- It is the number of times of deliveries by woman after the age of viability i.e, beyond 24wks. or baby wt. more than 500gms.

TPAL-

T= The no. of TERM deliveries i.e, G.A.> 37WKS.

P= The no.of PREMATURE deliveries i.e, G.A. > 20wks.but G.A.< 37 wks.

A= No. of spontaneous or theurapeutic ABORTIONS.

L= No.of LIVING CHILD.

GESTATION- It is the carrying of an embryo or faetus inside a female viviparous animal.

MULTIPLE GESTATION- More than one embryo or faetus in the uterus at single time pregnancy.

TRIMESTER- 3 months interval

Ist TRIMESTER- 1ST 3 months period of pregnancy i.e, until 12 to 13 wks of pregnancy.

IInd TRIMESTER- Middle 3 months of pregnancy i.e, from 12-13 wks of pregnancy to 28th wks of pregnancy.

III rd TRIMESTER- Last 3 months of pregnancy i.e, from 28th wks to time of delivery.
PRESENTATION- It is the anatomical part of faetus which is leading closet to pelvic inlet of birth canal just before birth.
e.g, vertex , breech, shoulder

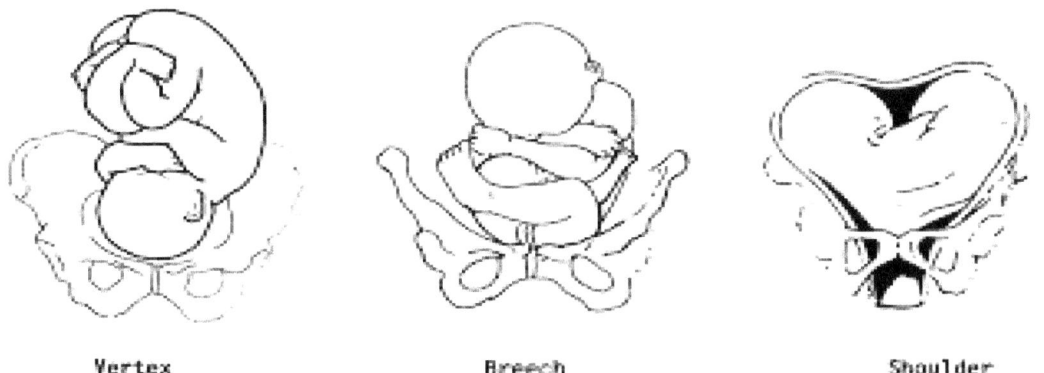

Vertex   Breech   Shoulder

Vertex is the normal presentation.
MALPRESENTATION- Any other presentation than the vertex presentation is called malpresentation.
LIE- Relationship of longitudinal axis of faetus to longitudinal axis of the maternal pelvis.

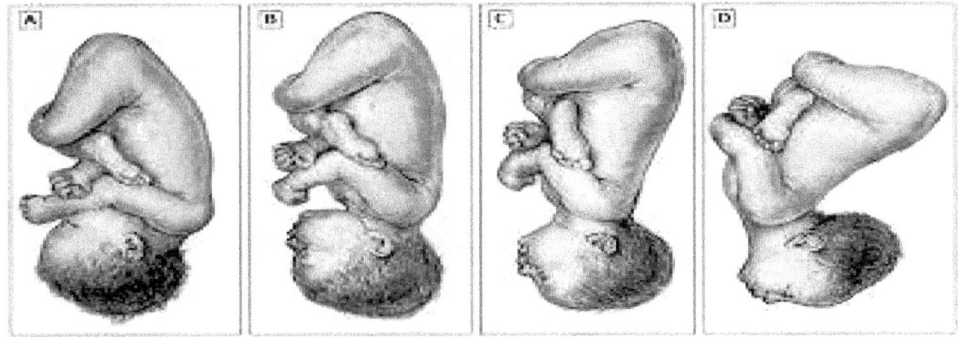

longitudinal lie- flexed ,deflexexed , extended and face
It is the most common lie of faetus.

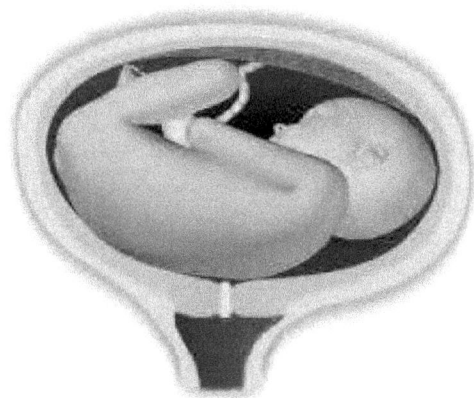

Transverse lie

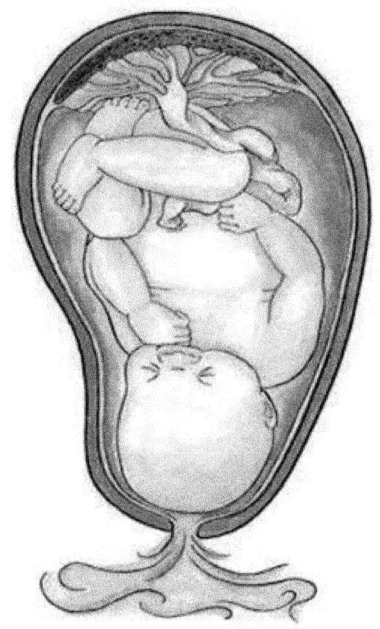

Oblique lie

Most common lie is longitudinal lie.

VARIETY-

The relation of the given portion of the presenting part to the anterior and /or posterior portion of mother's pelvis.

ATTITUDE-

It is the relationship of different parts of fetus to each other.

Normal is flexed attitude.

ENGAGEMENT-

When the widest part of presenting part of fetus has passed successfully through the pelvic inlet is called engagement.

If more than $2/5^{th}$ of fetal head is palpable abdominally the head is not yet engaged.

MOULDING-

Process of elective reduchan of diameter of fetal skull during process of vaginal delivery through maternal pelvis without harming the fetal brain.

EFFACEMENT-

Process of shortening of cervical os as it get included in lower segment of uterus.

EPISIOTOMY-

Surgically planned incision on perineum and posterior vaginal wall during II nd stage of labour just before fetal

head crowning.

CRL –

Crown to Rump length. Measurement from top of baby's head to buttocks.

CHADWICK'S SIGN-
Bluish or purple discolouration of vagina and cervix during pregnancy.

NSVD -
Normal spontaneous vaginal delivery.

CAESAREAN SECTION-
Delivary of boby through an abdominal incision.

*Primary Cesarean Section-
1st time a mother delivered by caesarean.

*Secondary Cesandin Section -
Mother has repeted caesarian section with H/O previous caesarian.

VBAC -Vaginal delivery after caesarian.

TOL- Trial of labour
Women who has previous H/O caesarian and wants VBAC called as she is going to trial of labour when her contractions starts.

VDD (VAD) – Voccum Assisted Delivery
When baby is low in pelvis, but mother is too exhausted to bear down during labour, the vaginal delivery assisted with application of suction cup to baby's head is called as VAD.

MISCARRIAGE / ABORTION-
Spontaneous end of pregnancy before viability i.e;before 24 wks.

*Threatened Abortion-
The process of abortion is started but yet not reach to conditions from where continuation of pregnancy is impossible.

*Inevitable Abortion-
The process of abortion is reached to a level from which continuation preg is impossible.

*Complete Abortion-
Where the whole conceptive product is aborted as a mass.

*Incomplete Abortion-
Abortion where the partial conceptive product is expelled out from uterus while partial remains inside.

*Missed Abortion-
Condition where the fetus is dead and yet not expelled out for more than 4 wks.

*Septic Abortion-Any process of abotion get complicated with secondary infections to female genitals is called septic abortion.

*Recurrent Or Habitual Abortion-
Three or more consequent miscarriages in mothers.

*Illegal Abortion-
Any abortion against MTP rules.

*Legal Abortion –

Any abortion according to MTP rules.

STILL BIRTH -

Baby without vital functions of birth though born after period of viability.

ECTOPIC PREGNANCY / (ECCYSIS)-

Pregnancy where embryo implants outside the uterine cavity.

*Tubal Pregnancy-

Ectopic type of pregnancy where embryo implants in follipian tubes.

*Non tubal Ectopic Pregnancy-

Ectopic pregnancy, where embryo implants other than follipian tubes.

*Heterotopic Pregnancy -

Twin pregnancy where one is intrauterine pregnancy and another is ectopic pregnancy.

*Persistant Ectopic Pregnancy-

Continuation of trophoblastic growth even after surgical intervention to remove an ectopic pregnancy.

HYPEREMESIS GRAVIDUM -

Severe type of vomiting during pregnancy which detoriates the maternal and faetal health.

SIMPLE VOMITTING-

Vomitting during pregnancy without any health detoriation of mother & child .

PRURITUS GRAVIDUM-

Itching during pregnancy.

POSTNATAL BLUES-

Mild depression after delivery.

POSTPAR DUM DEPRESSION-

Depression after delivery.

MONTAGOMERRY'S TUBERCLES-

Elevated sebaceous glands around nipples during pregnancy.

SECONDARY AERIOLA-

Pigmented aeriola development around primary aeriola of breast during pregnancy.

STRIAE GRAVIDUM-

Stretch marks during pregnancy.

LINEA NIGRA-

Dark brown verticle pigmentation from xyphisternum to pubic symphysis due to increased melanine synthesis during pregnancy.

Obstetrics (OB) Terminologies

1. **Abortion** - Termination of a pregnancy.
2. **Amniotic Fluid** - Fluid surrounding the fetus in the womb.
3. **Amniocentesis** - A procedure to extract amniotic fluid for testing.
4. **Antepartum** - The period before labor.

5. **Artificial Insemination** - Insertion of sperm into the female reproductive system for conception.
6. **Breech Presentation** - When the baby is positioned feet-first during birth.
7. **Cesarean Section (C-Section)** - Surgical delivery of the baby.
8. **Chorionic Villus Sampling (CVS)** - Prenatal test to detect genetic conditions.
9. **Conception** - The fertilization of an egg by sperm.
10. **Crowning** - The appearance of the baby's head at the vaginal opening during delivery.
11. **Eclampsia** - Severe complications of preeclampsia involving seizures.
12. **Ectopic Pregnancy** - Pregnancy occurring outside the uterus, typically in a fallopian tube.
13. **Elective Cesarean** - A scheduled cesarean without medical necessity.
14. **Endometriosis** - Condition where tissue similar to the uterus lining grows outside it.
15. **Episiotomy** - Surgical cut made in the perineum during childbirth.
16. **Fetal Heart Rate (FHR)** - The heartbeats per minute of the fetus.
17. **Fetal Movement** - The feeling of the baby moving inside the womb.
18. **Fetal Monitoring** - Watching the baby's heart rate and other vital signs.
19. **Gestation** - The period of pregnancy.
20. **Gestational Diabetes** - Diabetes that occurs during pregnancy.
21. **HCG (Human Chorionic Gonadotropin)** - A hormone produced during pregnancy.
22. **Hematoma** - A collection of blood outside blood vessels, commonly after labor.
23. **Hydatidiform Mole** - A type of molar pregnancy.
24. **Induction of Labor** - Stimulating labor before it starts naturally.
25. **Intrauterine Device (IUD)** - A contraceptive device placed in the uterus.
26. **Intrapartum** - The period during labor.
27. **Labor** - The process of childbirth involving contractions.
28. **Lactation** - Milk production after childbirth.
29. **Laparotomy** - Surgical procedure involving an incision in the abdomen.
30. **Low Birth Weight** - When a baby weighs less than 5.5 pounds at birth.
31. **Multiple Gestation** - Pregnancy involving more than one fetus.
32. **Nuchal Cord** - The umbilical cord wrapped around the baby's neck.
33. **Obstetrician** - A doctor specializing in pregnancy and childbirth.
34. **Oligohydramnios** - Low amniotic fluid levels during pregnancy.
35. **Placenta** - The organ that connects the fetus to the uterine wall.
36. **Placenta Previa** - A condition where the placenta covers the cervix.
37. **Placental Abruption** - Premature separation of the placenta from the uterus.

38. **Polyhydramnios** - Excessive amniotic fluid during pregnancy.
39. **Pre-eclampsia** - High blood pressure during pregnancy with organ damage.
40. **Premature Rupture of Membranes (PROM)** - Breaking of the water (amniotic sac) before labor begins.
41. **Preterm Birth** - A birth before 37 weeks of pregnancy.
42. **Prostaglandins** - Hormones that aid in labor contractions.
43. **Preeclampsia** - A pregnancy complication with high blood pressure.
44. **Postpartum** - The period after childbirth.
45. **Postpartum Hemorrhage** - Excessive bleeding after childbirth.
46. **Postterm Pregnancy** - Pregnancy that lasts longer than 42 weeks.
47. **Pregnancy Test** - A test to confirm pregnancy.
48. **Quickening** - The first movements of the fetus felt by the mother.
49. **Rh Factor** - A protein on red blood cells that can affect pregnancy if mismatched.
50. **Spontaneous Abortion** - A miscarriage or unplanned abortion.
51. **Tocolytics** - Medications to stop premature labor.
52. **Ultrasound** - An imaging technique to visualize the fetus in the womb.
53. **Umbilical Cord** - The cord that connects the fetus to the placenta.
54. **Urinary Tract Infection (UTI)** - A common infection during pregnancy.
55. **Vaginal Birth After Cesarean (VBAC)** - Vaginal delivery after a cesarean section.
56. **Vertex Presentation** - A position where the baby's head is down in the womb.
57. **Vernix Caseosa** - A protective coating on the skin of the fetus.
58. **Vulvar Varicosities** - Swollen veins around the vulva during pregnancy.
59. **Water Breaking** - The rupture of the amniotic sac before labor.
60. **Zygote** - A fertilized egg before it divides into multiple cells.
61. **Fetal Distress** - Abnormal signs indicating the fetus may not be coping well in the womb.
62. **Oxygenation** - The process of delivering oxygen to the fetus.
63. **Chorioamnionitis** - Infection of the amniotic sac and membranes.
64. **Cervical Ripening** - The process of softening and thinning the cervix before labor.
65. **Cord Prolapse** - When the umbilical cord slips into the vagina before the baby.
66. **Dilation and Curettage (D&C)** - A procedure to remove tissue from the uterus.
67. **Fertility Preservation** - Storing eggs or sperm for future use.
68. **Fetal Growth Restriction (FGR)** - Poor growth of the fetus in the womb.
69. **Induction of Labor** - Stimulating labor with medications.
70. **Meconium** - The first stool passed by a newborn.
71. **Morning Sickness** - Nausea and vomiting during pregnancy.
72. **Multigravida** - A woman who has been pregnant more than once.

73. **Nullipara** - A woman who has never given birth.
74. **Obstetric Ultrasound** - An ultrasound performed to monitor pregnancy.
75. **Oxytocin** - A hormone that triggers labor contractions.
76. **Postpartum Depression** - Depression occurring after childbirth.
77. **Preterm Labor** - Labor that occurs before 37 weeks of pregnancy.
78. **Prenatal Vitamins** - Supplements taken during pregnancy to support fetal development.
79. **Radial Cesarean** - A cesarean performed using a specific incision type.
80. **Sacrospinous Ligament** - Ligaments that support the uterus.
81. **Suture** - Stitches used to close incisions after a C-section.
82. **Term Pregnancy** - Pregnancy between 37 and 42 weeks.
83. **Thrombophilia** - A condition where blood clots form more easily.
84. **Vaginal Discharge** - Fluid secreted by the vagina during pregnancy.
85. **Vaginal Tears** - Tears that occur during vaginal delivery.
86. **Vertebral Deformities** - Abnormalities in the spine of a fetus.
87. **Wharton's Jelly** - The substance within the umbilical cord.
88. **Umbilical Artery Doppler** - A test measuring blood flow in the umbilical cord.
89. **Vasopressors** - Medications that constrict blood vessels, used in labor to manage low blood pressure.
90. **Vaginal Bleeding** - Bleeding during pregnancy or labor.
91. **Weight Gain** - Normal weight increase during pregnancy.
92. **Urinary Retention** - Difficulty urinating after childbirth.
93. **Transabdominal Ultrasound** - An ultrasound done on the abdomen.
94. **Transvaginal Ultrasound** - An ultrasound done through the vagina for better imaging.
95. **Preeclampsia Screening** - Tests to check for signs of preeclampsia.
96. **Apgar Score** - A system used to assess the health of a newborn immediately after birth.
97. **Maternity Care** - Health care provided to a pregnant woman before, during, and after birth.
98. **Labor Pain Management** - Methods to reduce pain during labor, such as epidurals or medication.
99. **Umbilical Vein** - The vein in the umbilical cord that carries oxygenated blood to the fetus.
100. **Placental Insufficiency** - When the placenta does not provide enough nutrients and oxygen to the fetus.

Gynecology (GYN) Terminologies

1. **Amenorrhea** - The absence of menstruation.
2. **Adenomyosis** - A condition where the inner lining of the uterus breaks through the muscle wall.
3. **Cervical Dysplasia** - Abnormal growth of cells on the cervix that could lead to cancer.
4. **Cervicitis** - Inflammation of the cervix.
5. **Colposcopy** - A procedure to examine the cervix using a magnifying instrument.
6. **Contraception** - Methods to prevent pregnancy.
7. **Dysmenorrhea** - Painful menstruation.
8. **Endometrial Biopsy** - A procedure to remove a small sample of tissue from the lining of the uterus.
9. **Endometriosis** - A condition where tissue similar to the uterine lining grows outside the uterus.
10. **Fibroids** - Noncancerous growths in the uterus.
11. **Hysterectomy** - Surgical removal of the uterus.
12. **Hysteroscopy** - A procedure to examine the inside of the uterus.
13. **IUD (Intrauterine Device)** - A device placed in the uterus to prevent pregnancy.
14. **Laparoscopy** - A minimally invasive surgery to view or treat the pelvic organs.
15. **Luteal Phase** - The phase in the menstrual cycle after ovulation.
16. **Menarche** - A woman's first menstrual period.
17. **Menopause** - The cessation of menstruation, typically occurring in the late 40s or early 50s.
18. **Menorrhagia** - Abnormally heavy menstrual bleeding.
19. **Metrorrhagia** - Abnormal bleeding between menstrual periods.
20. **Myomectomy** - Removal of uterine fibroids.
21. **Oophorectomy** - Surgical removal of an ovary.
22. **Ovarian Cyst** - A fluid-filled sac within or on an ovary.
23. **Pelvic Inflammatory Disease (PID)** - Infection of the female reproductive organs.
24. **Pelvic Ultrasound** - An imaging technique to visualize pelvic organs.
25. **Pap Smear** - A test to detect abnormal cells in the cervix.
26. **Polycystic Ovary Syndrome (PCOS)** - A condition where the ovaries develop cysts and hormonal imbalance occurs.
27. **Prolapsed Uterus** - When the uterus drops into the vaginal canal due to weakened pelvic muscles.
28. **Salpingectomy** - Removal of a fallopian tube.
29. **Sterility** - The inability to conceive.

30. **Tubo-Ovarian Abscess** - A collection of pus in the fallopian tube and ovary, usually due to infection.
31. **Ulcerative Vulvitis** - Inflammation and ulceration of the vulva.
32. **Urinary Incontinence** - Involuntary leakage of urine.
33. **Uterine Cancer** - Cancer that begins in the uterus, often the endometrium.
34. **Vaginitis** - Inflammation of the vagina, often due to infection.
35. **Vulvovaginal Atrophy** - Thinning of the vaginal and vulvar tissues, often due to menopause.
36. **Vulvodynia** - Chronic pain around the vulva without an identifiable cause.
37. **Menstrual Cycle** - The monthly process of ovulation and menstruation.
38. **Cystocele** - A condition where the bladder bulges into the vaginal space.
39. **Rectocele** - A bulging of the rectum into the vagina.
40. **Bartholin's Gland Abscess** - An infection of the Bartholin's gland near the vaginal opening.
41. **Bacterial Vaginosis** - An imbalance of vaginal bacteria leading to infections.
42. **Chlamydia** - A sexually transmitted infection.
43. **Genital Warts** - Growths caused by the human papillomavirus (HPV).
44. **HIV** - A virus that attacks the immune system and is transmitted sexually.
45. **Herpes Simplex Virus (HSV)** - A virus causing sores in the genital area.
46. **Lymphogranuloma Venereum** - A sexually transmitted disease caused by certain types of chlamydia.
47. **Papilloma** - A benign tumor of epithelial tissue.
48. **Perimenopause** - The transition phase before menopause, involving hormonal changes.
49. **Polycystic Ovarian Syndrome (PCOS)** - A hormonal disorder causing enlarged ovaries with cysts.
50. **Progestin** - A synthetic version of progesterone used in birth control.
51. **Sexually Transmitted Infections (STIs)** - Infections transmitted through sexual contact.
52. **Endometrial Cancer** - Cancer that develops in the lining of the uterus.
53. **Fibrocystic Breast Disease** - Noncancerous changes in the breast tissue.
54. **Bilateral Salpingectomy** - Removal of both fallopian tubes.
55. **Prolapse** - The downward displacement of an organ, such as the uterus.
56. **Vaginal Discharge** - Fluid secreted by the vagina, often indicating infection or hormonal changes.
57. **Vulvectomy** - Surgical removal of the vulva.
58. **Vulvar Cancer** - Cancer occurring in the external female genitalia.
59. **Cervical Cancer** - Cancer originating from the cervix, often linked to HPV infection.

60. **Dysfunctional Uterine Bleeding** - Abnormal bleeding not related to the menstrual cycle.
61. **Ovarian Cancer** - Cancer originating in the ovaries.
62. **Pelvic Exam** - A physical examination of the pelvic organs.
63. **Pessary** - A device inserted into the vagina to support the uterus or bladder.
64. **Progestogen** - A class of hormones that includes progesterone.
65. **Uterine Polyps** - Abnormal tissue growths in the uterus.
66. **Vulvar Disorders** - Conditions affecting the external female genitalia.
67. **Fertility Preservation** - Methods to save eggs, sperm, or embryos for future conception.
68. **Uterine Fibroids** - Non-cancerous tumors in the uterus.
69. **Fibrocystic Changes** - Breast changes that can cause lumps and pain.
70. **Chronic Pelvic Pain** - Long-lasting pain in the lower abdomen or pelvis.
71. **Menstrual Disorders** - Abnormalities in the frequency or characteristics of menstruation.
72. **Vulvar Infections** - Infections affecting the external genitalia.
73. **Endometrial Hyperplasia** - Thickening of the uterus lining, which can lead to cancer.
74. **Steroid Therapy** - The use of steroid hormones to treat various gynecological conditions.
75. **Laparotomy** - A surgical procedure involving a large incision to access abdominal organs.
76. **Vaginal Tightening** - Surgical or non-surgical methods to reduce vaginal looseness.
77. **Gonorrhea** - A bacterial sexually transmitted infection.
78. **Chronic Vaginal Infections** - Recurrent infections affecting the vaginal area.
79. **Cervical Polyp** - A growth on the cervix that can cause irregular bleeding.
80. **Pelvic Floor Dysfunction** - Difficulty controlling pelvic organs.
81. **Cystectomy** - Surgical removal of a cyst.
82. **Vaginal Atrophy** - Thinning and dryness of vaginal tissues, typically post-menopause.
83. **Endometrial Ablation** - A procedure to remove or destroy the uterine lining.
84. **Post-coital Bleeding** - Bleeding after sexual intercourse.
85. **Tubal Ligation** - A form of permanent birth control where the fallopian tubes are blocked or removed.
86. **Ovarian Reserve** - The number and quality of a woman's eggs.
87. **Fertility Treatment** - Medical interventions to help a woman conceive.
88. **In Vitro Fertilization (IVF)** - A process where eggs are fertilized outside the body and implanted in the uterus.

89. **Fertility Drugs** - Medications to stimulate ovulation.
90. **Uterine Artery Embolization** - A procedure used to treat fibroids.
91. **Pelvic Organ Prolapse** - When pelvic organs shift or bulge into the vaginal space.
92. **Torsion of the Ovary** - Twisting of the ovary, often causing severe pain.
93. **Endometrial Scraping** - Removal of tissue from the uterine lining for diagnostic purposes.
94. **Urinary Retention** - Difficulty in urinating.
95. **Cervical Insufficiency** - Weakness of the cervix that can lead to miscarriage or preterm birth.
96. **Interstitial Cystitis** - Chronic bladder pain syndrome.
97. **Fistula** - An abnormal connection between organs, such as between the vagina and rectum.
98. **Uterine Abnormalities** - Structural defects in the uterus, including septum or fibroids.
99. **Vulvar Dermatoses** - Skin disorders affecting the vulva.
100. **Neonatal Resuscitation** - Emergency procedures to assist newborns with breathing or heart function.

Benign Tumours Of Overies

DEF-Non malignant growth of overy.

Types of Benign Ovarian Tumors

Benign ovarian tumors can be classified into surface epithelial tumors, germ cell tumors, stromal tumors, and cystic tumors.

1. Surface Epithelial Tumors

These tumors arise from the epithelial lining of the ovarian surface. They are the most common type of ovarian tumor.

Types:

- **Serous Cystadenoma**: The most common type of benign ovarian tumor, often unilateral.
- **Mucinous Cystadenoma**: Characterized by mucus-producing cells. These tumors can grow large and may be bilateral.
- **Endometrioma (Chocolate Cyst)**: Caused by endometriosis, where endometrial tissue forms cysts on the ovaries.
- **Brenner Tumor**: Rare and typically asymptomatic, characterized by transitional cells.

Etiology:

- Genetic factors, hormonal influences, and a history of endometriosis can contribute to their development.

Clinical Features:

- Abdominal discomfort or bloating.
- Pelvic pain or pressure.
- Menstrual irregularities, especially with endometrioma.
- Unilateral mass felt on pelvic examination.

Complications:

- Torsion of the tumor (especially with large cysts).
- Rupture leading to peritonitis.
- Progressive enlargement can lead to infertility.

Diagnosis:

- **Ultrasound** (most common): Shows cystic nature, septation, and size of the tumor.
- **CT Scan/MRI**: For further assessment of complex tumors or large tumors.

- **CA-125**: A marker for ovarian cancers, though not typically elevated in benign tumors.

Management:
- **Surgical removal** (usually laparoscopic) if symptomatic or growing.
- Observation for smaller, asymptomatic cysts.
- In cases of endometrioma, hormonal therapy to prevent recurrence.

2. Germ Cell Tumors

Germ cell tumors originate from the reproductive cells of the ovary and are more common in younger women.

Types:
- **Teratoma (Dermoid Cyst)**: The most common type, containing various tissues (hair, teeth, fat).
- **Dysgerminoma**: A rare but important tumor that can be benign or malignant.
- **Endodermal Sinus Tumor**: Rare, typically found in younger women.
- **Embryonal Carcinoma**: Very rare, often malignant.

Etiology:
- Typically arise from abnormal development of the ovary's germ cells during fetal development.
- Associated with **gonadal dysgenesis** and **Turner syndrome** in some cases.

Clinical Features:
- **Teratomas**: Often asymptomatic, but large tumors may cause abdominal pain, distension, or torsion.
- **Dysgerminomas**: Can present with abdominal or pelvic pain, and often produce a palpable mass.

Complications:
- Torsion of teratomas.
- Rupture leading to peritonitis.
- Some germ cell tumors may have malignant potential (e.g., dysgerminoma).

Diagnosis:
- **Ultrasound**: Teratomas show a characteristic "tip of the iceberg" sign (solid and cystic components).
- Serum Tumor Markers: Elevated alpha-fetoprotein (AFP) and human chorionic gonadotropin (hCG) can be elevated in some germ cell tumors.
- **CT/MRI**: To evaluate the size, location, and complexity of the tumor.

Management:
- **Surgical removal** (typically cystectomy or oophorectomy).
- **Chemotherapy**: For certain malignant germ cell tumors (e.g., dysgerminoma).
- Fertility-sparing surgery may be an option, especially in young women.

3. Stromal Tumors

Stromal tumors arise from the ovarian stroma (the connective tissue and supporting structures).

Types:
- **Thecoma**: A hormone-producing tumor that secretes estrogen.
- **Fibroma**: A benign, solid tumor that is often asymptomatic.
- **Granulosa Cell Tumor**: Typically benign, produces estrogen, and can present with symptoms of estrogen excess.

Etiology:
- Hormonal imbalance, especially in granulosa cell tumors, which secrete estrogen.
- Genetic mutations, such as in **Leydig cell tumors** (which may secrete testosterone).

Clinical Features:
- **Granulosa Cell Tumors**: Menstrual irregularities, postmenopausal bleeding, and signs of estrogen excess (breast tenderness, endometrial hyperplasia).
- **Thecoma and Fibroma**: May present with abdominal pain or pressure, especially if large.

Complications:
- Torsion, especially in large fibromas or granulosa cell tumors.
- Hormonal effects (e.g., precocious puberty, endometrial hyperplasia).
- **Malignant transformation**: Rare but possible in granulosa cell tumors.

Diagnosis:
- **Ultrasound**: Solid or mixed solid/cystic masses with characteristic features.
- **Serum Inhibin A and B**: Elevated in granulosa cell tumors.
- **CA-125**: Elevated in some tumors, especially with large masses or in postmenopausal women.

Management:
- **Surgical removal** (oophorectomy or cystectomy).
- Hormonal therapy for symptomatic tumors (e.g., progesterone for estrogen-secreting tumors).
- **Follow-up**: Granulosa cell tumors require long-term follow-up due to the risk of recurrence.

4. Cystic Tumors

These are benign tumors that form cysts within the ovaries and may be filled with fluid or semi-solid material.

Types:
- **Follicular Cyst**: Develops when a follicle does not rupture during ovulation, leading to a cystic structure.
- **Corpus Luteum Cyst**: Develops when the corpus luteum (formed after ovulation) fills with fluid instead of degenerating.

Etiology:
- Hormonal imbalances, especially during the reproductive years.
- Common during the menstrual cycle (e.g., during ovulation or luteal phase).

Clinical Features:
- Often asymptomatic and detected incidentally on ultrasound.
- May cause pelvic pain if large or if rupture occurs.

Complications:
- Torsion, especially with larger cysts.
- Rupture, leading to bleeding and peritonitis.
- **Hemorrhagic cysts**: Can cause acute abdominal pain due to bleeding within the cyst.

Diagnosis:
- **Ultrasound**: Simple cysts are usually clear and unilocular, while hemorrhagic cysts may have internal echoes.
- **Serum hCG**: To rule out pregnancy (especially if the cyst is suspected to be corpus luteum cyst).

Management:
- **Observation** for smaller, asymptomatic cysts (many resolve spontaneously).
- **Surgical intervention** (cystectomy or oophorectomy) for large or symptomatic cysts.
- Hormonal treatment to prevent recurrence in some cases.

Common Key Points-
1. **Etiology**: Benign ovarian tumors are often due to hormonal imbalances, abnormal ovarian development, or genetic factors.
2. **Types**: Include surface epithelial tumors (e.g., serous cystadenomas), germ cell tumors (e.g., teratomas), stromal tumors (e.g., granulosa cell tumors), and cystic tumors (e.g., follicular cysts).

3. **Clinical Features**: Symptoms include pelvic pain, bloating, menstrual irregularities, and a palpable mass. Some tumors may be asymptomatic.
4. **Complications**: Torsion, rupture, bleeding, and hormone-related issues (e.g., endometrial hyperplasia or precocious puberty).
5. **Diagnosis**: Primarily done through ultrasound, CT/MRI, and serum markers (e.g., CA-125, AFP, hCG).
6. **Management**: Includes observation for small, asymptomatic tumors, and surgical removal (cystectomy or oophorectomy) for larger or symptomatic tumors. Fertility-sparing surgery is often an option in young women.

Common Homeopathic Remedies for Benign Ovarian Tumors

1. **Calcarea Carbonica**
   - **Indication**: Useful for patients who have **weak constitutions**, feel cold, and experience **heavy or dull aching** pain in the pelvic region. Often helpful in cases of **ovarian cysts** that are associated with **menstrual irregularities**, **obesity**, and **excessive perspiration**.
   - **Symptoms**: Large ovarian cysts, especially if they are painful and accompanied by **excessive weight gain**, **chronic fatigue**, and **anxiety**. There may be a tendency to **develop lumps** or **hard masses** in the pelvic area.
   - **Dosage**: 30C or 200C, depending on severity.

2. **Pulsatilla**
   - **Indication**: Typically indicated for **women who are emotional** and **changeable**, with a tendency to experience **irregular menstruation** or **delayed periods**. It is particularly helpful in cases of **benign cysts** and **hormonal imbalances**.
   - **Symptoms**: The ovarian tumors may be **soft** and **mobile**, and the patient may experience **painful periods** or **menstrual irregularities**. There can be a feeling of **heaviness** or **pressure in the abdomen**.
   - **Dosage**: 30C or 200C.

3. **Sepia**
   - **Indication**: Commonly used in cases of **hormonal disturbances**, such as **estrogen dominance**, and is often recommended for patients with **ovarian cysts** or **fibroids**. It is particularly useful when there are **premenstrual symptoms** or **feeling of heaviness in the abdomen**.
   - **Symptoms**: Ovarian masses that feel tender, with a sense of **bearing down** in the pelvic region. **Irritability** and a sense of **being overwhelmed** are also key features. This remedy is particularly indicated for **women who are exhausted**, and it helps in balancing **hormonal levels**.
   - **Dosage**: 30C or 200C.

4. **Lachesis**
   - **Indication**: Helpful in cases where the ovarian tumors are **painful** and **inflamed**, and the patient experiences a **sensation of fullness** or **congestion** in the pelvic region. **Lachesis** is often indicated when **hot flashes**, **irritability**, and **menstrual irregularities** are prominent.
   - **Symptoms**: A **feeling of tightness** in the pelvic region, which may be accompanied by **sharp pains**. Tumors may become more sensitive before menstruation, and the pain may **radiate to the thighs**. It is often used when tumors are suspected to be related to **hormonal imbalances** or **venous stasis**.
   - **Dosage**: 30C or 200C.

5. **Thuja Occidentalis**
   - **Indication**: A key remedy for wart-like growths, including benign tumors and cysts. Thuja is often recommended when there is abnormal cell growth or disordered tissue formation.
   - **Symptoms:** Benign ovarian tumors that feel lumpy or nodular, often accompanied by feeling of fullness or discomfort in the lower abdomen. It is also helpful when the tumors cause irregular periods or hormonal disturbances.
   - **Dosage:** 30C or 200C.

6. **Conium Maculatum**
   - **Indication**: Typically used for **benign cysts**, particularly when they are **hard**, **indurated**, and **painful** to the touch. It is effective for **hormonal cysts** and **tumors** that are caused by **chronic inflammation** or **congestion**.
   - **Symptoms**: Tumors that cause **sharp, aching pains** in the pelvic region, often aggravated by **pressure** or **movement**. It may also help in **fibroids** that are associated with a **feeling of weight** in the lower abdomen.
   - **Dosage**: 30C or 200C.

7. **Natrum Muriaticum**
   - **Indication**: Used when the ovarian tumors are related to **emotional trauma**, especially **grief** or **sadness**. It is often recommended for women who have **chronic menstrual issues** or who experience **water retention**.
   - **Symptoms**: The tumors are often accompanied by **abdominal bloating** and **irregular periods**, and the patient may have a tendency to **withhold emotions**. **Fatigue** and **mood swings** are common.
   - **Dosage**: 30C or 200C.

8. **Aconitum Napellus**
   - **Indication**: Aconitum is useful in the **acute** stages of any ovarian condition, especially if there is sudden **severe pain** or **inflammation** in the pelvic region,

possibly due to torsion or rupture of a cyst. It is also helpful if the patient is **anxious** and **restless**.
- Symptoms: Sudden onset of sharp, stabbing pain in the ovaries, along with restlessness, fever, and thirst for cold drinks.
- **Dosage**: 30C or 200C for acute symptoms.

9. **Belladonna**
    - **Indication**: Belladonna is recommended when there is a **sudden, intense, throbbing pain** in the ovaries, often accompanied by **redness** or **swelling**. It can be useful for **inflammatory conditions** such as **ovarian cysts** with **hot, congested feeling**.
    - **Symptoms**: Sudden sharp pains, fever, hot flashes, and sensitivity to light. The patient may experience pain relief when lying on the affected side.
    - **Dosage**: 30C or 200C.

10. **Caulophyllum**
    - **Indication**: Caulophyllum is commonly used for female reproductive issues, especially those related to menstrual irregularities and ovarian cysts. It is helpful for painful periods or when ovulation is irregular.
    - **Symptoms**: Pain in the lower abdomen during ovulation, heavy or painful periods, and aching in the pelvic area. The pain may be sharp and cramp-like.
    - **Dosage**: 30C or 200C, as prescribed by a homeopath.

11. **Cinchona Officinalis (China)**
    - **Indication**: This remedy is typically used when ovarian cysts or tumors are associated with **fluid accumulation**, such as **ascites** (abdominal fluid). It is particularly helpful when there is **weakness** or **fatigue** from **blood loss** or **chronic disease**.
    - **Symptoms**: Weakness, **bloating**, and **swelling** in the abdomen. The patient may experience **gastrointestinal symptoms** like **diarrhea** or **constipation**, and feel **exhausted** after exertion.
    - **Dosage**: 30C or 200C.

12. **Kali Carbonicum**
    - **Indication**: Kali carbonicum is a remedy for **female reproductive problems** involving **congestion** and **inflammation** in the **pelvic area**. It is often used in cases of **ovarian cysts** that are tender to touch or have **pressure** symptoms.
    - **Symptoms**: A sensation of **heaviness** or **fullness** in the **lower abdomen**, with **pain** when walking or during physical exertion. There may be **sharp** or **stitching pain** around the ovaries.
    - **Dosage**: 30C or 200C.

13. **Silicea**
    - **Indication**: Silicea is particularly helpful when the **benign tumors** are **hard** or **indurated** in nature. This remedy is often used when there is a **tendency to develop lumps** or **nodular growths**, such as ovarian cysts that are fibrous or calcified.
    - **Symptoms**: Hard, **painful cysts** or **tumors** in the ovaries. The patient may have a tendency to **develop abscesses** or **pus-filled lumps** in various parts of the body.
    - **Dosage**: 30C or 200C.

14. **Baryta Carbonica**
    - **Indication**: Baryta carbonica is often prescribed for individuals with **delayed development** or **growth issues**, particularly those who have a **history of ovarian cysts** or tumors that develop during **puberty** or **early adulthood**.
    - **Symptoms**: Tendency to form **benign cysts**, especially in younger women. There may also be **weakness**, **fatigue**, and **mental sluggishness**.
    - **Dosage**: 30C or 200C.

15. **Conium Maculatum**
    - **Indication**: Conium is particularly useful for **benign tumors** or **cysts** that are **hard**, **painful**, or associated with **chronic inflammation**. It may help with tumors that involve **hormonal disturbance** or have **congestive** properties.
    - **Symptoms**: Hard, indurated tumors or painful lumps in the ovaries, often with sharp or stitching pain. There may be pelvic fullness or heavy pressure in the lower abdomen.
    - **Dosage**: 30C or 200C.

16. **Phytolacca**
    - **Indication**: Phytolacca is useful in cases where there are **benign tumors** associated with **fibrosis**, **induration**, or **nodule-like growths**. It may also help with **painful breasts** or **fibrocystic changes**.
    - **Symptoms**: **Hard, fibrous** ovarian masses or **nodules** that are painful. The patient may have **tightness** or **congestion** in the pelvic region.
    - **Dosage**: 30C or 200C.

17. **Lilium Tigrinum**
    - **Indication:** Lilium Tigrinum is helpful when ovarian cysts or tumors are associated with pelvic congestion and a feeling of heaviness in the abdomen. It is also beneficial when the patient experiences irregular menstruation or uterine displacement.
    - **Symptoms:** Fullness or pressure in the lower abdomen, with bearing down sensations. The patient may have mood swings, irritability, and difficulty concentrating.
    - **Dosage:** 30C or 200C.

18. Nux Vomica

- **Indication**: Nux vomica is indicated when **irritability**, **indigestion**, and **liver congestion** accompany **ovarian cysts**. It is often recommended for those who have a **tendency to develop cysts** related to **stress** and **unhealthy lifestyle**.
- **Symptoms**: Bloating, abdominal cramps, and pelvic discomfort, often accompanied by digestive disturbances such as constipation or nausea.
- **Dosage**: 30C or 200C.

Breast Lump

Defination-

Breast lump is a localised swelling or protuberance or bulge or bump in the breast that feel different from the breast tissue around it.

Breast Anatomy-

IT IS THE LARGEST SWEAT GLAND.

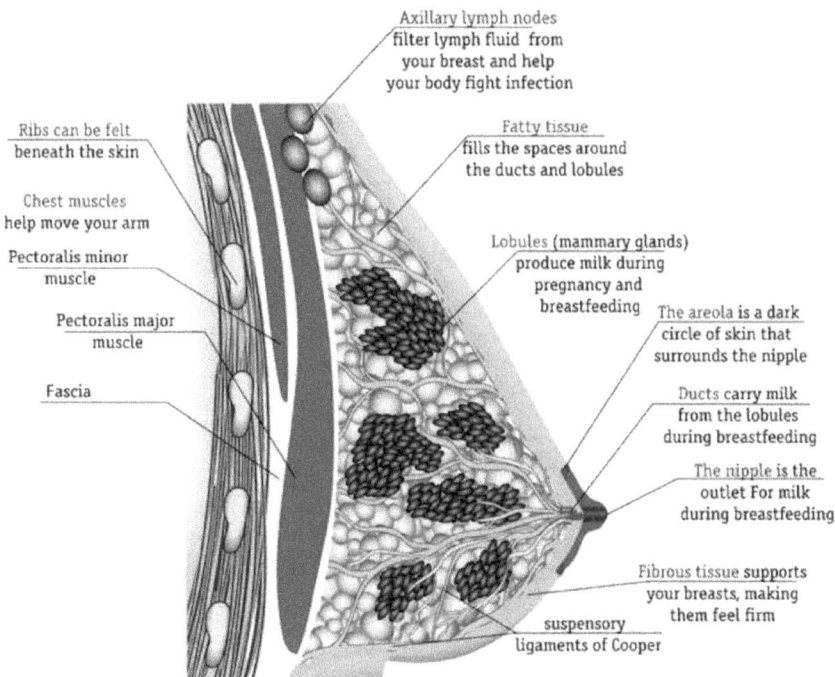

Breast tissue contains different types of tissues-

NIPPLE
AERIOLA
LACTATING GLANDS
LACTACTING TUBULES
SEBASCEOUS AND SWEAT GLANDS
ADIPOSE TISSUE
FIBROUS TISSUE
SUSPENSORY LIGAMENTS
MUSCLES
LYMPHNDES..CENTRALLY PARASTERAL AND LATERALLY AXILLARY GROUP

Aetiology-

2 Types, Benign And Malignant

I] Benign causes are,
- Breast cyst
- Sebaceous cyst
- Milk cyst
- Abscess
- Adenoma
- Intraductal papilloma
- Fat necrosis
- Lipoma
- Injury

II] Malignant lumps

Breast cyst-

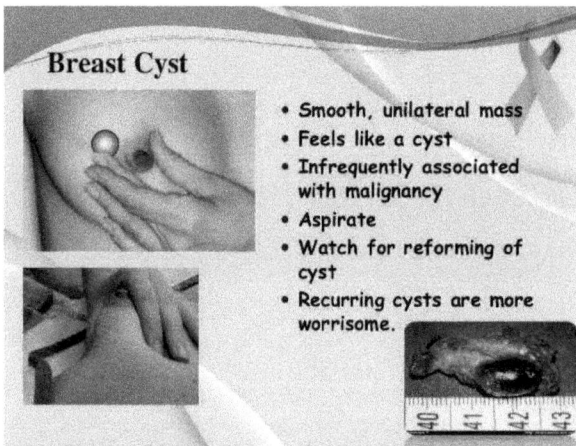

- It is a non cancerous fluid-filled lump in the breast.
- It is a smooth rubbery under skin.
- Painless or painful
- It is rare over the age of 50.
- As it is under control of the hormones especially during menstruation the patient may complaints the pressure symptoms during menstruation.

Sebaceous Cyst-

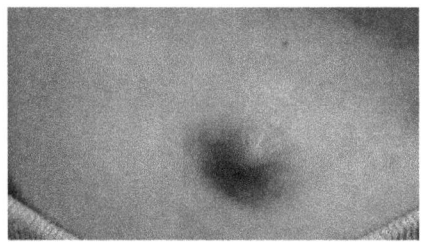

- Caused due to it occurs due to blockage of sebaceous or oil glands always develops below the skin
- It is a result of injury or hormone stimulation.
- Most of the cases did not required any treatment.
- If it is a painful due to the compression of the nerve required to be removed.

Breast Abscess-

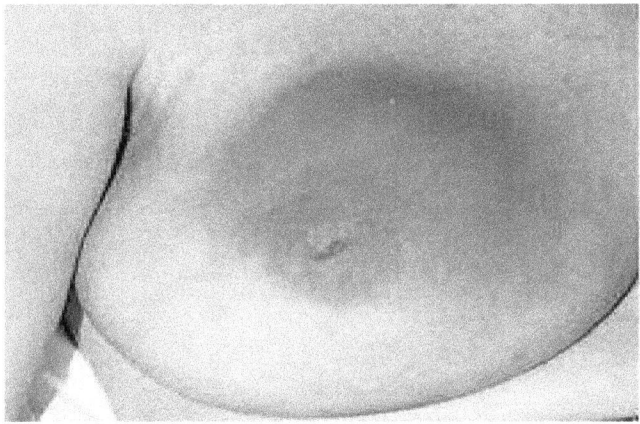

- These are due to infectious inflammation caused especially by bacterias
- Show all signs of inflammation-redness, congestion, local hotness, pain and tenderness,exudation with collection.
- May causes local discharges.
- It is common in feeding women.

Adenoma-

- Is a non cancerous abnormal growth of glandular tissue in the breast fibroadenoma.

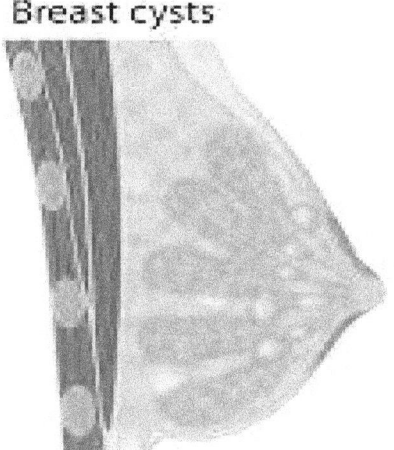
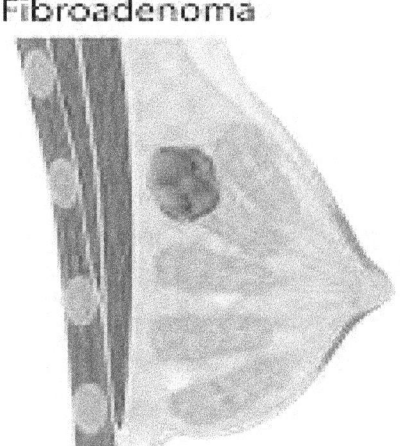

- Have smooth regular margins
- Always movable like the mouse in the chest.
- Round in shape and firm in border.

- Are common in reproductive age group.
- In some condition these are related to the hormones.

Intraductal Papilloma-

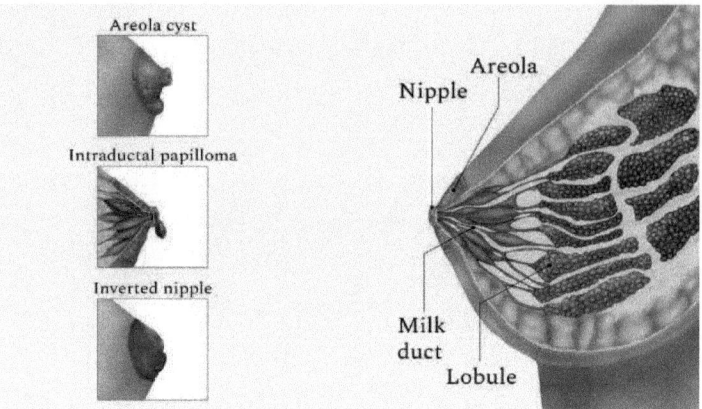

- These are wart like growths which develops in MILK duct of the breast.
- Is specially developed under the nipple so produces bloody discharges.
- Young woman prone to multiple growth while females nearing the Menopause usually develops less.

Fat Necrosis-

- It is a lump due to damage of fatty tissue of the breast as a result of trauma, crush injuries.
- It is painful with nipple discharges and dimpling of the skin over the lump.
- Skin discolouration always coexist.

Lipoma

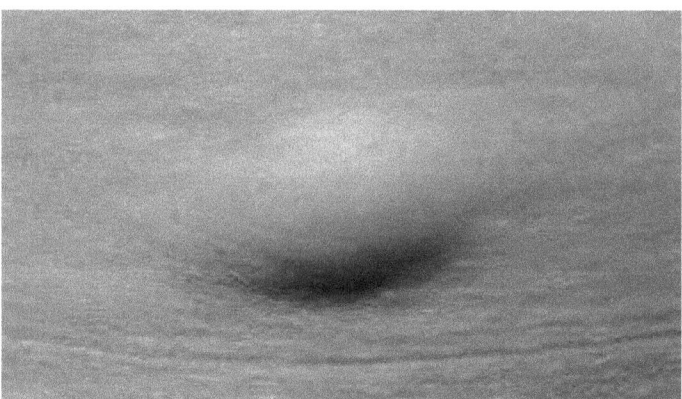

- It is a benefit tumor under the skin, a tumor of fatty or adipose tissue.
- Soft non cancerous lump with his movable and painless, harmless.

Cancerous/ Malignant Lumps-

- These are the fixed to mass.
- Irregular in shape.

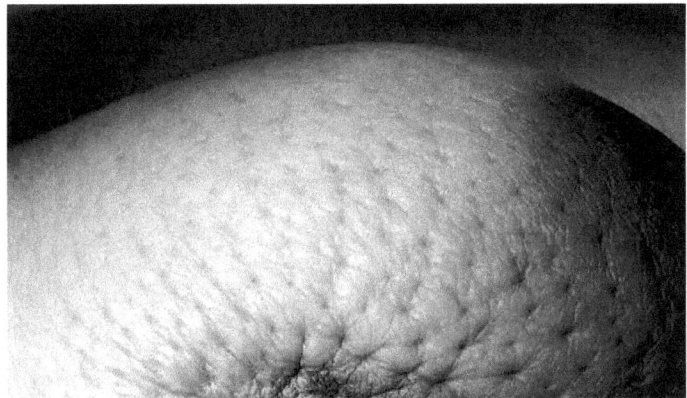
Fig.1 peel of orange skin

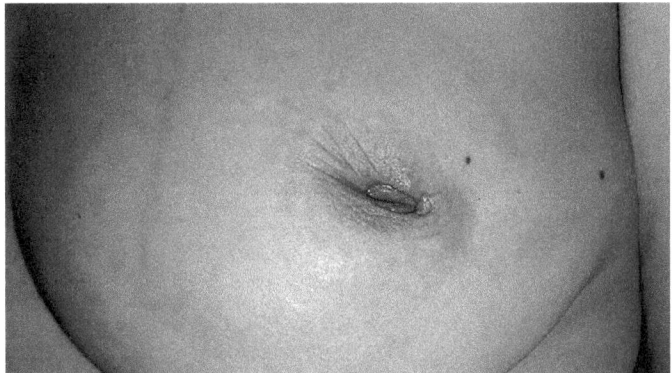
Fig.2 inverted nipple with discharges & red spots

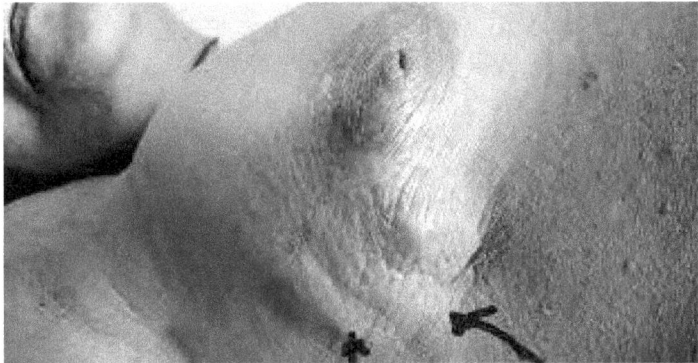
Fig.3 Dimpling of breas

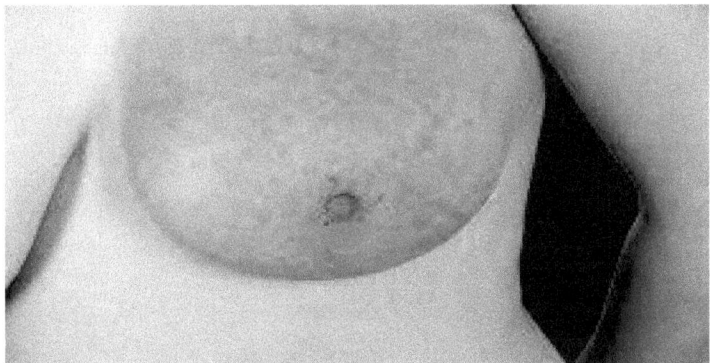
Fig .4 prominent vessels and discolouration of skin

- Hard and usually restricted to the bones breast.
- Is not usually painful in the early stages.
- Becomes painful in later stage.
- Peeled Orange peel skin like structure.
- Along with the bloody nipple discharges.
- Along with that there are palpable group of lymph nodes.
- Breast cancers in early stage they are not have any palpable symptoms or noticeable symptoms but as the tomorrow grows the breast looks heavy and feels something changes and those cancer right changes are crying in the breast especially in the underarm area.
- pulling inside the breast skin.

Diagnosis-

Mammogram-A mammogram is an X-ray of the breast that helps identify breast abnormalities.

It can rule out smallest as 1.1cm tumour.

Ultrasound-An ultrasound is a noninvasive, painless procedure to rule out lump.

Magnetic Resonance Imaging (MRI)-

This test uses a magnetic field and radio waves to take detailed pictures of your breast.

Fine-Needle Aspiration-

Fluid from a breast lump can be removed with a needle. In some cases, an ultrasound is used to guide the needle. Noncancerous cysts go away when the fluid is removed. If the fluid is bloody or cloudy, the sample will be analyzed by a laboratory for cancer cells.

Biopsy-

This is a procedure to remove a sample of tissue for analysis under a microscope. There are several types of breast biopsy:

- fine-needle aspiration biopsy-a tissue sample is taken during a fine-needle aspiration.
- core needle biopsy-uses an ultrasound for guidance; a larger needle is used to get a tissue sample.
- vacuum-assisted biopsy-a probe with a vacuum is inserted into a small incision in the skin and a tissue sample is removed using an ultrasound for guidance.
- stereotactic biopsy-a mammogram takes images from different angles and a tissue sample is taken with a needle.
- surgical biopsy (excisional biopsy)-the whole breast lump, along with surrounding tissue, is removed.
- surgical biopsy (incisional biopsy)-only part of the lump is removed

Management-

Rule out the cause treat it.

Breast infection, abscess- aspiration biopsy ,culture and corresponding antibiotics.
Dranage of abscess under local anaesthetia.
Cyst- In some cases, cysts do not need to be treated and may disappear on their own.
Some requires local drainage.
Fibroadenoma,lipoma doesn't require treatment or exision until wide in size to produce pressure symptoms.
Breast cancer- treatment can include:
- lumpectomy, or removing the lump
- mastectomy, which refers to removing your breast tissue

chemotherapy, which uses drugs to fight or destroy the cancer radiation, a treatment that uses radioactive rays or materials to fight the cancer.

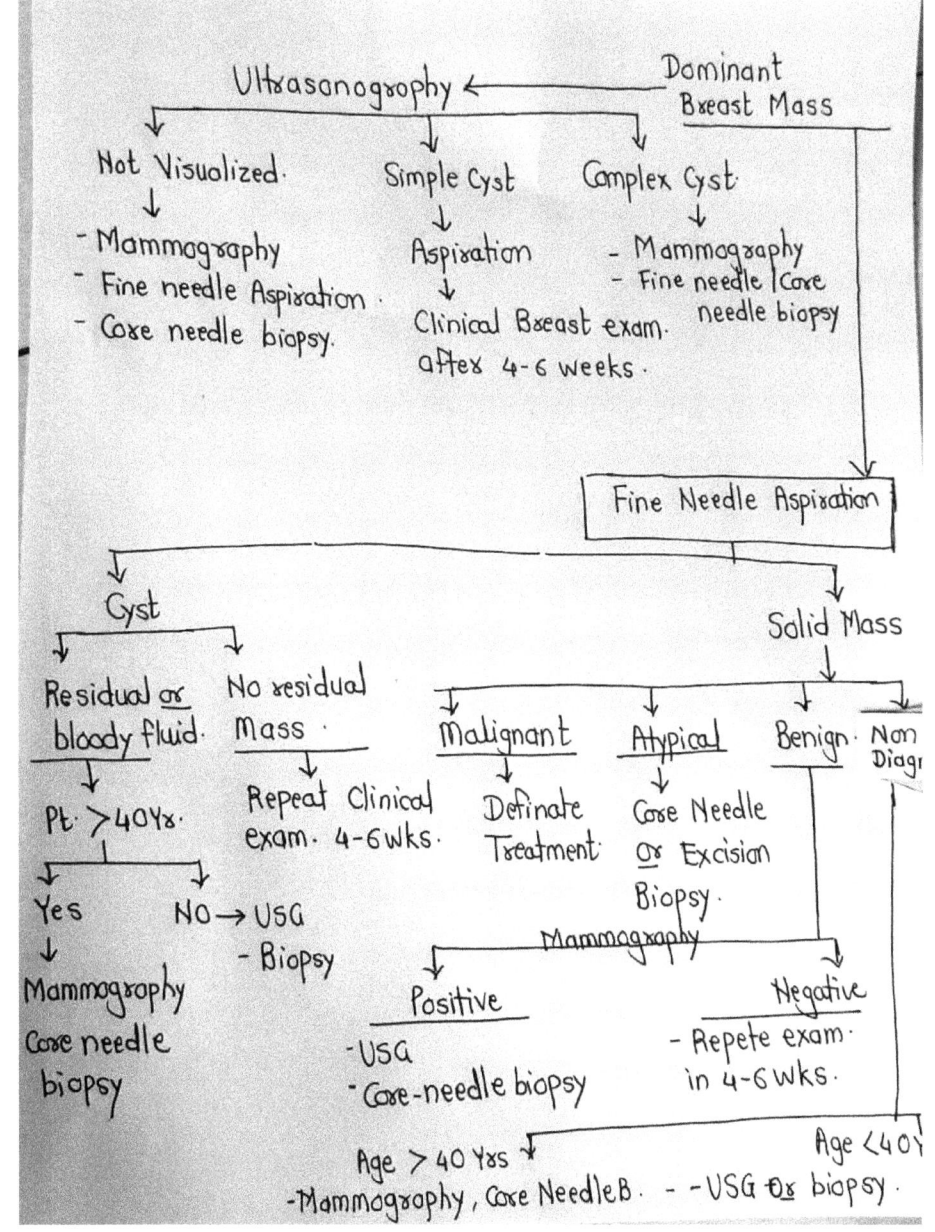

Homoeopathic Management

Conium maculatum	Best suited for hard, immovable lumps in the breast, especially in women with a history of trauma or suppressed sexual desire. The pain is stitching or stinging and worsens before menstruation. Often used in cases of fibrocystic breast disease.
Calcarea fluorica	This remedy is highly effective for stony-hard tumors in the breast. It helps in the resolution of glandular indurations, nodules, and cysts. It is particularly useful for slow-growing, painless lumps.
Phytolacca decandra	Indicated when the breasts are painful, swollen, and tender. The pain radiates from the breast to other parts of the body. Often used in nursing mothers with mastitis and fibrous lumps. Symptoms worsen during lactation.
Silicea	Suitable for breast tumors that tend to suppurate or form abscesses. It helps in the expulsion of pus and promotes healing in cases of chronic breast lumps and indurations.
Scrophularia nodosa	A specific remedy for breast tumors, particularly nodular swellings. It helps dissolve glandular enlargements and is especially beneficial for scrofulous or tubercular constitutions.
Thuja occidentalis	Used for left-sided breast lumps that feel like warty growths. Suitable for women with hormonal imbalances, particularly after long-term use of contraceptives. It is also effective in fibrocystic breast disease.
Carcinosin	Recommended for women with a family history of breast cancer or multiple small nodules in the breast. It is particularly helpful for highly sensitive and perfectionist personalities with a history of prolonged grief or stress.
Lapis albus	Best for glandular enlargements with a tendency to harden. It is indicated in cases where tumors show scirrhous (hard, fibrous) changes. It helps prevent malignancy in long-standing breast lumps.
Pulsatilla nigricans	Indicated for soft, movable lumps in the breast, especially in young women with menstrual irregularities. Symptoms worsen before menstruation and improve with open air and gentle motion.
Bellis perennis	Useful for breast trauma or injury-related lumps. It helps in the resolution of deep-seated bruises and indurations in the breast tissue. It is particularly effective for women who develop lumps after surgery or childbirth.

Comparison Points	Conium Maculatum	Phytolacca Decandra	Calcarea Fluorica	Silicea	Thuja Occidentalis
Type of Lump	Hard, indurated, painless at first	Painful, inflamed, nodular	Stony-hard, slow-growing nodules	Deep-seated, tendency to suppurate	Multiple fibrocystic lumps
Pain Characteristics	Dull pain, worse before menses	Radiating pain, worse during lactation	Mild pain, feels heavy	Sensitive lumps, tender to touch	Sharp, stitching pains
Aggravation Factors	Pressure, touch, before menses	Suckling, movement, cold exposure	Cold, damp weather	Cold, drafts, emotional stress	Hormonal changes, vaccination history
Other Indications	History of trauma or injury	Mastitis, lymph node involvement	Glandular indurations, slow resolution	Weak immunity, prone to abscess formation	Warts, skin issues, cystic tendencies
Best Suited For	Women with history of trauma	Lactating women with painful lumps	Hard, slowly developing tumors	Suppurative tendencies, low vitality	Hormonal imbalances, multiple cysts

Breast examination in breast lump

Cancer Of Cervix

DEF- Malignancy of cervix.

Aetiology-

Most cervical cancer cases are caused by the sexually transmitted **human papillomavirus (HPV)**. This is the same virus that causes genital warts.

— There are about 100 different strains of HPV.

— The two types that most commonly cause cancer are HPV-16 and HPV-18.

Being infected with a cancer-causing strain of HPV doesn't mean you'll get cervical cancer. Your immune system eliminates the vast majority of HPV infections, often within two years.

HPV can also cause other cancers in women and men. These include:

- vulvar cancer
- vaginal cancer
- penile cancer
- anal cancer
- rectal cancer
- throat cancer

Other Risk Factors-

HPV is the biggest risk for cervical cancer. Other factors that can also increase your risk include:

SPERMS MAY BE THE STIMULATING CAUSE FOR CA CERVIX.SO commonly found in

— Younger girls who expose to sex in earlier life span

— Women with multiple sexual parteners

— In prostitutes

— Womken with multiple pregnancies as compare to nulliparous.

— RACE- Nigros having more percentage of occurance

Other Factors-

- human immunodeficiency virus (HIV)
- chlamydia
- smoking
- obesity
- a family history of cervical cancer
- a diet low in fruits and vegetables

- taking birth control pills
- having three full-term pregnancies
- being younger than 17 when you got pregnant for the first time

Clinical Features-

Typical cervical cancer symptoms are:
- MENSTRUAL ABNORMALITIES-

Unusual bleeding, such as in between periods, after sexual intercourse or after menopause. Slightest touch to cervix causes p/v spotting

- LEUCORRHEA-

Vaginal discharge that looks or smells different than usual. Profuse cervical discharges mostly blood staining.

- ABDOMINAL PAINS-

Constant dull aching abdominal pains.

- BACKACHE-

Constant low backache always with pain in the pelvis.

- DYSPARENIA-

Painfull sexuall intercourse f/b p/v bleeding.

- RECURRENT URINARY TRACT INFECTION-

Frequent urination

Dysuria

Haematuria

Staging Of Ca Cervix- Cin [Cervical Intraepithelial Neoplasm]

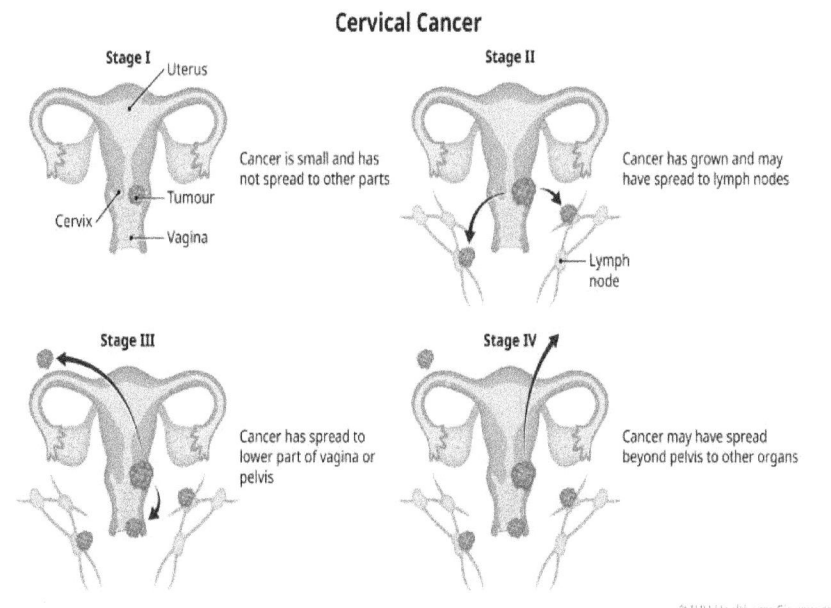

- **Stage 1:** The cancer is small. Limited to cervix only.z

1 A- Lesion less than 3-5mm x 7mm,only microscopic diagnosis.Invoves only superficial layer of cervix.

1B1- Lesion is visible under microscope only but > 5 x 7 mm

1B2- Lesion is visible without microscope and > 2 cm

1B3- Lesion > = 4cm

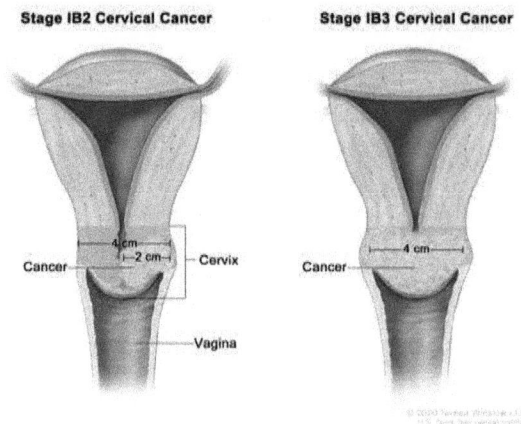

- **Stage 2:** The cancer is larger. It spreads to cervix, upper 2/3 rd of vagina in downward spread and parametrium in outward direction spread. It still hasn't reached other parts of your body.

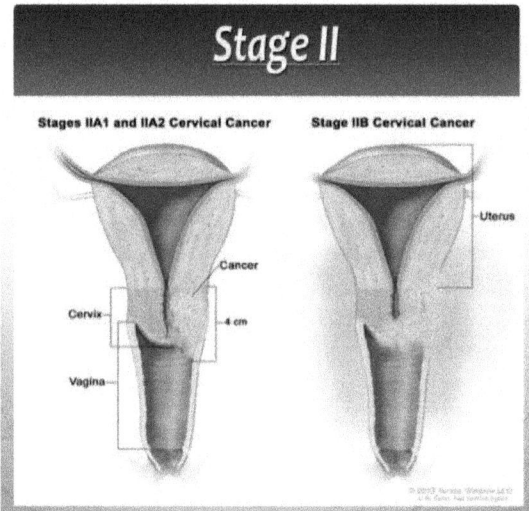

STAGE II A- Cancer invades upper 2/3 rd of vagina but not involves tissues around uterus i.e, no parametrial involvement.

STAGE II B-Cancer involves both upper 2/3rd of vagina and parametrium.

- **Stage 3:** The cancer has spread to the lower 1/3rd of the vagina . It spread all over genital organs ,pelvic ligaments,PELVIC WALL ,lymphnodes .It involves to ,ureter ,kidneys.It may be blocking the ureters.may causes ureteric obstructions.

STAGE III A- Cancer spread to lower 1/3rd of vagina and whole female genital system but not involve Pelvic wall

STAGE III B – Cancer invoves pelvic wall, adjusant kidneys, lymphnodes and ureters.

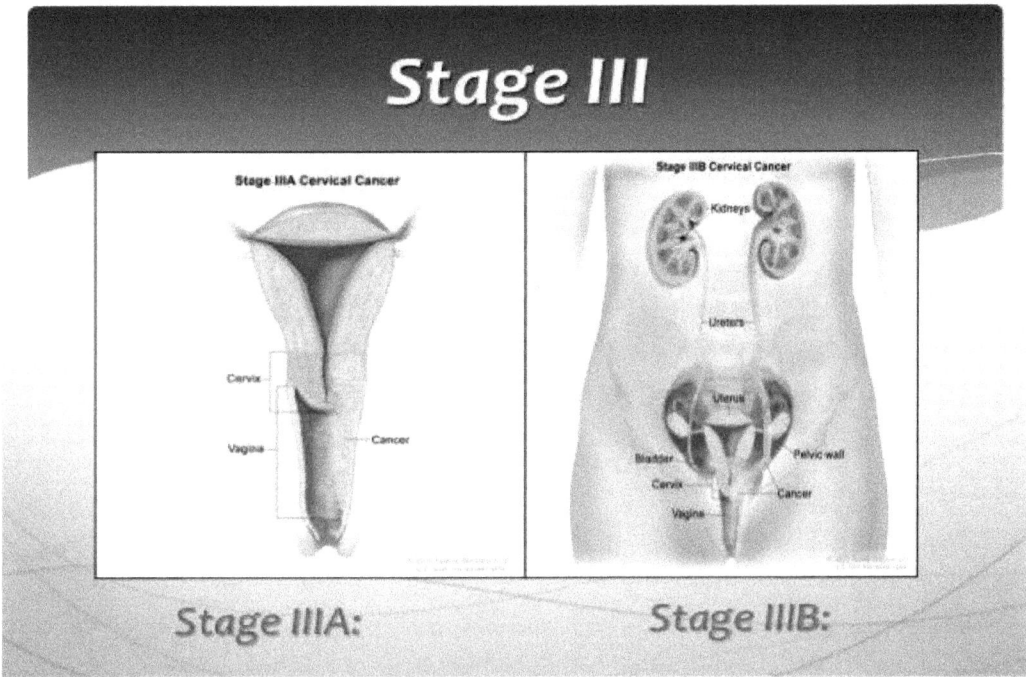

- **Stage 4:** The cancer may have spread outside of the pelvis to the distant organs like your lungs, liver, heart, brain and breast. It also involves distant group of lymphnodes.

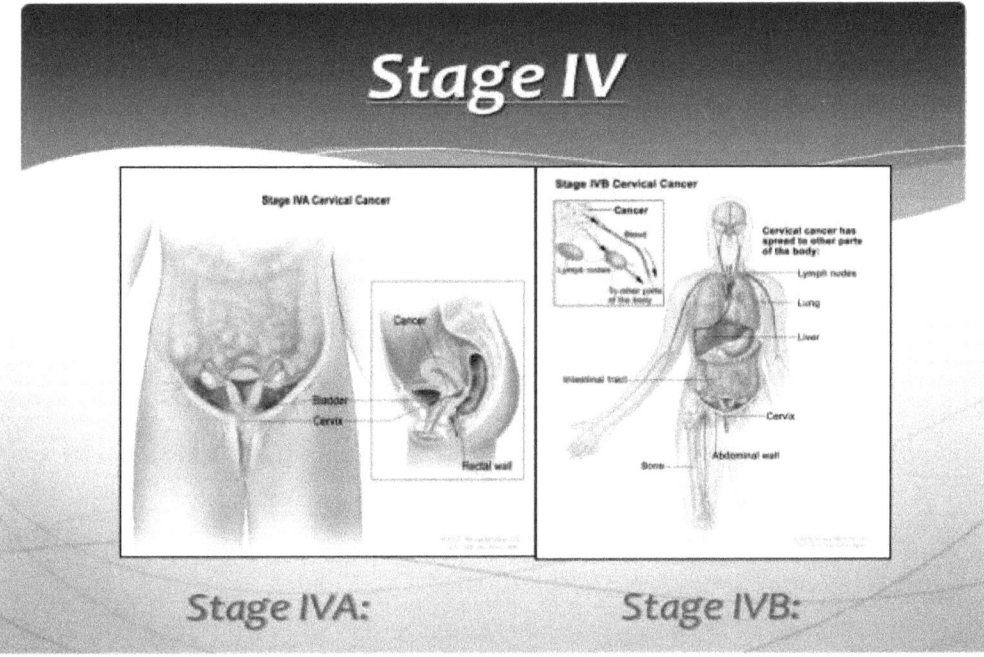

STAGE IV A- Involvement of adjacent organs like bladder and rectum.

STAGE IV B- Spread to distant organs and lymphnodes.

Complications of cervical cancer can occur as a side effect of treatment or as the result of advanced cervical cancer.

Side effects

Early menopause

If your ovaries are surgically removed or are damaged during treatment with radiotherapy, it will trigger an early menopause if you haven't already been through it. Most women experience the menopause naturally in their early fifties.

Symptoms of the menopause include:
- no longer having monthly periods or your periods becoming much more irregular
- hot flushes
- vaginal dryness
- loss of sex drive
- mood changes
- leaking urine when you cough or sneeze (stress incontinence)
- night sweats
- thinning of the bones, which can lead to brittle bones (osteoporosis)

These symptoms can be relieved by taking a number of medications that stimulate the production of the hormones oestrogen and progesterone. This treatment is known as hormone replacement therapy (HRT).

Narrowing of the vagina

Radiotherapy to treat cervical cancer can often cause your vagina to become narrower, which can make having sex painful or difficult.

There are 2 main treatment options if you have a narrowed vagina. The first is to apply a hormone cream to your vagina. This should increase moisture within your vagina and make having sex easier.

The second is to use vaginal dilators, sometimes called vaginal trainers. These are tampon-shaped plastic tubes that come in many different sizes. You insert one into your vagina, usually starting with the smallest size.

Dilators are designed to help stretch the vagina and make it more supple. As you get used to the smaller sizes, you can work your way up to slightly larger ones.

It's usually recommended to use dilators for 5 to 10 minutes at a time on a regular basis during the day over the course of 6 to 12 months.

Your specialist cancer nurse or radiographers in the radiotherapy department should be able to give you more information and advice.

You may find that the more times you have sex, the less painful it becomes. However, it may be several months before you feel emotionally ready to be intimate with a sexual partner.

Macmillan has more information about sexuality and cancer.

Lymphoedema

If the lymph nodes in your pelvis are removed, it can sometimes disrupt the normal workings of your lymphatic system.

One of the functions of the lymphatic system is to drain away excess fluid from the body's tissue. A disruption to this process can lead to a build-up of fluid in the tissue, called lymphoedema. This can cause certain body parts to become swollen – usually the legs, in cases of cervical cancer.

There are exercises and massage techniques that can reduce the swelling. Wearing specially designed bandages and compression garments can also help.

Read more about treating lymphoedema.

Emotional impact

The emotional impact of living with cervical cancer can be significant. Many people report experiencing a "rollercoaster" effect.

For example, you may feel down when you receive a diagnosis but happy when removal of the cancer has been confirmed. You may then feel down again as you try to come to terms with the after effects of your treatment.

This type of emotional disruption can sometimes trigger depression. Typical signs of depression include feeling sad and hopeless, and losing interest in things you used to enjoy.

Contact your GP if you think you may be depressed. There are a range of effective treatments available, including antidepressant medicationand talking therapies, such as cognitive behavioural therapy (CBT).

Read more about coping with cancer.

Advanced cervical cancer

Some of the complications that can occur in advanced cervical cancer are discussed in the following sections.

Pain

If the cancer spreads into your nerve endings, bones or muscles, it can often cause severe pain, which can usually be controlled with painkilling medications.

These painkillers can range from paracetamol and non-steroidal anti-inflammatory drugs (NSAIDs), such as ibuprofen, to more powerful opiate-based painkillers, such as codeine and morphine, depending on pain levels.

Tell your care team if the painkillers you're prescribed aren't effective. You may need to be prescribed a stronger medication. A short course of radiotherapy may also be effective in controlling the pain.

Macmillan nurses, who work both in hospitals and in the community, can also provide expert advice about pain relief.

Kidney failure

In some cases of advanced cervical cancer, the tumour can cause a build-up of urine inside the kidneys (hydronephrosis), which can lead to loss of most or all of the kidneys' functions. This is called kidney failure.

Kidney failure can cause a wide range of symptoms, including:
- tiredness
- swollen ankles, feet or hands, caused by water retention
- shortness of breath
- feeling sick
- blood in your pee (haematuria)

Treatment options for kidney failure associated with cervical cancer include draining urine out of the kidneys using a tube inserted through the skin and into each kidney, or widening the ureters by placing a small metal tube, called a stent, inside them.

Blood clots

As with other types of cancer, cervical cancer can make the blood "stickier" and more prone to forming clots. Bed rest after surgery and chemotherapy can also increase the risk of developing a clot.

Large tumours can press on the veins in the pelvis. This slows the flow of blood and can lead to a blood clot developing in the legs.

Symptoms of a blood clot in your legs include:
- pain, swelling and tenderness in one of your legs (usually your calf)
- the skin of your leg being warm and red

A major concern in these cases is that the blood clot from the leg vein will travel up to the lungs and block the supply of blood. This is known as a pulmonary embolism and can be fatal.

Blood clots in the legs are usually treated using a combination of blood-thinning medication, such as heparin or warfarin, and compression garments designed to help encourage blood flow through the limbs.

Read more about treating deep vein thrombosis.

Bleeding

If the cancer spreads into your vagina, bowel or bladder, it can cause significant damage, resulting in bleeding. Bleeding can occur in your vagina or back passage (rectum), or you may pass blood when you pee.

Minor bleeding can often be treated using a medication called tranexamic acid that encourages the blood to clot and stop the bleeding. Radiotherapy can also be highly effective in controlling bleeding caused by cancer.

Major bleeding may be temporarily treated by using gauze to stem the bleeding and, later, by surgery, radiotherapy or cutting off blood supply to the cervix.

Fistula

A fistula is a rare but distressing complication of advanced cervical cancer.

In most cases involving cervical cancer, the fistula is a channel that develops between the bladder and the vagina. This can lead to a persistent discharge of fluid from the vagina. A fistula can sometimes develop between the vagina and rectum.

Surgery is usually required to repair a fistula, although it's often not possible in women with advanced cervical cancer because they're usually too frail to withstand the effects of surgery.

In such cases, treatment often involves using medication, creams and lotions to reduce the amount of discharge and protect the vagina and surrounding tissue from damage and irritation.

Diagnosis-

— Pap smear, collection of a sample of cells from the surface of anterior and posterior lips of cervix. These cells are then sent to a lab to be tested for precancerous or cancerous changes.

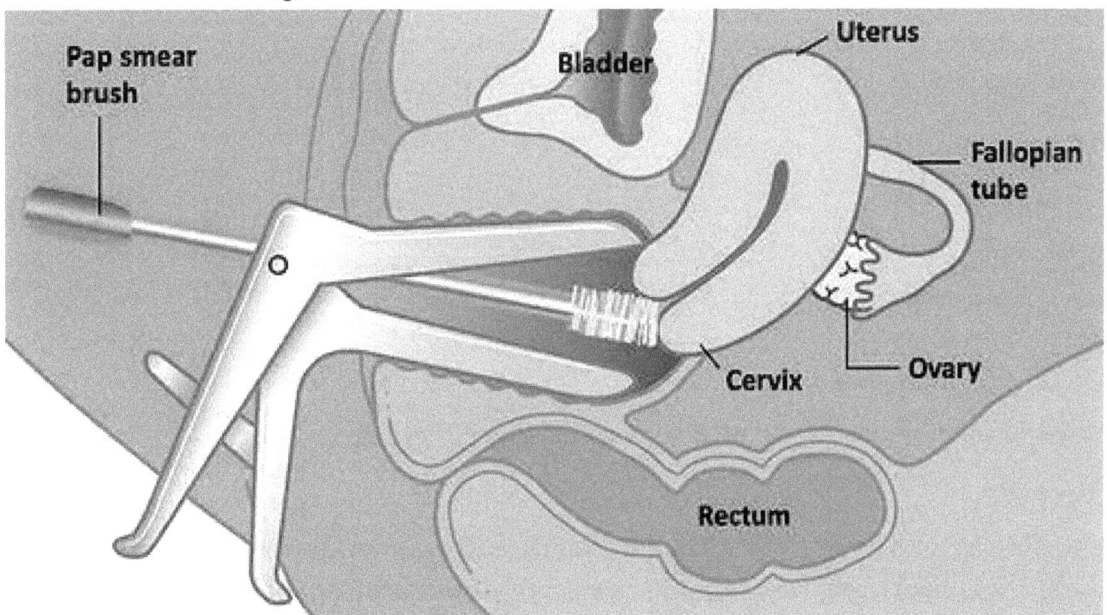

— A colposcopy, a procedure for examining cervix. WE CAN TAKE THE TISSUE SAMPLE FOR BIOPSY FOLLOWING SCHILLER'S IODINE TEST.

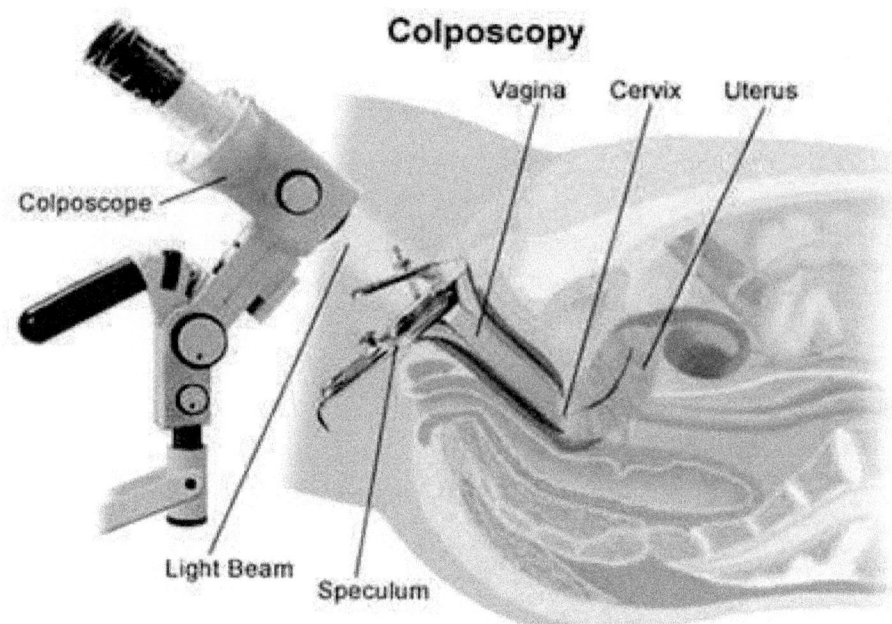

- **Ages 21 to 29:** Get a Pap smear once every three years.
- **Ages 30 to 65:** Get a Pap smear once every three years, get a high-risk HPV (hrHPV) test every five years, or get a Pap smear plus hrHPV test every five years.

Management-

Cervical cancer is very treatable if you catch it early. The four main treatments are:

- surgery
- radiation therapy
- chemotherapy
- targeted therapy

Sometimes these treatments are combined to make them more effective.

Surgery

The purpose of surgery is to remove as much of the cancer as possible. Sometimes the doctor can remove just the area of the cervix that contains cancer cells. For cancer that's more widespread, surgery may involve removing the cervix and other organs in the pelvis.

— Partial hysterectomy
— Subtotal hysterectomy
— Total hysterectomy
— Wertheim's hysterectomy

Some different Cervical cancer surgeries-

Several different types of surgery treat cervical cancer. Which one your doctor recommends depends on how far the cancer has spread.

- Cryosurgery freezes cancer cells with a probe placed in the cervix.

- Laser surgery burns off abnormal cells with a laser beam.
- Therapeutic Conization removes a cone-shaped section of the cervix using a surgical knife, laser, or a thin wire heated by electricity.

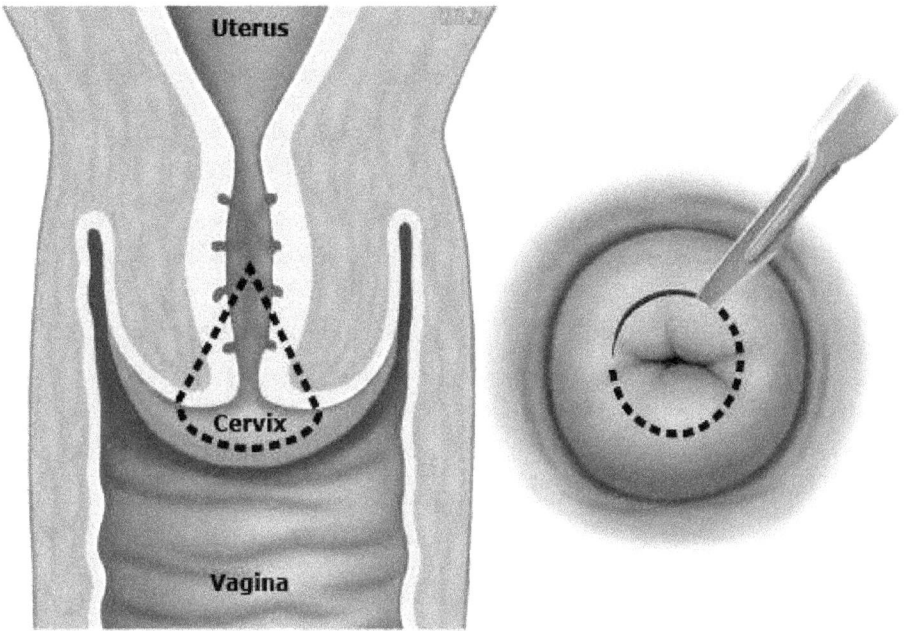

- Hysterectomy removes the entire uterus and cervix. When the top of the vagina is also removed, it's called a radical hysterectomy.
- Trachelectomy removes the cervix and the top of the vagina, but leaves the uterus in place so that a woman can have children in the future.
- Pelvic exenteration may remove the uterus, vagina, bladder, rectum, lymph nodes, and part of the colon, depending on where the cancer has spread. Also called as Wertheim's Hysterectomy

Radiation therapy

Radiation kills cancer cells using high-energy X-ray beams. It can be delivered through a machine outside the body. It can also be delivered from inside the body using a metal tube placed in the uterus or vagina.

Chemotherapy

- Chemotherapy uses drugs to kill cancer cells throughout the body. Doctors give this treatment in cycles. You'll get chemo for a period of time. You'll then stop the treatment to give your body time to recover. e.g. paclitaxel, carbopastin

Targeted therapy

- Bevacizumab (Avastin) is a newer drug that works in a different way from chemotherapy and radiation. It blocks the growth of new blood vessels that help the cancer grow and survive. This drug is often given together with chemotherapy.

Prevention-

One of the easiest ways to prevent cervical cancer is by getting screened regularly with a Pap smear and/or hrHPV test. Screening picks up precancerous cells, so they can be treated before they turn into cancer.

HPV infection causes most cervical cancer cases. The infection is preventable with the vaccines Gardasil and Cervarix. Vaccination is most effective before a person becomes sexually active. Both boys and girls can be vaccinated against HPV.

Here are a few other ways you can reduce your risk of HPV and cervical cancer:
- limit the number of sexual partners you have
- always use a condom or other barrier method when you have vaginal, oral, or anal sex

An abnormal Pap smear result indicates you have precancerous cells in your cervix.

Diagnosis of Cervical Cancer

Diagnostic Test	Purpose
Pap Smear (Cytology)	Screening test for precancerous lesions
HPV DNA Test	Detects high-risk HPV strains
Colposcopy + Biopsy	Confirms cervical dysplasia/cancer
MRI Pelvis	Locoregional spread evaluation
CT Scan (Chest/Abdomen/Pelvis)	Detects metastasis
PET-CT Scan	Staging and metastasis detection
Cystoscopy/Proctoscopy	Evaluates bladder and rectal involvement

FIGO Staging & Treatment Approach

FIGO Stage	Extent of Disease	Treatment
Stage 0 (CIN III, Carcinoma in situ)	Pre-invasive	LEEP, Cryotherapy, Conization
Stage I (Confined to Cervix)	IA1: ≤3 mm deep IA2: 3-5 mm deep IB1: ≤4 cm IB2: >4 cm	Radical hysterectomy (IA2-IB2), Pelvic Lymphadenectomy ± Radiation
Stage II (Beyond Uterus but Not to Lower Vagina or Pelvic Wall)	IIA: Upper vagina involvement IIB: Parametrial invasion	Chemoradiotherapy (Cisplatin + Radiation) ± Brachytherapy

FIGO Stage	Extent of Disease	Treatment
Stage III (Pelvic Sidewall/Vaginal Involvement or Hydronephrosis)	IIIA: Lower vagina IIIB: Pelvic wall/Hydronephrosis	Definitive Chemoradiotherapy (Cisplatin + External Beam Radiation + Brachytherapy)
Stage IV (Metastatic Disease)	IVA: Bladder/Rectum IVB: Distant Metastases (Lungs, Liver, Bones)	Palliative Chemotherapy (Platinum-based), Immunotherapy, Palliative Radiation

Modern Treatment Modalities for Cervical Cancer

1. **Surgery (For Early-Stage Disease, Stage IA2-IB1)**
   - Cone Biopsy/LEEP – For CIN III and microinvasive cancer
   - Radical Hysterectomy with Lymphadenectomy – Standard for localized cervical cancer
   - Fertility-Preserving Surgery (Trachelectomy) – For early-stage cancer in young women

2. **Radiotherapy (Definitive or Adjuvant Therapy)**
   - External Beam Radiation Therapy (EBRT) – Treats primary tumor & regional nodes
   - Brachytherapy (Intracavitary Radiation) – Delivers high-dose radiation to the cervix

3. **Chemotherapy (For Advanced, Recurrent, or Palliative Care)**

Drug	Indication	Dose
Cisplatin	Standard for chemoradiotherapy	40 mg/m² IV weekly
Carboplatin + Paclitaxel	Metastatic/Recurrent Disease	AUC 5 + 175 mg/m² IV q3 weeks
Bevacizumab (Anti-VEGF mAb)	Advanced/Recurrent Disease	15 mg/kg IV q3 weeks
Pembrolizumab (PD-1 Inhibitor)	PD-L1 positive cases, recurrent/metastatic	200 mg IV q3 weeks

Targeted Therapy & Immunotherapy
- Bevacizumab (Avastin): Inhibits tumor angiogenesis, used in metastatic cases
- Pembrolizumab (Keytruda): Immunotherapy for PD-L1 positive recurrent/metastatic cancer

Palliative & Supportive Care
- Pain management (NSAIDs, opioids for severe pain)
- Blood transfusions for anemia
- Psychological support, counseling
- Nutritional support for cachexia

Conclusion
- Early-stage cervical cancer (Stage I-IIA) is treated with surgery or chemoradiation.
- Locally advanced cases (Stage IIB-IVA) require definitive chemoradiotherapy.
- Metastatic cases (Stage IVB) benefit from palliative chemotherapy, targeted therapy, and immunotherapy.
- HPV vaccination and screening programs play a vital role in prevention.

Cervical Carcinoma In Situ / 'O' Stage Cancer

Carcinoma in situ (CIS) is a general term for

— An early stage cancer.

— Stage 0 cervical cancer.

— Noninvasive,

which means the cancerous cells are confined to the surface of your cervix and haven't penetrated more deeply into the tissues.

— VISIBLE UNDER MICROSCOPE ONLY.

Aetiology-

HPV is the main risk factor for developing cervical CIS. There are hundreds of strains of HPV, which are divided up into either low risk or high risk. There are 10 high-risk strains that are associated with abnormal cell changes in the cervix that can lead to cancer, but two of the strains (HPV 16 and HPV 18) are responsible for 70 percentTrusted Source of cases of cervical cancer.

Other risk factors may also play a role in the development of cervical CIS including:
- having multiple sexual partners
- smoking cigarettes
- having a weakened immune system
- having sexual intercourse at an early age
- having a diet low in fruits and vegetables
- using birth control pills for an extended period
- being infected with Chlamydia

Clinical Features-

Cervical cancer typically doesn't cause symptoms until its later stages, so you may not have any symptoms with cervical CIS. That's why having regular Pap smears are important for catching any abnormal cell changes early.

Diagnosis-

A Pap smear can collect abnormal cells that are then identified in a lab. An HPV test may be performed on the sample to check for the virus and to see whether high-risk or low-risk strains are present.

A colposcopy is an in-office procedure that allows your doctor to view your cervix with a special magnifying tool called a colposcope. Your doctor will apply a solution to the surface of your cervix to show any abnormal cells. They can then take a small piece of tissue called a biopsy. They'll send this to a lab for a more definitive diagnosis.

If the biopsy shows CIS, your doctor might want to remove a larger piece of your cervix. If they remove the area with abnormal cells, they'll also remove a surrounding margin of healthy tissue.

Management-

The treatment for cervical CIS is similar to that for cervical dysplasia. Although it's called carcinoma in situ, it's often treated like a precancerous growth because it's not invasive. Possible treatments include the following:

- A hysterectomy is an option for women who don't want to preserve their fertility.
- Cryosurgery, or freezing the abnormal cells, can be done in your doctor's office.
- Laser surgery or loop electrosurgical excision procedure are surgical options that are done on an outpatient basis. They involve removing the abnormal tissue with lasers or an electrically charged wire loop.
- Conization, another outpatient procedure, is used less often. It involves removing a larger, cone-sized piece of the cervix to ensure removal of the entire abnormal area.

Your treatment will depend on your age, desire to preserve your fertility, general health, and other risk factors.

Follow-Up Care for Cervical CIS

After you have treatment for cervical CIS, your doctor will want to see you for follow-up visits and Pap smears every three to six months. Cervical cancer can come back, but regular Pap smears and checkups will allow your doctor to catch and treat abnormal cells early.

— USG WHOLE ABDOMEN AT specific interval

— MRI –to rule out secondaries at regular interval.

Your doctor will also address any concerns you may have about your cervical health.

Homoeopathic Management-

Remedies For Cervical Erosion / Ulceration / Overgrowth
- MERC. SOL
- NIT.ACID
- THUJA
- SYPHILLINUM

Remedies Of Ematiation In Cancer
- PHOS.
- SILICEA
- ARS.ALB
- ABROTANUM
- CARCINOSIN

Remedies For Bloody Cervical Discharges
- PHOS
- MERC.SOL
- HYDROCOTYLE
- HYDRASTASIS
- CARCINOSIN
- KREOSOTUM
- NITRIC ACID
- FLUORIC ACID

MERC SOL-
It is called human barometer as sensitive to all exernal impressions. Very sensitive to weather changes,temp.changes, emotional up and downs.all complaints aggravated sunset to sunrise.EASILY FRIGHTENED AND SPEAKS HURRIED AND RAPID.All type of mucus membranes esp.apathae AND CANCER. Cervical erosions, ulcerations with BLOODY, SLIMY HORRIBLY OFFENSSIVE DISCHARGES.

Nitric Acid-
CRACKS AND FISSURES AT CERVIX WITH SPLINTER LIKE PAINS.Easily bleeding ulcers of cervix ON SLIGHTEST TOUCH.Profuse, yellowish-greenish, brownish ACRID ,OFFENSSIVE discharges . Penduculated,condylaamatous growth of vagina, cervix. INVOLVEMENT OF BLADDER IN Ca cervix with pungent, HORSE SMELLING URINE.All complaints aggravated in evening or night, better only by riding on carriage.

Fluoric Acid-

SYPHILITIC OR PSORIC ULCERS, even of bones.Ca Cx with rodent, decubotus ulcers with profuse, acrid vaginal discharges with characyteristic LIGHTNING PAINS remains for short time.Red, round edged, open cervical ulcers with bloody discharges. ACRID SWEAT. PATIENT HAS INCREASED HER EXERCISE ABILITY WITHOUT DANGER.

Thuja-

CANCEROUS OVERGROWTH OVER CERVIX.King of sycosis.DIRTY ,brownish look of skin with multiple moles,mottled spots and dry scaly eruptions.URETHRITIS WITH CHRONIC INCONTENECE OF URINE. Cancer of cervix with involvement of lt.ovary, lt.follipian tubes, lt.ureter and lt.kidney .NEWMOON –FULLMOON AGGRAVATION, 3AM 3PM AGGRAVATION.DAMP WEATHER AGGRAVARION Multiple hallucinations, illusions and dilusions e.g, something live is moving inside the abdomen.

Syphilinum-

COPPER COLOURED ERUPTIONS.Ca with family history of syphilis or cancer.Craving for alcohol in any form with family tendency for alcoholism.Sunset to sunrise aggravation.pains appears gradually, goes gradually. Shifting type of pains-wandering here and there.

Phosphorus-

Progressive Ematiation All Over Body With Anaemia.

INDICATIVE IN PROGRESSIVE AND LATER STAGE OF CA CERVIX.Involvement of adjusaant and distant organs with bleeding from all orifices.e.g, haemoptysis with lung involvement,haematemesis with stomach involvement,malaena with rectal involvement, haematuria in bladder involvement. THIN,PROFUSE,WATERY,BRIGHT RED AND YET NON-COAGUABLE BLLEDING. Cervical ulcerstion with bloody discharges and excessive burning ,rubbing or magnetism gives reliefe.

Hydrocotyle-

EXCELLENT REMEDY FOR FUNGUS GROWTH AND ULCERATION OF UTERUS,NECK AND LIPS OF CERVIX.profuse watery ,transperant leucorrhea with violent itching.Also applicable for leprosy.

Hydrastasis-

Suited to old ladies with all gone feeling ,in cancerous or precancerous conditions of vulva,with profuse, thick, yellowish ropy, viscid leucorrhea, HANGING DOWN IN LONG STRINGS.EXCORIATION AND EROSION OF CERVIX WITH knife like sharp cutting pains. LIVER AND STOMACH INVOLVEMENT IN CANCER with disturb metabolism DEPRESSED AND WAITING FOR HER DEATH.

Carcinosin-

CA CERVIX with family h/o cancer. FAIR, healthy lady with MULTIPLE MOLES OR BIRTH MARKS ON BODY AND afterwards goes through progressive ematiation of body. GOES THROUGH both apposite conditions, e.g, very jolly, happy enjoys music, party while sometimes extremely depressed with suicidal tendency. Intelligent, artistic or dull idiotic. EITHER FASTIDIOUS OR WITH VERY FILTHY HABITS. ENJOYS THUNDERSTORMS, MAKES POEM, HAVE SENSE OF RHYTHM.

Cervical Erosion (Cervical Ectropion)

Cervical erosion, also referred to as **cervical ectropion**, is a benign gynecological condition where the columnar epithelium (glandular cells) of the endocervical canal is exposed on the outer surface of the cervix. It is common in women of reproductive age and is often mistaken for more serious conditions due to similar symptoms.

Definition

Cervical erosion is a condition characterized by the replacement of the squamous epithelium of the ectocervix (outer layer of the cervix) with columnar epithelium, typically found in the endocervical canal. This results in an area of redness around the external os, which may be misinterpreted as an ulceration.

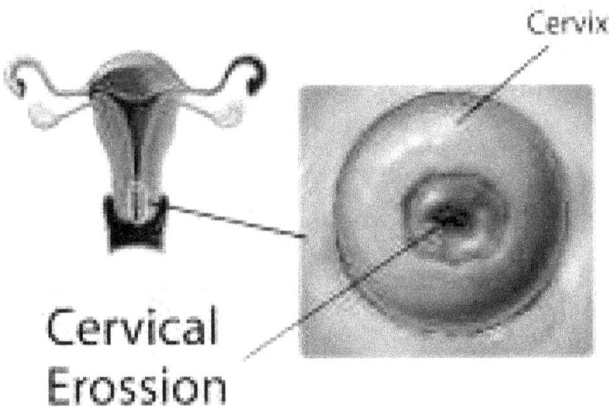

Types

Cervical erosion can be classified into the following types:

1. **Congenital Erosion:**
    - Occurs in newborns or young girls due to maternal hormonal influence.
    - Resolves spontaneously after a few weeks or months.

2. **Inflammatory Erosion:**
    - Caused by chronic infections or irritation of the cervix (e.g., sexually transmitted infections).

3. **Traumatic Erosion:**
    - Results from mechanical injury to the cervix due to childbirth, abortion, or insertion of intrauterine devices (IUDs).

4. **Hormonal Erosion:**
      - Common in women taking oral contraceptives or during pregnancy due to high estrogen levels.

Etiology (Causes)

1. **Hormonal Changes:**
   - High estrogen levels during pregnancy, oral contraceptive use, or puberty.
2. **Infections:**
   - Chronic cervicitis caused by bacterial, fungal, or viral infections (e.g., Chlamydia, Trichomonas, or HPV).
3. **Mechanical Trauma:**
   - Injury to the cervix due to childbirth, surgical procedures, or frequent vaginal douching.
4. **Chemical Irritation:**
   - Exposure to irritants like contraceptive creams or vaginal hygiene products.
5. **Lifestyle Factors:**
   - Multiple sexual partners, early onset of sexual activity, or poor genital hygiene.
6. **Congenital:**
   - Hormonal stimulation in neonates or young girls.

Clinical Features

1. **Symptoms:**
   - Vaginal discharge (white or yellowish, sometimes blood-tinged).
   - Postcoital bleeding (bleeding after sexual intercourse).
   - Irregular bleeding or spotting between periods.
   - Pain or discomfort during sexual intercourse.
   - Burning or itching sensation in the vaginal area (rare).
2. **Signs (on physical examination):**
   - Red, inflamed area around the external cervical os.
   - Mucopurulent discharge from the cervix.
   - Cervical tenderness (in case of associated infection).

Complications

1. **Chronic Cervicitis:**
   - Persistent inflammation of the cervix leading to secondary infections.

2. **Infertility:**
   o Chronic infections and cervical stenosis may interfere with conception.
3. **Increased Risk of STIs:**
   o The exposed columnar epithelium is more susceptible to infections like HPV, increasing the risk of cervical dysplasia and carcinoma.
4. **Cervical Polyps:**
   o Recurrent irritation may lead to the formation of cervical polyps.
5. **Preterm Labor:**
   o In pregnant women, cervical erosion may increase the risk of complications during pregnancy.

Diagnosis

1. **History:**
   o Detailed medical and sexual history to identify potential causes.
2. **Physical Examination:**
   o Visualization of the cervix using a speculum reveals a red, inflamed area around the external os.
3. **Diagnostic Tests:**
   o Pap Smear:
     ▪ To rule out cervical dysplasia or malignancy.
   o Colposcopy:
     ▪ Detailed examination of the cervix to differentiate benign erosion from precancerous lesions.
   o Biopsy:
     ▪ If malignancy is suspected.
   o Culture and Sensitivity:
     ▪ To identify and treat underlying infections.
   o HPV Testing:
     ▪ To detect high-risk strains of the human papillomavirus.

Modern Medicine Management

1. **Medical Treatment:**
   o Antibiotics:
     ▪ Used for infections like bacterial vaginosis, Chlamydia, or gonorrhea.
   o Antiviral or Antifungal Agents:
     ▪ For viral or fungal infections, respectively.
   o Hormonal Therapy:

- Adjusting oral contraceptive pills or using progesterone-only pills in cases of hormonal erosion.

2. **Surgical Treatment:**
   - Cryotherapy:
     - Freezing the affected area to promote healing.
   - Electrocautery (Diathermy):
     - Burning the eroded area to remove the abnormal cells.
   - Laser Ablation:
     - Using laser energy to destroy the affected area.
   - LEEP (Loop Electrosurgical Excision Procedure):
     - Removing the affected tissue with an electrically heated wire loop.

3. **Supportive Measures:**
   - Maintaining good genital hygiene.
   - Avoiding irritants like douching or harsh chemicals.

Lifestyle and Supportive Care

1. **Maintain Hygiene:**
   - Use gentle, non-irritating hygiene products.

2. **Avoid Douching:**
   - Douching may worsen irritation and disrupt the natural vaginal flora.

3. **Diet and Nutrition:**
   - Eat a balanced diet rich in vitamins (A, E, and C) to support healing.

4. **Stress Management:**
   - Practice yoga, meditation, or relaxation technique

Remedy	Key Indications	Physical Symptoms	Mental/Emotional Symptoms	Modalities
Pulsatilla Nigricans	Changeable symptoms: irregular menses, PMS, and PCOS.	Delayed or suppressed periods, white or yellow discharge, mild cramping.	Weepy, seeks consolation, feels better in open air.	**Better:** Open air. **Worse:** Warm rooms.
Sepia Officinalis	Hormonal issues: amenorrhea,	Bearing-down sensation, scanty periods,	Indifference to loved ones, irritable, depressed.	**Better:** Vigorous

Remedy	Key Indications	Physical Symptoms	Mental/Emotional Symptoms	Modalities
	menopause, infertility.	or complete suppression of menses.		exercise. **Worse:** Rest.
Calcarea Carbonica	Hormonal imbalance with obesity or thyroid dysfunction.	Profuse, prolonged menses, cold intolerance, excessive sweating.	Anxious, overwhelmed, fearful of disease or insanity.	**Better:** Warmth. **Worse:** Cold.
Lachesis Muta	Severe PMS, menopause, or suppressed periods.	Pain worsens before flow starts and improves after. Swollen ovaries.	Jealous, talkative, intense emotions.	**Better:** Free flow. **Worse:** Tight clothing.
Natrum Muriaticum	Stress or grief-related menstrual issues, scanty periods.	Vaginal dryness, migraines with menses, salty cravings.	Reserved, avoids consolation, emotional, holds grudges.	**Better:** Alone. **Worse:** Consolation.
Belladonna	Sudden, violent menstrual pain with heat and redness.	Flushed face, throbbing pain, sensitivity to light and noise.	Restless, irritable, oversensitive.	**Better:** Rest. **Worse:** Noise, light.
Magnesia Phosphorica	Spasmodic or cramping menstrual pain relieved by warmth.	Severe cramps radiating to back and thighs, relief with pressure or heat.	Nervous, oversensitive, dislikes confrontation.	**Better:** Warm applications. **Worse:** Cold air.
Ignatia Amara	Emotional trauma, grief, or stress-induced menstrual problems.	Cramping uterine pain, sighing, lump in throat.	Moody, hysterical, easily offended.	**Better:** Deep breathing. **Worse:** Grief.

Remedy	Key Indications	Physical Symptoms	Mental/Emotional Symptoms	Modalities
Silicea	Delayed menses in undernourished or weak individuals.	Cold hands and feet, late puberty, poor stamina, sweating profusely.	Shy, timid, easily discouraged.	**Better:** Warmth. **Worse:** Cold drafts.
Thuja Occidentalis	PCOS, irregular periods, warts, and cystic growths.	Oily skin, hirsutism, suppressed or irregular cycles, ovarian cysts.	Fixed ideas, secretive, low self-esteem.	**Better:** Warmth. **Worse:** Damp weather.
Cimicifuga Racemosa	Painful menstruation or menopausal symptoms with mood swings.	Radiating pelvic pain to back and thighs, spasmodic contractions.	Fear of impending illness, depression, restlessness.	**Better:** Open air. **Worse:** Movement.
Phosphorus	Heavy, prolonged menses leading to anemia or weakness.	Bright red blood, weakness, craving for cold drinks.	Friendly, emotional, oversensitive to others' emotions.	**Better:** Lying down. **Worse:** Fasting.
Hydrastis Canadensis	Chronic infections and cervical erosion with discharge.	Thick, tenacious yellow discharge.	Weakness, irritability, fatigue.	**Better:** Rest. **Worse:** Cold weather.
Murex Purpurea	Increased libido with painful or irregular menses.	Pelvic pain, profuse bleeding, and sensitivity.	Excitable, energetic, emotionally expressive.	**Better:** Rest. **Worse:** Movement.
Helonias Dioica	Uterine prolapse and menstrual irregularities from exhaustion.	Weakness, dragging sensation in pelvis, excessive bleeding.	Irritable, depressed, feels overworked and unappreciated.	**Better:** Rest. **Worse:** Overexertion.

Remedy	Key Indications	Physical Symptoms	Mental/Emotional Symptoms	Modalities
Sabina	Profuse bleeding with bright red clots and severe back pain.	Pain extending to thighs, worse from movement.	Nervous, sensitive to noise, dislikes music.	**Better:** Rest. **Worse:** Warm room.

Modern Medicine vs. Homeopathic Medicine for Cervical Erosion:

Category	Modern Medicine (Allopathy)	Homeopathic Medicine
Antibiotics (for infections)	Metronidazole, Doxycycline, Azithromycin, Ciprofloxacin.	Homeopathic remedies are not antibiotics but work to boost immunity; examples: **Mercurius Solubilis**, **Kreosotum**, **Nitric Acid** (for foul discharge).
Anti-inflammatory Agents	Ibuprofen, Diclofenac (NSAIDs) for pain and inflammation.	**Belladonna**, **Apis Mellifica**, **Sepia** (for redness, swelling, and pain).
Antiseptic/Vaginal Washes	Povidone-Iodine (Betadine), Chlorhexidine vaginal wash.	**Calendula**, **Hydrastis Canadensis**, **Echinacea** (as natural antiseptic remedies).
Hormonal Therapy (if needed)	Estrogen cream (for atrophic cervical erosion).	**Sepia**, **Pulsatilla**, **Oophorinum** (for hormonal imbalance-related cervical erosion).
Tissue Healing Agents	Silver nitrate, Cryotherapy, Laser therapy for cauterization.	**Kreosotum**, **Silicea**, **Graphites** (to promote healing of cervical tissue).
Pain Relief	Local anesthetics (Lidocaine), NSAIDs for pain relief.	**Chamomilla**, **Hypericum**, **Belladonna** (for pain management).

Category	Modern Medicine (Allopathy)	Homeopathic Medicine
Immune Boosters	Multivitamins, probiotics, zinc supplements.	**Thuja Occidentalis**, **Echinacea**, **Sulphur** (to enhance immunity and prevent recurrence).
Anti-Fungal (if Candida infection present)	Fluconazole, Clotrimazole, Nystatin.	**Borax**, **Kreosotum**, **Sepia** (for white discharge and fungal infections).

Cervical Polyp

Definition

Cervical polyps are benign, finger-like growths that arise from the surface of the cervical canal (endocervix) or ectocervix. These growths are usually small, pedunculated, and vascular, often protruding through the external cervical os.

Types of Cervical Polyps

1. **Endocervical Polyps:**
   - Originating from the glandular tissue of the endocervix.
   - Commonly found in premenopausal women.
   - Associated with hormonal changes and inflammation.

2. **Ectocervical Polyps:**
   - Arise from the squamous epithelium of the ectocervix.
   - More common in postmenopausal women.

Aetiology (Causes)

1. **Chronic Inflammation:**
   - Repeated infections or irritation of the cervix can trigger polyp formation.

2. **Hormonal Imbalance:**
   - High estrogen levels, as seen during pregnancy or with the use of estrogen-based medications, can lead to polyp growth.

3. **Congestion of Cervical Blood Vessels:**
   - Stagnation or pooling of blood in the cervical veins contributes to the development of polyps.

4. **Infections:**
   - Long-standing cervicitis caused by infections like *Chlamydia*, *HPV*, or *Trichomonas*.

5. **Trauma:**
   - Physical injury to the cervix, e.g., due to childbirth or mechanical devices like IUDs.

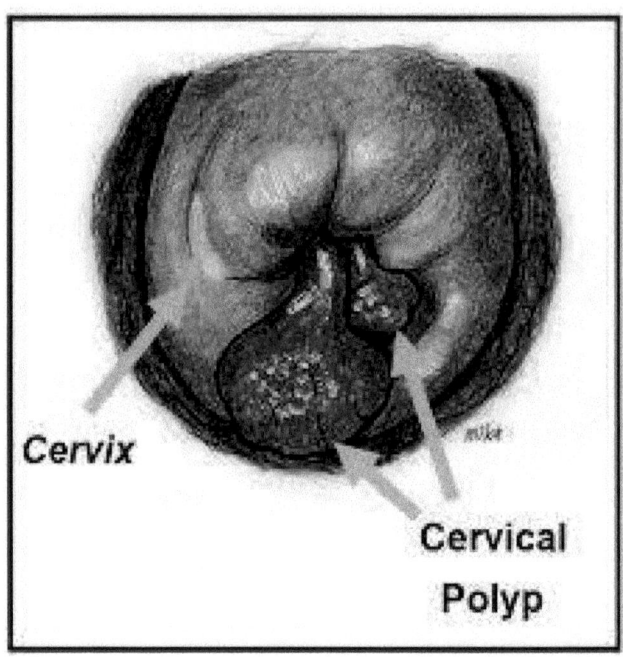

Clinical Features

1. **Symptoms:**
    - Asymptomatic in most cases (incidentally found during pelvic exams).
    - Abnormal vaginal discharge (may be blood-streaked or foul-smelling).
    - Postcoital bleeding (bleeding after intercourse).
    - Intermenstrual bleeding (bleeding between periods).
    - Heavier or irregular menstrual cycles in some women.

2. **Signs (on Examination):**
    - Small, reddish, or purplish growths visible at or protruding through the cervical os.
    - Polyps may be soft, smooth, and pedunculated.

Complications

1. **Bleeding:**
    - Persistent postcoital or intermenstrual bleeding.

2. **Infections:**
    - Cervical polyps may become infected, leading to chronic cervicitis.

3. **Infertility:**
    - Large polyps may interfere with sperm movement or implantation.

4. **Malignant Transformation:**
    - Rare (<1% of cases); endocervical polyps are slightly more prone to malignancy than ectocervical polyps.

Diagnosis

1. **History Taking:**
   - Detailed menstrual, sexual, and reproductive history to identify symptoms.

2. **Pelvic Examination:**
   - Visualization of polyps using a speculum.

3. **Colposcopy:**
   - To assess the vascularity and structure of the polyp for further evaluation.

4. **Pap Smear:**
   - To rule out cervical dysplasia or malignancy.

5. **Ultrasound:**
   - Transvaginal or pelvic ultrasound may help identify associated conditions (e.g., uterine or endometrial polyps).

6. **Biopsy:**
   - Essential to rule out malignancy, especially in postmenopausal women.

Modern Medicine Management

1. **Medical Treatment:**
   - **Antibiotics**: For infected polyps.
   - **Hormonal Therapy**: For polyps associated with hormonal imbalance.

2. **Surgical Treatment:**
   - Polypectomy:
     - The most common treatment where the polyp is twisted off or removed with forceps.
   - Electrocautery:
     - To cauterize the polyp base and prevent recurrence.
   - Cryotherapy or Laser Ablation:
     - In cases of multiple or recurrent polyps.
   - Hysteroscopy:
     - To identify and remove polyps higher up in the cervical canal.

3. **Follow-Up:**
   - Regular Pap smears and pelvic exams to monitor for recurrence or malignancy.

Comparative Table: Cervical Polyp vs. Endometrial Polyp

Aspect	Cervical Polyp	Endometrial Polyp
Origin	Arises from the cervical canal or ectocervix.	Arises from the lining of the uterus (endometrium).
Location	Visible on the cervix during a pelvic exam.	Located inside the uterus; diagnosed via ultrasound or hysteroscopy.
Aetiology	Chronic inflammation, trauma, high estrogen.	Hormonal imbalance (e.g., estrogen dominance), obesity.
Symptoms	Vaginal discharge, postcoital bleeding, intermenstrual bleeding.	Heavy or irregular periods, infertility, pelvic pain.
Complications	Infection, infertility, rare malignancy (<1%).	Endometrial hyperplasia, infertility, rare malignancy (1-3%).
Diagnostic Methods	Pelvic exam, colposcopy, biopsy.	Ultrasound, hysteroscopy, biopsy.
Management (Modern)	Polypectomy, electrocautery, hormonal therapy.	Hysteroscopic polypectomy, hormonal therapy.
Homeopathic Remedies	Thuja, Kreosotum, Calcarea Carbonica, Sepia.	Sabina, Calcarea Fluorica, Aurum Metallicum, Phosphorus.

Comparative Table of Homeopathic Therapeutics for Cervical Polyps

Remedy	Key Indications	Vaginal Discharge	Bleeding Symptoms	Mental/Emotional Symptoms	Modalities
Thuja Occidentalis	Soft, pedunculated polyps; linked with history of warts or genital infections.	Offensive, greenish, or yellow discharge.	Bleeding on slight touch or irritation.	Fixed ideas, low self-esteem, aversion to company.	**Better:** Warmth. **Worse:** Damp weather.

Remedy	Key Indications	Vaginal Discharge	Bleeding Symptoms	Mental/Emotional Symptoms	Modalities
Kreosotum	Cervical polyps with offensive, acrid, and irritating discharge causing itching or burning.	Offensive, yellowish, or watery discharge.	Profuse, irregular, or postcoital bleeding.	Irritability, restlessness, and anxiety about health.	**Better:** Warmth. **Worse:** Cold or wet weather.
Calcarea Carbonica	Polyps in overweight individuals with hormonal imbalances; tendency to profuse perspiration.	White or yellow discharge; sour-smelling.	Heavy, prolonged bleeding during menstruation.	Anxiety, fear of illness, and fatigue.	**Better:** Warmth. **Worse:** Cold and exertion.
Sepia Officinalis	Polyps with bearing-down sensation in the pelvis, aversion to intercourse, and hormonal irregularities.	Yellowish, milky, or offensive discharge.	Irregular menses; spotting between cycles.	Indifferent to loved ones, irritability, and fatigue.	**Better:** Vigorous exercise. **Worse:** Rest.
Lachesis Muta	Bluish or dark-colored polyps; sensitivity to touch; intense bleeding and irritability.	Dark, offensive, or blood-streaked discharge.	Bleeding worsens before menses and improves afterward.	Jealousy, talkativeness, and emotional extremes.	**Better:** Free flow. **Worse:** Tight clothing.
Medorrhinum	Polyps associated	Thick, acrid, and fishy-	Bright red bleeding;	Nervousness, irritability, and	**Better:** Evening.

Remedy	Key Indications	Vaginal Discharge	Bleeding Symptoms	Mental/Emotional Symptoms	Modalities
	with a history of sexually transmitted infections or suppressed gonorrheal discharge.	smelling discharge.	tendency to hemorrhage.	desire for stimulants.	**Worse:** Damp weather.
Phosphorus	Bleeding polyps; anemia from chronic blood loss; craving for cold drinks.	Profuse, watery, or mucopurulent discharge.	Bright red, profuse bleeding; worsens with exertion.	Warm, friendly, and highly emotional.	**Better:** Lying down. **Worse:** Cold air.
Silicea	Polyps in weak, undernourished individuals prone to chronic infections.	Offensive, purulent, or yellowish discharge.	Occasional spotting or bleeding after exertion.	Shy, timid, and emotionally fragile.	**Better:** Warmth. **Worse:** Cold drafts.
Murex Purpurea	Polyps with increased libido and pelvic sensitivity.	Bloody, offensive, or irritating discharge.	Profuse, bright red bleeding; pain in the pelvis.	Excitability, emotional outbursts, and hypersensitivity.	**Better:** Rest. **Worse:** Motion.
Sabina	Large polyps with bright red, clotted bleeding and severe back pain.	Foul-smelling or blood-streaked discharge.	Profuse bleeding during or after menstruation.	Nervousness and hypersensitivity to noise.	**Better:** Cool, fresh air. **Worse:** Warm rooms.
Hydrastis Canadensis	Chronic cervicitis with polyps	Thick, ropy, or mucopurule	Spotting after exertion;	Weakness, irritability, and fatigue.	**Better:** Rest. **Worse:**

Remedy	Key Indications	Vaginal Discharge	Bleeding Symptoms	Mental/Emotional Symptoms	Modalities
	and thick, tenacious, yellowish discharge.	nt discharge.	occasional hemorrhage.		Cold, damp weather.
Helonias Dioica	Weakness and dragging sensation in the pelvis; polyps due to uterine congestion.	Thin, watery, or yellowish discharge.	Bleeding associated with uterine prolapse or congestion.	Depressed, irritable, and feels unappreciated.	**Better:** Rest. **Worse:** Overexertion.

Chemotherapy And Radiotherapy In OB/GYN

Chemotherapy involves the use of drugs to kill or stop the growth of cancer cells. In OB/GYN cancers, chemotherapy is used in several scenarios:

1. **Ovarian Cancer:**
    - **First-Line Treatment**: Ovarian cancer is one of the most common gynecological cancers, and chemotherapy is the cornerstone of treatment, especially after surgery. The combination of platinum-based drugs (such as carboplatin or cisplatin) and taxanes (like paclitaxel) is commonly used.
    - **Adjuvant Therapy**: After surgery, chemotherapy may be used to eliminate any remaining cancer cells, reducing the risk of recurrence.
    - **Recurrent Ovarian Cancer**: If the cancer recurs, chemotherapy is used to control symptoms and prolong survival, often involving different agents or combinations than those used initially.

2. **Cervical Cancer:**
    - **Neoadjuvant Chemotherapy**: In cases of locally advanced cervical cancer, chemotherapy may be used before surgery (neoadjuvant chemotherapy) to shrink the tumor and make surgery more successful.
    - **Chemoradiation**: For advanced or recurrent cervical cancer, chemotherapy is combined with radiation therapy (chemoradiation) to improve the treatment outcome.

3. **Endometrial Cancer:**
    - **Advanced Stages**: For endometrial cancer (uterine cancer) that is in an advanced stage or has spread, chemotherapy is typically given as a part of a multi-modality treatment approach.
    - **Recurrence**: In recurrent endometrial cancer, chemotherapy may be used to control the cancer, although the response rate is generally lower compared to other cancers.

4. **Vulvar and Vaginal Cancer:**
    - **Advanced or Metastatic Disease**: In cases of advanced vulvar or vaginal cancers, chemotherapy may be used to control the spread of cancer. Chemotherapy can also be used when surgery is not an option.

5. **Chemotherapy Regimens:**
    - Common chemotherapy drugs include cisplatin, carboplatin, paclitaxel, docetaxel, etoposide, and cyclophosphamide.

- o **Combination Therapy**: Chemotherapy is often combined with radiation (chemoradiation) or surgery to improve the overall treatment outcome.

Radiotherapy in OB/GYN Cancers

Radiotherapy involves using high-energy radiation to destroy cancer cells. It can be used as a standalone treatment or in conjunction with chemotherapy and surgery.

1. **Cervical Cancer:**
   - o **Primary Treatment**: For patients with locally advanced cervical cancer, radiotherapy is a primary treatment. External beam radiation is commonly used along with intracavitary brachytherapy (radiation placed directly at the tumor site).
   - o **Chemoradiation**: This is the standard treatment for locally advanced cervical cancer. Chemotherapy sensitizes the tumor to radiation, improving the effectiveness of both treatments.
   - o **Post-Surgical Treatment**: After surgery for cervical cancer, radiation may be used to eliminate any residual tumor cells and reduce the risk of recurrence.

2. **Endometrial Cancer:**
   - o **Adjuvant Radiation**: For patients with high-risk endometrial cancer (such as those with deep myometrial invasion or lymphovascular space involvement), radiation therapy may be recommended post-surgery, especially if the cancer has spread beyond the uterus.
   - o **Pelvic Radiation**: Radiation may also be used in cases of recurrent disease, particularly for those with regional pelvic recurrence.

3. **Ovarian Cancer:**
   - o **Palliative Radiation**: In advanced ovarian cancer that is no longer curable, radiotherapy can be used for symptom relief, such as reducing tumor size to alleviate pain or pressure.
   - o **Rarely Used as Primary Therapy**: Radiotherapy is not commonly used as a primary treatment for ovarian cancer, except in specific cases of localized recurrence.

4. **Vulvar and Vaginal Cancer:**
   - o **Local Treatment**: In cases of early-stage vulvar or vaginal cancer, radiation therapy may be used either alone or after surgery to ensure complete removal of cancer cells.
   - o **Advanced or Recurrent Disease**: For more advanced or recurrent vulvar or vaginal cancers, radiation is a key component of treatment, sometimes combined with chemotherapy.

5. **Pelvic Radiotherapy:**
   - For many OB/GYN cancers, particularly those of the cervix, uterus, and vagina, radiation therapy is targeted at the pelvic region, and the goal is to treat the tumor while minimizing the exposure of healthy tissues.

Role of Chemotherapy and Radiotherapy in Combination

In certain situations, chemotherapy and radiotherapy are used together:

1. **Chemoradiation for Cervical Cancer**: This combination is standard for treating locally advanced cervical cancer. Chemotherapy agents (usually cisplatin) are used to enhance the effectiveness of radiation therapy.
2. **Ovarian Cancer Recurrence**: If ovarian cancer recurs, chemotherapy is the mainstay, and radiation may be used for specific localized recurrences.
3. **Neoadjuvant Therapy**: Chemotherapy or chemoradiation may be given before surgery to shrink tumors and improve surgical outcomes, especially in advanced cases of cervical or endometrial cancer.

Side Effects and Considerations

Both chemotherapy and radiotherapy come with potential side effects, which vary depending on the type of cancer and the individual patient. Common side effects include:

1. **Chemotherapy Side Effects:**
   - Nausea and vomiting
   - Fatigue
   - Hair loss
   - Lowered immunity (increased risk of infections)
   - Anemia and low platelet count
   - Peripheral neuropathy (nerve damage)

2. **Radiotherapy Side Effects:**
   - Skin irritation and redness at the site of treatment
   - Fatigue
   - Nausea and bowel problems (in pelvic radiation)
   - Vaginal dryness or changes in sexual function (in pelvic radiation)
   - Potential for secondary cancers in the long term

Colposcopy

Colposcopy is a diagnostic procedure used to closely examine the cervix, vagina, and vulva for signs of disease, particularly premalignant and malignant lesions. It is performed using a colposcope, which is a specialized magnifying instrument with a light source, enabling a detailed evaluation of the epithelial surfaces.

Indications for Colposcopy

1. **Abnormal Cervical Screening Results:**
   - Atypical squamous cells (ASC-US, ASC-H).
   - Low-grade squamous intraepithelial lesion (LSIL).
   - High-grade squamous intraepithelial lesion (HSIL).
   - Atypical glandular cells (AGC).
   - Presence of high-risk human papillomavirus (HPV).

2. **Evaluation of Abnormalities Detected Clinically:**
   - Visible cervical lesions.
   - Persistent postcoital or intermenstrual bleeding.
   - Unexplained abnormal vaginal discharge.

3. **Suspicion of Vulvar or Vaginal Lesions:**
   - Abnormal growths, pigmentation, or nonhealing ulcers.

4. **Follow-Up of Treated Cervical Lesions:**
   - After cryotherapy, LEEP, or conization for cervical intraepithelial neoplasia (CIN).

5. **Assessment of DES (Diethylstilbestrol) Exposure:**
   - For structural abnormalities and adenosis.

6. **Investigation of Unexplained Infertility:**
   - To identify cervical stenosis or structural abnormalities.

Preoperative Management

1. **Patient Counseling:**
   - Explain the purpose of the procedure, expected outcomes, and potential findings.
   - Reassure the patient about minimal discomfort during the procedure.

2. **Informed Consent:**
   - Obtain consent after explaining risks and benefits.

3. **Preparation Instructions:**
   - Advise the patient to avoid:

- Vaginal douching, tampons, or vaginal medications for 48 hours before the procedure.
- Sexual intercourse for 24–48 hours before the procedure.
  - Schedule the procedure when the patient is not menstruating, as blood may obscure the findings.

4. **Medications:**
   - Mild analgesics (e.g., ibuprofen or paracetamol) may be prescribed preemptively to minimize discomfort.
   - Antibiotics if there's a risk of infection.

5. **Physical Preparation:**
   - Ensure the patient empties their bladder prior to the procedure.

Procedure for Colposcopy

1. **Positioning:**
   - The patient is positioned in the lithotomy position.

2. **Preparation of Equipment:**
   - Ensure the colposcope is functional and properly adjusted.
   - Prepare 3%–5% acetic acid and Lugol's iodine solution.

3. **Examination Process:**
   - Initial Inspection:
     - Visualize the cervix and vaginal walls with a speculum.
     - Note any visible abnormalities (e.g., lesions, ulcers, discharge).
   - Application of Acetic Acid:
     - Apply 3%–5% acetic acid to the cervix using a cotton swab or sponge.
     - Observe for acetowhite changes, which indicate areas of high nuclear density, often seen in dysplasia.
   - Examination Under Magnification:
     - Focus on the transformation zone (area of squamous and columnar epithelium) for abnormal patterns.
   - Application of Lugol's Iodine:
     - Apply iodine to stain glycogen-rich squamous epithelium (normal tissue stains brown).
     - Dysplastic or cancerous tissue (glycogen-deficient) will appear as unstained areas (Schiller's test).
   - Targeted Biopsy (if indicated):
     - Take a biopsy from suspicious areas for histopathological evaluation.

Findings in Colposcopy

1. **Normal Findings:**
   - Uniformly pink epithelium.
   - Staining with Lugol's iodine (glycogen-rich tissue turns brown).

2. **Abnormal Findings:**
   - Acetowhite Epithelium:
     - White areas after acetic acid application, suggesting dysplasia.
   - Punctation:
     - Small red dots representing dilated capillaries in dysplastic areas.
   - Mosaicism:
     - Abnormal capillary networks seen in CIN or early malignancy.
   - Atypical Vessels:
     - Irregular, coarse, or non-branching vessels, often indicative of invasive cancer.
   - Unstained Areas with Lugol's Iodine:
     - Areas that fail to stain brown, suggesting glycogen depletion (dysplasia or cancer).
   - Ulcerations, Growths, or Keratosis:
     - Seen in advanced lesions or invasive cancer.

Complications of Colposcopy

1. **During the Procedure:**
   - Mild discomfort or pain during biopsy or application of acetic acid/iodine.
   - Vasovagal reaction (e.g., dizziness or fainting).

2. **Post-Procedure:**
   - Light spotting or bleeding (normal after biopsy).
   - Vaginal discharge (may occur if acetic acid or iodine is applied).

3. **Rare Complications:**
   - Infection (rare but possible if biopsy is performed).
   - Prolonged bleeding from biopsy sites.
   - Scarring (extremely rare).

Congenital Uterine Anomalies

Congenital uterine anomalies (CUAs) are malformations of the uterus resulting from improper development, fusion, or resorption of the Müllerian ducts during embryogenesis. These anomalies can affect reproductive, obstetric, and gynecological health.

Classification of Congenital Uterine Anomalies

The American Society for Reproductive Medicine (ASRM) and European Society of Human Reproduction and Embryology (ESHRE) classify these anomalies into the following types:

1. **Hypoplasia or Agenesis (Class I)**
   - Complete or partial absence of uterine tissue.
   - Example: Mayer-Rokitansky-Küster-Hauser (MRKH) syndrome.

2. **Unicornuate Uterus (Class II)**
   - One Müllerian duct fails to develop.
   - May or may not have a rudimentary horn.

3. **Uterus Didelphys (Class III)**
   - Failure of fusion of both Müllerian ducts, resulting in two separate uteri and often two cervices.

4. **Bicornuate Uterus (Class IV)**
   - Incomplete fusion of the Müllerian ducts.
   - Two endometrial cavities, but a single cervix or two cervices.

5. **Septate Uterus (Class V)**
   - Incomplete resorption of the medial septum between the two Müllerian ducts.
   - The cavity is divided by a fibrous or muscular septum.

6. **Arcuate Uterus (Class VI)**
   - Mild indentation of the uterine cavity due to incomplete resorption of the septum.
   - Considered a normal variant.

7. **Diethylstilbestrol (DES)-Related Uterus (Class VII)**
   - T-shaped uterine cavity resulting from in utero exposure to diethylstilbestrol.

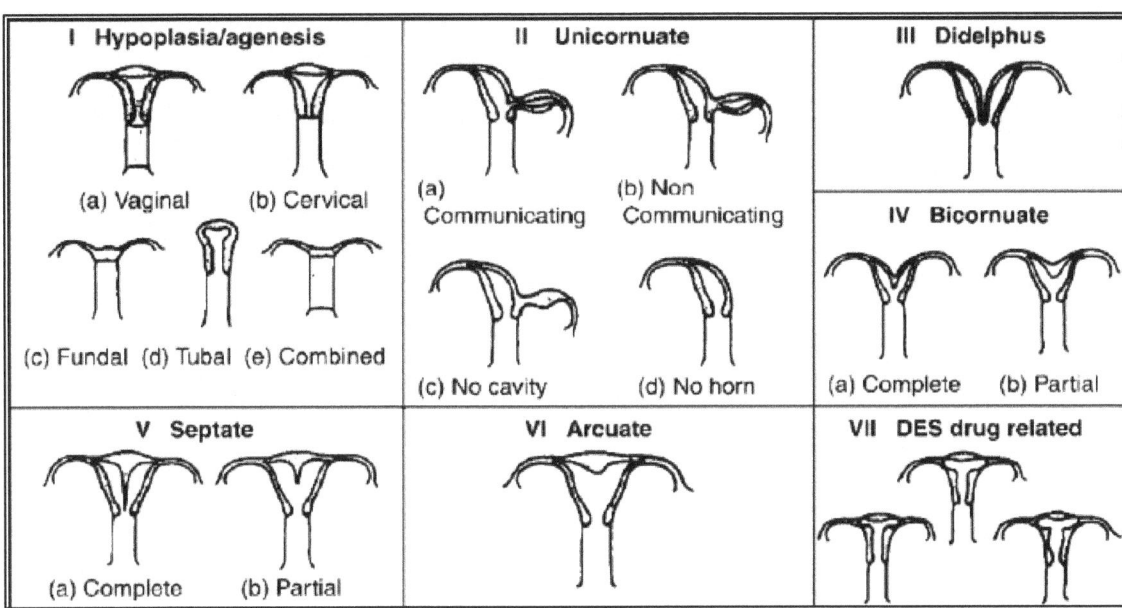

T-shaped uterine cavity resulting from in utero exposure to diethylstilbestrol.

Causes

1. **Genetic Factors**
   - Mutations in genes regulating Müllerian duct development (e.g., WNT4, HOXA10).
   - Familial occurrence in some cases.

2. **Teratogens**
   - In utero exposure to substances like diethylstilbestrol (DES).

3. **Environmental Factors**
   - Radiation, infections, or medications during fetal development.

Clinical Features

Symptoms vary based on the type and severity of the anomaly.

1. **Hypoplasia or Agenesis**
   - Primary amenorrhea.
   - Normal secondary sexual characteristics.
   - Infertility.

2. **Unicornuate Uterus**
   - Asymptomatic in some cases.
   - Dysmenorrhea, recurrent pregnancy loss.
   - Infertility.

3. **Uterus Didelphys**
   - Dysmenorrhea.

- Dyspareunia.
- Menstrual irregularities and recurrent miscarriages.

4. **Bicornuate Uterus**
   - Irregular menses, recurrent miscarriage.
   - Preterm labor, malpresentation of the fetus.

5. **Septate Uterus**
   - Recurrent pregnancy loss.
   - Menstrual irregularities.
   - Infertility.

6. **Arcuate Uterus**
   - Usually asymptomatic.
   - Associated with occasional pregnancy loss.

7. **DES-Related Uterus**
   - Infertility.
   - Increased risk of miscarriage and ectopic pregnancy.

Complications

- **Reproductive**: Infertility, recurrent pregnancy loss, implantation failure in IVF.
- **Obstetric**: Preterm labor, abnormal fetal presentation, intrauterine growth restriction (IUGR), uterine rupture.
- **Gynecological**: Dysmenorrhea, endometriosis due to menstrual outflow obstruction.

Diagnosis

1. **Clinical Examination**
   - Primary amenorrhea or abnormal menstrual patterns prompt investigation.

2. **Imaging Techniques**
   - **Ultrasound (USG)**: 2D or 3D transvaginal ultrasound to assess uterine morphology.
   - **MRI**: Gold standard for detailed evaluation of uterine anatomy.
   - **Hysterosalpingography (HSG)**: Outlines the uterine cavity and fallopian tubes.
   - **Sonohysterography**: Adds detail to the cavity evaluation.

3. **Endoscopic Techniques**
   - **Hysteroscopy**: Direct visualization of the uterine cavity.
   - **Laparoscopy**: Used to confirm external uterine morphology.

4. **Karyotyping**
   - To rule out chromosomal abnormalities like Turner syndrome.

Management

Management depends on the type of anomaly, associated symptoms, and reproductive goals.

1. Non-Surgical Management

- For mild anomalies (e.g., arcuate uterus) or asymptomatic cases.
- Psychological counseling for amenorrhea or infertility.

2. Surgical Management

- **Septate Uterus**: Hysteroscopic metroplasty to remove the septum.
- **Unicornuate Uterus**: Removal of a non-communicating rudimentary horn to prevent hematometra.
- **Uterus Didelphys/Bicornuate Uterus**: Metroplasty (Strassman procedure) to unify the cavities if recurrent pregnancy loss occurs.
- **MRKH Syndrome**: Vaginal reconstruction surgery (e.g., Vecchietti procedure) for functional sexual intercourse.
- **DES-Related Uterus**: No specific surgical correction; supportive reproductive care.

3. Reproductive Assistance

- IVF for infertility if surgery is not feasible.
- Cerclage for cervical incompetence in bicornuate uterus.

4. Obstetric Management

- Close monitoring for preterm labor, fetal growth restriction, and malpresentation.

Prognosis

- Early diagnosis and appropriate management improve fertility outcomes.
- Women with repaired septate uterus or bicornuate uterus often achieve term pregnancies.
- Severe anomalies like hypoplasia or agenesis have limited reproductive potential but may benefit from advanced reproductive technologies (e.g., surrogacy).

Contraception

Definition

Contraceptions are the all measures temporary or permonant designed to prevent pregnancy due to coital act.

Contraceptives - Metiods used for contraception.

Crieteria For Ideal contraceptive -
- Widely acceptable
- Non expensive
- Simple to use
- Safe
- Highly effective
- Required minimal motivation
- Low maintainance
- Low supervision
- Less reactions or adverse effects.

Various Methods Of Contraception-

1] Temporary

2] Permanent

1] Temporary Methods-

Methods which one used to postpone or to space births.

-i] Barrier Methods (e.g, condom,spermicidal jelly, sponge etc.)

- ii] Natural Methods (Rhythm method ,Coitus inturptus)

-iii] IUCD 's (hormonal/non hormonal)

-iv] Steroidal contraception(Oral, Parenteral, Devices).

2] Permanent Methods -

-A] Female Tubal Occlusion

-B] Male Vasectomy

Temporary methods

i] Barrier Methods-

Methods of contraception where objective is achieved by mechanical devices or by chemical means...which produces sperm immobilization and to prevent sperm deposition or penetration in cervical canal.

*Mechanical

Male - Condom.
Female -Condom
— Diaphragm
— Cervical ring

*Chemical (vaginal contraceptive)
— Vaginal Creams e.g; Delfen.
— Jelly - Preceptin,Volpar paste
— Foam Tab-e.g,Aerosol foams, Chlarimin T, Sponge Today
— Combination use of both mechanical & chemical

MALE CONDOM

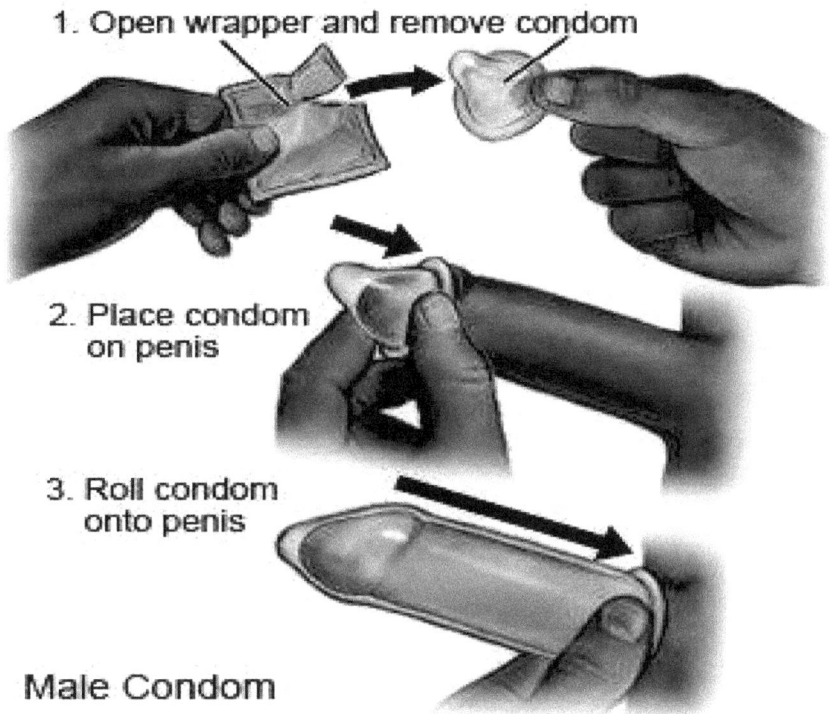

Most widely practiced method.
Available in latex & polyurethane.
Comparitively polyurethane is thinner have less reactions & allergies.

Usefull in;

— Spacing child bath
— Who have infrequent intercourse
— Who are sensitive or contradict for other methods of contraception.
— Before new IUD fitted.
— During treament of sexually transmitted diseases
e.g;vaginitis, cervicitis.

— In management of immunnological male infertility adviced to use for 3 months.

Advantages-
- Cheaper
- Easily available
- No side effects.
- Easy to carry & disposible with simple to use
- Give protection against Sexually transmitted diseases e.g, gonorrhea, Chlamydia, HPV, HIV
- Protection against PID.
- Poor incidence of tubal or ectopic pregn.

Disadvantages -
- -Chances of rupture so failure rate is high.
- Inadequate sexual pleasure.
- Skin reactions
- Only single use.

FEMALE CONDOM

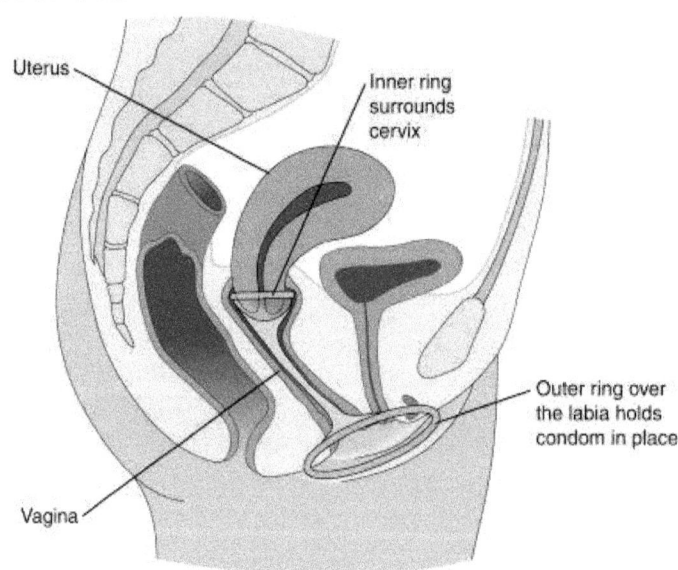

- 5 cm in length.
- Made up of polyurethane.
- Other all disadvantages & uses are same to that of male condom.

DIAPHRAGM
- Intravaginal rubher device with flexible metal or spring ring at margins.
- Size is variable.

- Device need to introduced 3hrs. before intercourse & tobe kept at least 6hrs. after last coital act.
- Ill fitting, accidental displacement & ascent of sperms along with the margins of devices increases the failure rate. Additional chemical spermicides are required to be use.

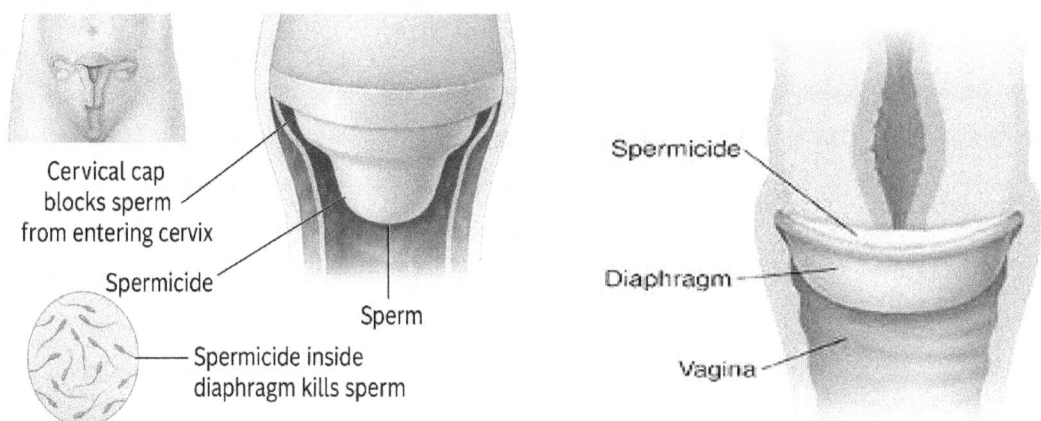

Advantages-
- Cheap.
- Can use repetedly for long time.
- Used with spermicide reduces incidence of PID & STD.

Disadvantages -
- Required size determination by medical, paramedical
- Person.
- Risk of vaginal irritation, allergic reactions.
- Chances of UTI.
- Contradictory to women with uterine prolapsed.

Chemical Vaginal Contraceptives
Action-
These agents are spermicidal to action .
Same extends produces sperm immobilization.
Prevents Sperm penetration in Cervix.
e.g; Cream, jelly, foam tablets.
Advantages-
- Less local, vaginal & vulval allergic reactions.
- Increases efficacy of condom.
- Less failure rate.

When to introduce - 5 min or soon before coitus

Disadvantages-
Mostly need to use with other barrier method.

Vaginal Contraceptive Sponge (Today)
Action-
— Polyurethane filled with monoxynol 9 (a spermicidal)
— Moisten with clean water & intraduce just before coitus. -It releases Speamicide during coitus & kills the sperms.
— Obstuct the cervical enterence with absorption of ejaculation.

Advantages-
— Easy to apply, not required 2 nd person.

Disadvantages-
— Single use (only for 24 hrs.)
— Shouldn't be removed for 6 hrs after intercourse.
— Less effective
— More Expensive
— High failure date:
— Allergic reaction
— Chances of vaginal soreness is high.

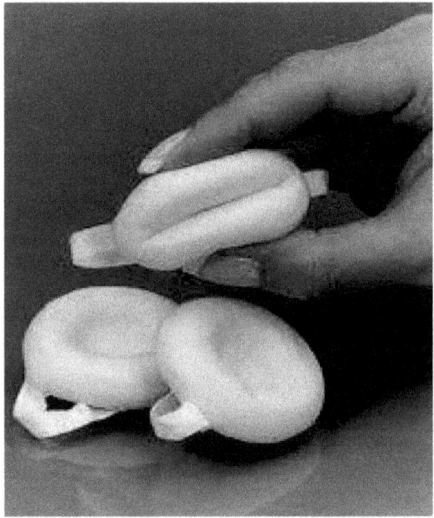

ii] Natural Contraception
DEF-
Contraception without any mechanical aid.

Rhythm Method
The method is based on identification of the fertile period of cycle and obstain from sexual intercourse in that period i.e;around the time of ovulation.

Those r-
1. Calender rhythm
2. Temperature rhythm
3. Mucus rhythm
4. Symptomothermal method
5. Ovulation indicator testing

1. Calendax rhythm-

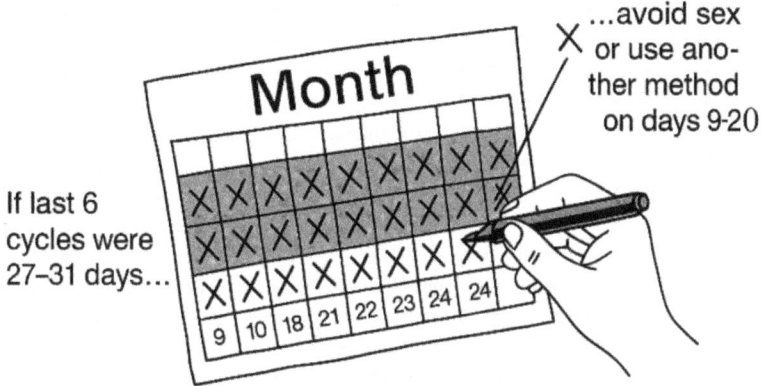

The period of abstinence is calculated from previ0us twelve menstrual cycles records.
— 1st unsafe day is obtained by shortest period length - 20 dys & last unsafe day is by longest period duration - 10 dys.

Advantages-
Contraception can achieve without ony mechanical or chemical aid in women with regular menstruation cycle.

Disadvantages-
— Twelve ovulation cycle study record needed.
— Failure rate is more in women with irregular menstruation.

2. Basal body temp method-
— The period of sexual obstinance is calculated by BBT records of women.
— The fact is based upon a women's temp drops 12 to 24 hrs before ovolution & increases again after ovulation.
— The temp difference is less than 1°F at body rest so require very carefull accurate mouth temp with sensitive thermometer.
— Every early morning mouth temp should he record by women before she gets out of bed.
— Daily temp variation noted.9-20

Iii] Mucus Rhythm Method /Ovulation Mucus Method

- At different times of month, the vaginal secreation change in colour & consistency. Fertile mucus i.e; around ovulation is copious, clear & stretchy like row of egg white .Infertile mucus is scanty, thick & opaque.
- This method involves abstaining from sexual intercourse in dys of fertility derived from observations of cervical mucus.
- During dys of ovulation, this fertile mucus is thin & slippery that helps the sperm travelling from cervix to uterus to tubes to meet female gamette & hence fertilization

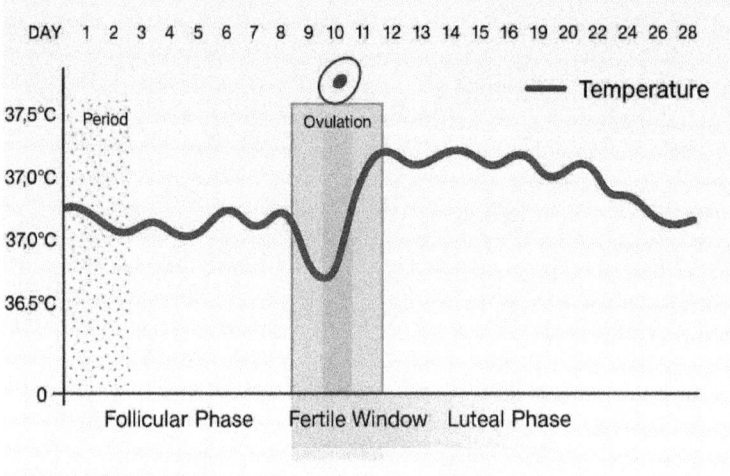

Advantages-
- No side effects
- No mechanical or chemical device used
- Easy to stop & conceive
- No cost

Disadvantages-
- kean observation of mucus changes needed.
- Failure rate is high
- Sexual abstinence is necessary

Iv] Symptomothermal Method -
Combination of all 3 methods to rule out dys. of ovulation; fertility period of women f/b sexual obstinence during that fertility period.
Period of Sexual Obstinance –
 Ovulated egg has max 72 hrs. capacity of festilization while spasms can remain live max. 5 dys after intrauterine ejaculation. So even unprotected sexual intercourse 4-5 dys before ovulation may causes festization.
So for natural contraception 5. dys before and 3 dys after Ovulation is the duration of Sexual obstinance.

*Coitus Interuptus-
- -Withdrawal of penis short before ejaculation is called coitus interuptus.
- -Requires sufficient self controll of man to withdrawal of penis before ejaculation.

Advantage –
- No applicance required.
- No cost
- No mechanical or chemical aid required.

Disadvantages-
- Poor sexual satisfaction
- Requires self controll by man
- Pregnancy can accur as precoital secretions or accidental sperm deposition in vagina during withdrawal.
- Women may develop anxiety neurosis, vaginismus or pelvic congestion.

*Breast Feeding-
- Prolonged & sustained breast feeding causes maintaining of high prolactine levels thal supresses ovulation hence gives natural protection against pregnancy.
- Method is more effective in post- delivery Lamenashaic women than in menstauating women.
- Addition barrier methods along with breast feeding provide complete contraception.

*FAB methods-
[Fertility awareness based methods]

- Natural contraception (Rhythm method, coitus interruptus & lactational amenorrhea)

    +

Barrier Methods. [condom, diaphragm, spermicides]

Iii] Intrauterine Contraceptive Devices -

Classification :
- Open and closed
- Medicated [bioactive] Hormonal & Non harmonal
- Non- medicated
- Open IUCD's-

have very small aperture < 5mm.

so thal if accidentally uterine perforation occurs, intestine loop or omentum containt can"t strangulated.

e.g, CuT, Cu7 Multiload 250/375.cte

Lippe's loop

— Closed IUCD's -

They have potential of causing gut strangulation if accidentally enters uterine cavity.

eg, Grafenberg Ring

Birnberg bow

— Medicated IUCD's-

Harmonal;

Either releasing progesteron (progestasert). or levonorgestrel e.g; Progestasert, LNG-IUS

Non hormonal -

Contains metal like copper which is spesmicidal in action e.g;CuT 200,Multiload 250, Multiload 375, CuT 380

Non-medicated IUCD's- No any harmone or melal used.

Only causes obstruction to sperm travelling and engadement of fertilised product – not in used today.

eg, Lippes loop

Duration of Each Medicaled IUCD's actions -

The number in name of CuT suggest surface area accupied by copper in device. As the surface area increases ,the duration for replacent also increases.

CuT 200   -3 to 4 yrs.

Multiload 250 - 3Yrs.

CuT 380.   -10 Yrs.

Multiload 375   - 5. Yrs.

Progestasert   - 1yr.(Not manufactured today)

LNG- IUS   - 5 Yrs.

Lippes loop- No longer used in India

Mode of Action –

Actual antifertility role is unknown.

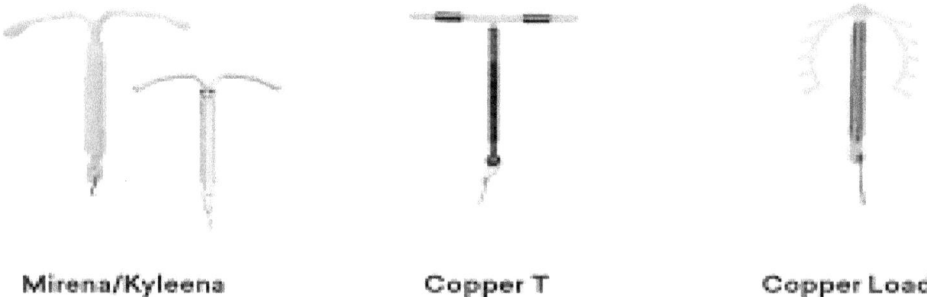

Mirena/Kyleena   Copper T   Copper Load

Probable Actions are;

- Non specific endometrial inflammation & bio chemical changes decreases sperm motility & vitality.
- Gametotoxic & spermicidal in action.
- Increases cervical mucus thickness & production as result of inflammatory action which causes obstruction to sperms to enter into cervix to uterus.
- It increases tubal motility which leads to quick migration of fertilized ovum in urine cavity before desirable endometrial changes occurs. Thus obstructs the engadgement of fertilized ovum.
- Copper Action-
- Ionised copper itself has local infertility in action.
- LNG –IUS-

As it is hormonal device, it produces anovulatory cycles & causes endametrial hypoplasia.

Time of Insertion –

- 2-3 days after menstruation bleed over.
- Any time in lactational amenorhoea.
- In late abortion, following D&C, D&E, S&E
- In late abortion, post delivery at least 6 wks later i.e; ofter uterine involution so that CuT will not expelled out.

Time to Remove –

- 2 to 4 dys prior menstral cycle.
- Can remove any y time of menstruation cycle.

Contraindications of Insertion-

- Fibroid Uterus
- PID
- DUB
- Congenital uterine anomalies
- Prolapsed Uterus
- Pregnancy
- H/O dysmenorrhea
- P/H ectopic pregnancy
- Nulliparous
- PID
- Suspected Ca Cx
- HIV + ve mother

— within 6wks of LSCS

Indications of Removal-
— Persistant DUB
— Suspected Ca Cx
— 1 yr. after menopause
— Flariing up of salpingitis
— Device action expire
— Perforation Of uterus
— Partial expulsion of CuT
— Desire for pregnancy
— Missing thread

Complications-

Immediate
— Abdominal Pains
  Sudden, transient and cramps lasting for 1hr. relieved by analgesics or antispasmodics.
— Syncopal shock with sudden pain esp. when device is insesled in comparitively small uterus.
  e.g; in nulliparous woman
— Perforation of uterus.
  Partial or complete perforation of uterus due to faulty methods of cuT Insestion.
— P/V spotting
  Slight P/V bleeding may occure. Menses may appear if inserted just before expected day of menstruation.

Remote
— Abdominal Pains
  It is proportionate to degree of myometrial distension .
  May be minimised with choice of proper sized CuT
  Dull aching lower abd pains, aggr. before, during menses and after coitus.
— Menstrual Abnormalities
  Menorrhagia, Metrorrhagia, epimenorrhea, DUB causes anaemia. Rate of occurance is less in 3rd generation IUCD,s (Hormonal IUCD's)
— Pelvic Infection (PID)
  Comman in multipara
— Spontaneous Expulsion

It is common when inserted in distended uterus. e.g; post abortal, puerperal insertion

Expultion is common during menstruation.

Diagnosed by failure to palpate the thread in vagina.

— Perforation Of The Uterus

Due to migration of CuT with subsequent myometrial contractions.

— -Pregnancy

Pregn rate is about 2%

The risk of ectopic pregnancy, abdominal pregnancy is high.

3rd generation IUCD's decreases risk of ectopic pregnancy.

Advantages-

— Free of cost in government hospitals.
— Opd simple technique of insertion and removal.
— Prolonged contaceptive protection on single insertion.
— Applicable in Women with systemic illness like

Hypertension, epilepsy.

— No Systemic side effects.
— No any permanent effect on fertility.
— Easy to conceive after removal of device.
— Use can be discontinue any time.

Disadvantages -

— Required motivation
— Adverse local reactions like menstrual abnormalities eg;PID, dysmenorrhea, menorrhagea, metrorrhagia, backache, pelvic pains.
— Contraindications in intrauterine space ocupying lesions e.g;fibroids, Ca endometrium, polyp etc.
— Risk of ectopic pregnancy is high.
— Required annually checking for proper placing by USG.

*Hormonal IUCD'S-

Advantages -

— Prolonged contraceptive protection. (5yrs.)
— Reduction in rate of CuT complications like metro,
— Menorrhagia, dysmenorrheal, PMS.
— Applicable in adenomyosis, leomyomas, Ca endometrium, endometrial hyperplasia.

— It is advisable as HRT at perimenopausal age.

— It can be used alternative to hysterectomy for menorrhagia

Disadvantages-
— Not provided by government.

— Costly

— Deposition of Calcium on device hampers diffusion of

— copper on prolonged use.

— Steroidal Contraception-

Route of administration-

A] Oral- Single Preparations e.g; Progestin Only Pill (mini pill),oestrogen only (emergency contraceptive pills)

-Combined Preperations e.g ;Monophasic, Biphasic, Triphasic, Post coital or emergency)

B] Parenteral-Injectables [e.g; DMPA , NET- EN.
Once a month injection]

- Implants [e.g, Norplant, Implants]

C] Devices -IUD (LNG IUS) Hormone releasing

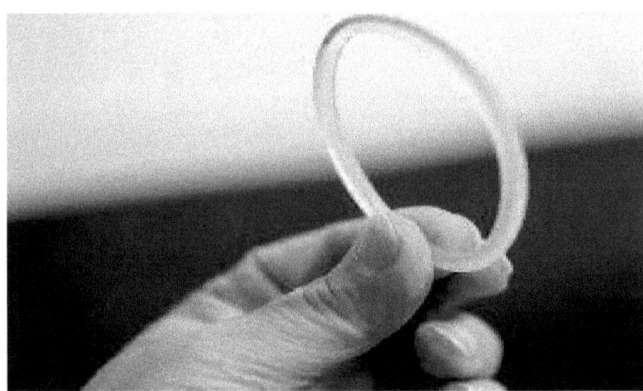

Vaginal Ring

Common and Combined Preparations-
— Progestins - levonorgestrel / norethisteron/desogestrel

— Oestrogens-ethyl oestradiol/menstranol

— The amount of E (ethinyl estradiol & P (Progestin) goes on decreasing as drug generation increases.

I st generation OCpills- 50 Microgram or more

II nd generation OC pills- 30-35 Microgram or more

III rd generation OC pills.-20-30 Microgram

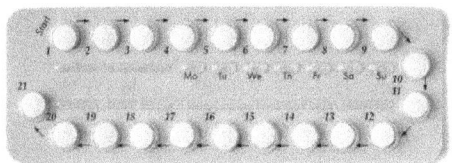
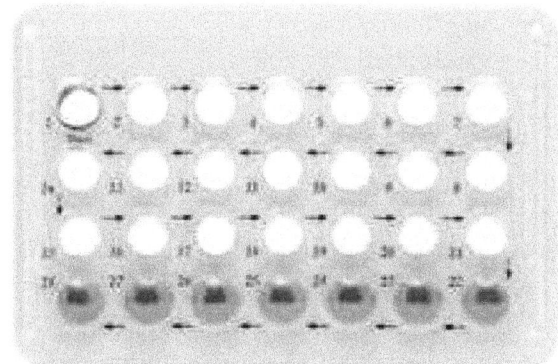

Made of Action-

— Both harmones supresses Gonadotropin Releasing hormone causes no FSH& LH Peak which causes failure of follicular growth & ovulation, i.e; anovulatory cycles

— Causes endometrial hypoplasia with regression of endometrial glands & their secretary functions.

— Makes the cervical mucus more thick, viscid, scanty that prevents sperm entry.

— Alters the follipian tube mobility & secretions so prevents conception in accidental ovulation.

Contraindications-

I] Absolute-

H/O or present cardiovascular diseases

e.g; Hypertension

— Angina and IHD

— Arterial or venous thrombosis

— Valvular heart diseases

— Focal migraine

Liver diseases

e.g:in Jaundice during pregnancy

— Gallbladder diseases

— Liver adenoma

— Granuloma of Liver

— Other active liver diseases

Other diseases

e.g ; breast cancer

- G.I. Tract bleeding disorders

II] Relative-

- Obesity
- Epilepsy
- Bronchial Asthma
- Depression & mood swinging
- Above age 35 yrs.
- 1st 6 months ofter delivery in lactating mother.
- Varicosities
- Smoking
- Alcoholism

Advantages-

- Prevention of unwanted pregnancy with rare failure.
- Menstrual regularization.
- Reduction of menstrual disorders like menorrhagia, metrorrhagea, dysmenorrhea
- Reduction of PMS (pre menstrual syndrome)
- Reduction of Mittle schmerz syndrome
- Protection against iron deficiency anaemia
- Protection against PID
- Ectopic Pregnancy
- Fibroid uterus
- Endometroisis
- Hirsuitism, acne
- Begin breast diseases
- Autoimmune thyroid disorders
- Rheumatoid arthritis
- Osteopania & podmenopausal osteoporotic fractures
- Endometrial & cervical cancer
- Colorectal cancer

Disadvantages/ Adverse Effects -

Some effects are temporary while some are permanent.

- Nausea, Vomiting, headache.
- Mastalgia- breast heaviness and tenderness
- Weight gain (increased fally deposition).
- Oedema (Increased Na- water retention)

- Chloasma & Acne.
- Menstrual abnoamalities due to missing pill or drug interactions which decreases contraceptive absorption (e.g; broad sprectrum antibiotics, enzymes, antiepileptic drugs, antituberculin drugs, Grisoflavins)
- Post pill amenorrhea & Hypomenorrhea.
- Loss of libido (due to dryness of vagina).
- Leucorrhea (due to increased mucus secretions.)
- Depression, mood swinging ,sleep disturbances & other psychiatric manifestations (give pyridoxine 50mg to reduce these symptoms.
- Increases pre-existing system diseases like e.g,Hypertension
- Cholestatic jaundice
- Cervical cancers
- Thrombo embolism
- Haemmorrhagic /ischemic myocardial infarction
- Increased insulin resistance hence hyperglycemia.
- Increased sex hormone binding harmones.
- Increased total cholesterol & triglycerides, increased plasma lipids & lipoproteins
- Decreased level of vit. B6, B12, folic acid ,calcium,

Maganeses, zinc, ascorbic acid

- Increased vit. A & Vit k levels
- Decreased level of LH & FSH. produces anovulatory cycles
- Fibrosis of Ovaries
- Endometrial oedema
- Thick cervical secretions with ectopy & glandular

Hyperplasia.

- Bulky uterus
- Ulcerative colitis
- Increased UTI & sexual activities.
- Depressed liver functions
- Small risk of congenital anomalies in children.
- Lactational suppression.

How to use when to withdraw –

New Users - Start the pill on 1st day of m.c for 21 dys f/b 8 dys. break (when pack is of 21 tab) .No need of break if pack is.of 28 tab .

After menstruation- 2 nd pocket should start an 8th day irrespective of m.c bleeding (in pack of 21 tab.)

To avoid this confusion, we can start each packet on 5th day of menstruation with advice to use condom for next 7 dys.

If 1 pill missed - take as remember early in the morning & continue the schedule.

If 2 pills missed, she should take 2 pills on each of next 2 dys & continue the rest schedule.

Extra precautions-e.g; condom should used atlest for next 7 dys. following missed pills.

Withdrawal indications -

— Cramps & pains in leg.
— Sudden excessive weight.gain
— Visiual disturbances
— Severe migraine
— Chest pains
— Severe depression.
— Prior to surgery (atleast 6 weeks before surgery to avoid vascular complications)
— Desire of pregnancy.

Injectable-

Common used drugs –

DMPA (Depo-medroxy-progesterone acetate.) & (NET -EN) i.e; Norethisterone enanthate.

Route of Inj - Intramuscular

Dose - DMPA =150 mg/3mnths or 300 mg/ 6 mnths
  -NET EN 200mg /2 mnths.

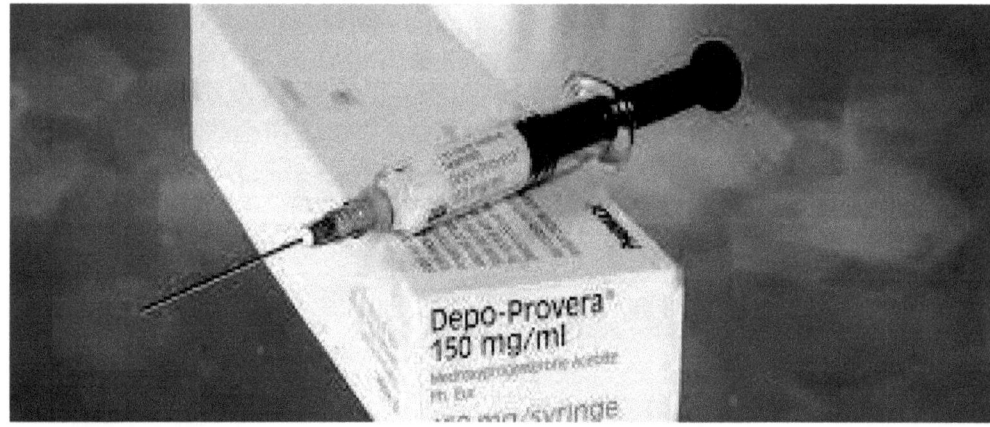

Mode of action -

— Suppression of LH & inhibition of ovulation.
— Increased cervical mucus secretions &thickness hence inhibits sperm penetration.

— Endometrial atrophy & hence prevent implantation of conceptive product.

Advantages -
- Safe in lactation.
- Increases milk secretions without alteration in composition.
- Can used as intermit method of contraception before vasectamy becaomes effective.
- No oestrogenic side effects.
- Decreases menstrual c/o menorrhagia,dysmenorrhea.
- Protect against endometrial Ca,Ovarian Ca
- Decreased PID, endometriosis, ectopic pregnancy.
- No need of daily mediacation as in OCpills, so no problem of missing pill.

Disadvantages-
- Chances of irregular bleeding, prolonged amenorrhea
- Return of fertility delayed for several months (4-8 mnths)

Contraindications-
- Same

Implants-
- Drug used- Progestin –levonorgestrel

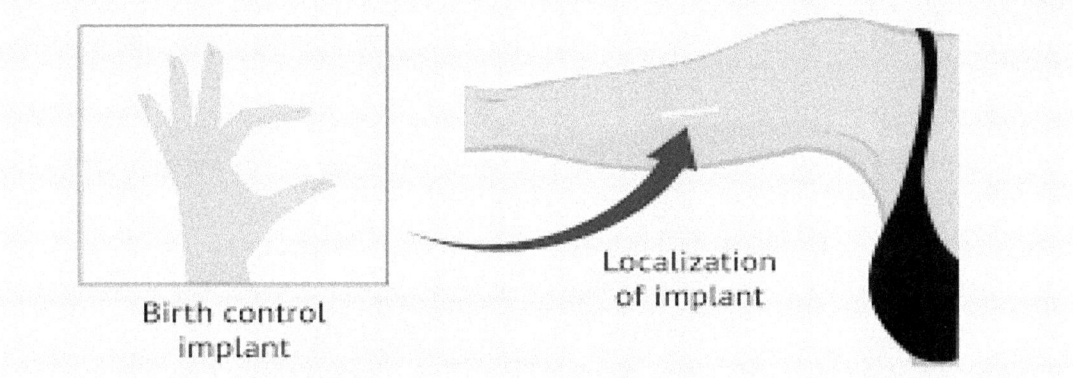

Route of administration-
- 6 flexible closed capsules containing 36mg,leonorgestrel each are inserted subdermally or non- dorminant arm, about 6-8 cm above elbow fold under LA on 1 st day of menstruation.

Time of insertion-
— 1st day of menstruation.
— Immediately after abortion.
— Three wks. following delivery.

Mode of Action -
— Decreases LH and hence supression of ovulation.
— Endomebrial atrophy & hence prevents pregnancy
— cervical mucus thickness hence prevents sperm penetration.

Advantages-
— Long term contraception (5Yrs) in one insertion.
— No complications of missing pills.
— Helpful in women who are not ready for permonant sterilization.
— Loss of contraceptive action immediate after removal.

Disadvantages-
— Chances of frequent p/v spotting, intermenstrual bleed or long term amenorrhea.
— Difficult removal

Implanon-
Drug used - Etanogestrel
Route-
Same to implant, but single 4cm long rod containing 60mg .
Duration of action- 3yrs.
All other informations are same to that of implants.only that insertion and removal is comparatively easy.

EMERGENCY CONTRACEPTION-(Post Coital Contraception)

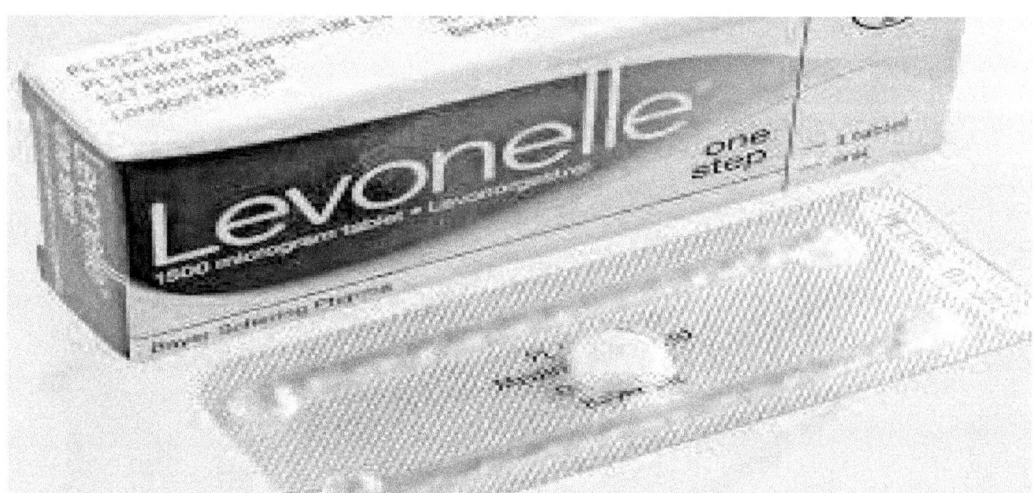

Indications-
- Unprotected intercourse
- 1st time intercourse (Mostly unplanned)
- Condom rupture.
- Missed o .c pills
- Sexual Assault
- Rape
- Unprotected sex around ovulation.

Drug & Dose-
- Ethinyl oestradiol : 2.5mg BD for 5 days.
- Conjugated oestrogen : 15mg x 5 dys
- Ethynyl oestrediol 5omg + Norgestrel 0.25mg:
- 2 tab stat 2 aftes 12 hrs
- Levonorgestrel(emergency) : 0.75mg stat & after 12hrs.
- Mifepristone : 600mg single dose
- All tab should start within 72 hrs. following unprotected sex.

Mode of Action -
- Prevention or delayed ovulation.
- Interfere fertilization
- Unfavourable endometrium for implantation.
- Interfares corpus luteum function causes luteolysis.

Drawbacks-
- 1% failure rate
- Induct of abortion should offer if drug fail.
- Nausea & vomiting so advice antiemetics.
- V]Permonant Contraception. (sterilization)

Def"-It is a surgical method whear by the reproductive function of individual (male or female) is purposefully & permananly destroyed.

Surgery in male is vasectomy in female is tubal acclussion on tubectomy.

Vasectomy-
DEF-
Permonant sterilisation of male by resectioning and ligation of bilateral segment of vas deference.

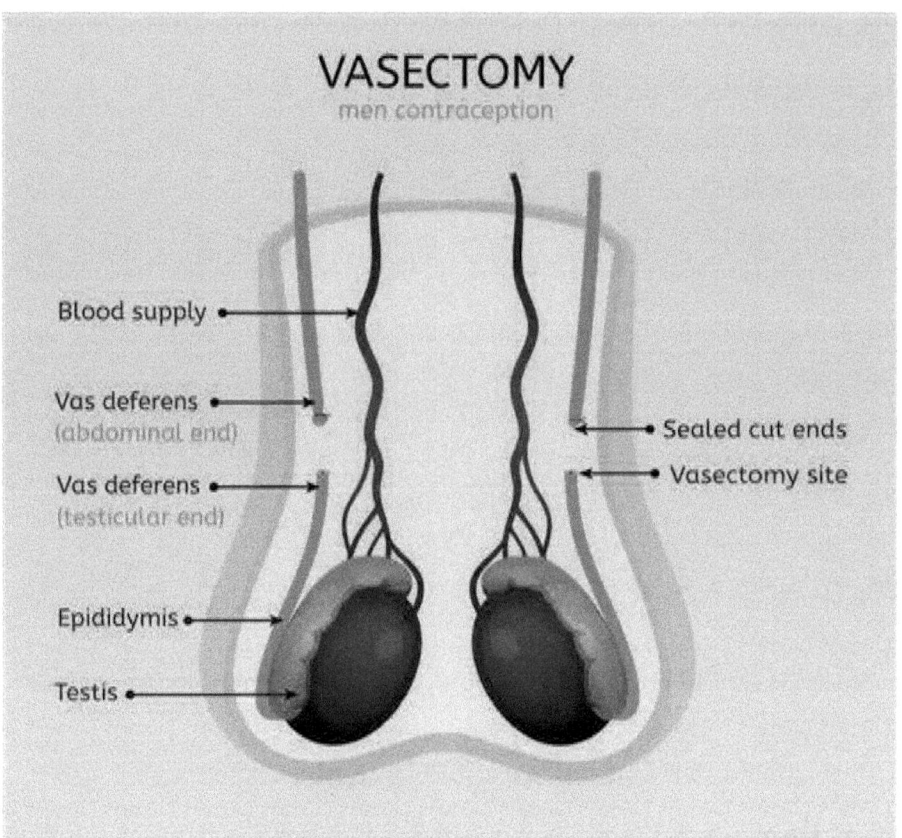

Advantages-
— Simple
— Less expenses.
— Less hospital stay
— Complications are low.
— Success of reversal anastomosis operation is 50%
— Can done as outdoor procedure in mass camp.
— Hydrocele or inguinal hernia can also be corrected during surgery.

Disadvantages-
— Psychological impotency or frigidity.
— 2:3 mnths required following operation to semen become sperm free.
— Eczema or scabies on scrotal area are temperory contraindications.
— Restriction of heavy worl,lifting heavy weight,cycling atleast for 2 wks.

Procedure-
— Writtten consent of person.
— Local area shaving & antiseptic dressing to maintain surgical asepsis.
— Pre operative medication is not necessary.

- Vas is palpate out at base of scrotum, lift it with fingers
- Small verticle incision is taken under local anaesthetia on

scrotum.
- By secting surrounded structures, vas deferens catch Allies forceps / Backock's forceps.
- Vas is ligated at 2 sites, 1cm apart with catgut & middle segment should cut out.
- Same procedure with other sided vas.
- Skin is sutured by catgut.
- Scotal suspensory dressing is given for discharge patient after 30 min. of operation.
- Antibiotics & analgesics are given at least for 5 dys.

Advice.
- Restrict weight lifting, heavy work, cycling at least for two wks.
- Additional contraceptive use 2-3 mnthe following
- surgery as 20 ejaculations are required to empty the stored semen.
- Sterilily should confirm by semen analysis after 2-3 mths.

Complications-
- Wound sepsis.
- Scrotal cellulitis or abscess.
- Scrotal haematoma.
- Psychological frigidity or impotency.
- Increased sperm agglutinin in circulation.
- Spontaneous recanalisation

Other methods-
*Non-scalpel vasectomy-
- Scalpel is not used for incision, it taken by tip of forceps under L.A same to that of regular vasectomy.

*Open ended vasectomy-
Abdamınal end of resected vas coagulated and
testicular end is left open.

*Percutaneous Vasocclusion-
- Reversible method
- Polyurethane elastmere is injected in vas which get
solidified & block the sperm passage.
In reversible method, this black can be removed under LA.

Female Sterilisation/ Tubectomy/ Tubal occlusion-

DEF-
Resection of a segment of both the fallopian tubes to achieve permanent sterilization.

Types-
— Abdominal & Vaginal
— Open & Laparoscopic

Conventional (laparotomy)& Minilaparotomy.

Comparision-

Points	Abdominal	Vaginal
surgeon	Any surgeon can perform	Surgeon with plaqstic surgeory knowledge required
Time of operation	Any time	Uterus should be less than 12 wks.contraindication in purperium
contraindications	Not specific	-purperium, -t.o.mass
complications	-Easy to tackle -wound infection -incisional hernia -rarely peritonitis	-difficult to handle -haemorrhage -ligamental haematoma -rectal injuries -dysparenia
anaesthetia	Local anaesthetia	General anaesthetia Or spinal anaesthetia
Hospital stay	5-6 dys	1-2dys
Failure rate	Less	More
-	Minilaparotomy	Laparoscopic sterilization
Cost	Minimal	Expensive
Person	Any surgeon	Special training
Assistance	Nil or minimum	Team work required

Time of operation	Any time with MTP	Can't within 6 wks of delivery or in enlarged uterus.
Contraindications	Not specific	Lung infection, heart diseases, intra abdominal adhesions, obesity
Complications	No life threatening	Fetal bowel injuries, surgical emphyma, blood vessel injuries
Hospital stay	3-5 dys	3-4hrs.
Failure rate	0.1-0.3%	0.2-0.6%
Reversibility	Difficult due to multiple adhesions & short length tube left behind.	Easier & effective Only 4mm tube get destroyed.

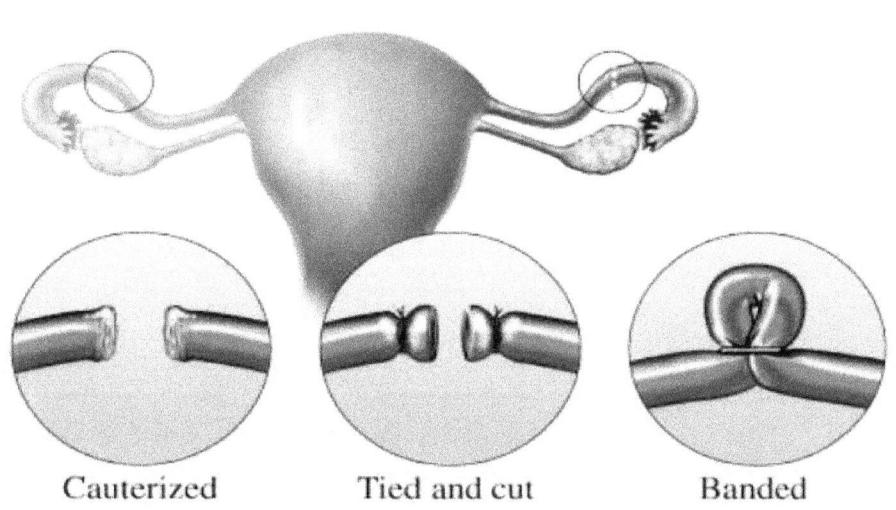

Indications-
— Family planning-to control the population.

— According to socio-economic status of family.
— If mother having following illness aggravated during pregnancy e.g, Heart diseases

    Diabetes Melitus

    Chronic renal failure

    Hypertension

    3rd time LSCS

    Post repair of prolapsed uterus.

Complications-

— Wound infection
— Incisional hernia
— peritonitis
— ligamental haematoma
— blood vessel injuries
— bowel perforation
— rectal injuries
— dysparenia
— occlusional obesity
— psychological upset
— chronic pelvic pain
— menstrual abnormalities
— dysmenorrhagea
— hypomenorrhea
— irregular menses
— post ligation syndrome
— cystic ovaries
— Alteration in libido

https://youtu.be/5qMl7czLmGU

FEMALE CONDOME

https://youtu.be/_yGh1rBV-kU

DIAPHRAGM AND CAP

ACTION OF COPPER T

CUT INSERTION AND REMOVAL

IMPLANTS

TUBECTOMY

VASECTOMY

Dilatation And Curettage

DEF-
This operation comprises of dilatation of internal cervical os and curettage of the uterine cavity.

INDICATIONS-

I] Diagnostic Indications-

1. Infertility
   — Detection of ovulation
   — Diagnosis of Endometrial Tuberculosis
   — Secretory status of endometrium
2. DUB & Menorrhagia-
   — To exclude organic uterine pathology, e.g. carcinoma endometrium
   — To differentiate between ovular and anovular dysfunctional uterine bleeding
   — Suspicion of Endometrial Tuberculosis
3. Post Menopausal Bleeding –
   — To exclude or diagnose endometrial carcinoma, fractional curettage is performed.
4. Follow up of Vesicular Mole-
   — In case of irregular bleeding
   — To diagnose Choriocarcinoma

II] Therapeutic Indications-

Gynaecological-
   — Dysfunctional Uterine Bleeding
Removal of endometrium helps to arrest the bleeding
   — Infertility
Some patients may conceive after D&C
   — Only Dilatation of internal os is indicated for Spasmodic Dysmenorrhoea
   — Drainage of the pyometra
   — Radium insertion
   — Initial step in Fothergill's operation
   — Cervical polyp
   — Endometrial polyp
   — Endometrial biopsy in premalignant and malignant conditions.
   — Intrauterine adhesions in Asherman's syndrome and endometriosis

- Intrauterine foreign body
- submucous myoma

Obstrectrical indications-
- Abortion, 1st tm termination
- Retained placenta
- Excessive bleed following delivery
- Hydatidiform mole

When to perform operation

- Usually, curettage is performed premenstrually, in secretary phase of menstruation for detection of ovulation in infertile patients and for studying endocrine status of the woman.
- Curettage is performed on the first day of menstruation in women having irregular or infrequent menses. It has an additional advantage of definitely excluding the pregnancy
- Curettage may be performed on any day for therapeutic purpose to arrest the bleeding

Anaesthesia-

Usually performed under General Anaesthesia, sometimes under local anaesthesia.

Pre-operative preparations-

- The patient is to be kept nil by mouth for at least 6 hours --The bowels should be completely emptied either by enema or by purgatives taken at last night
- Emptying of bladder immediately before operation.
- Perineum should be shaved and cleaned.
- Proper consent for the operation should be obtained
- Surgical Principles- paracervical block by Inj. Lignocaine 1%

NECESSARY INSTRUMENTS-

- Sponge holding forceps
- Sim's or Auvard's speculum
- Anterior vaginal wall retractor
- Volsellum Playfair's probe
- Uterine Sound
- Set of cervical dilators
- Uterine Curette
- Ovum forceps sos

Steps of Operation-
1. Patient in Lithotomy position .
2. Perineum is painted and vagina cleaned thoroughly by antiseptic solutions.
3. Suitable anaesthesia is given
4. Vaginal examination is done under anaesthesia to confirm position and size of uterus
5. Sim's or Cusco's vaginal speculum is inserted in the vagina to expose cervix.
6. Anterior vaginal wall is retracted by anterior vaginal wall retractor to visualize cervix.
7. Anterior lip of the cevix is held by Volsellum forceps.
8. Cervical canal is disinfected by Playfair's probe, soaked in iodine.
9. The length and the position of the uterus is assessed by uterine sound.
10. Depending upon the size of the curette the cervical canal is dilated with dilators set.
11. The cavity is curetted out with the help of sharp end of the curette. Endometrial debris collected with ovum forceps sos.
12. The curetted endometrium is collected over a piece of gauze and is sent for histopathological study to the

Laboratory where sample has to kept in formalin for all other indications and in normal saline for suspected cases of endometrial tuberculosis.

FRACTIONAL CURETTAGE

DEF-

It is a procedure in which sectional endometrium is collected separately for focal histopathological study.

INDICATIONS-

Abnormal uterine bleeding in menopausal or postmenopausal women.
- To diagnose or exclude
  — Possibility of malignancy.
  — stage of cancer
  — to locate the site of malignancy.

Steps of Operation-other procedure is same to that of regular D& C,

Sites for collection of sample for testing-
- Endocervical curettage is done:
  — Sample 1 • Length of the uterine cavity is measured.
  — Area 1 cm above the level of the internal os is curetted
  — Sample 2 = Anterior uterine wall

— Sample 3 = Posterior uterine wall
— Sample 4= Fundal region

COMPLICATIONS OF D&C

— Cervical Lacerations : When cervix resists in forced dilatation and curettage.
— Fallure to dilate the Cervix : If cervix is too much stenosed.
— Uterine Perforation
— Heavy p/v bleeding
— Septicemia
— PID
— Tubal blockages due to adhesion and hence secondary infertility.
— Cervical laceration
— Cervical incompetence & hence cervical incompetence.
— Asherman's Syndrome
— Psychological trauma
— Rh isoimmunisation in Rh – ve mother where anti D has missed.

Video regarding D & C

Dysfunctional Uterine Bleeding (DUB)

Definition
DUB refers to abnormal uterine bleeding without any identifiable structural or organic cause, typically related to hormonal imbalances.

Types
1. **Anovulatory DUB**: Common in adolescents and perimenopausal women, caused by lack of ovulation.
2. **Ovulatory DUB**: Normal ovulation but abnormal bleeding due to corpus luteum dysfunction or endometrial disorders.

Causes
1. **Hormonal Imbalances**: Estrogen-progesterone dysregulation.
2. **Systemic Conditions**: Thyroid disorders, polycystic ovary syndrome (PCOS).
3. **Medications**: Contraceptives, anticoagulants.
4. Other Causes: Obesity, stress, excessive exercise Causes of Dysfunctional Uterine Bleeding (DUB)

DUB occurs due to hormonal imbalances affecting the normal menstrual cycle. The causes can be broadly classified into **hormonal**, **systemic**, and **external factors**. Below is a detailed breakdown:

1. Hormonal Causes
Hormonal dysregulation is the most common cause of DUB, especially in anovulatory cycles.

  a. **Anovulation**

  Occurs when the ovary fails to release an egg.

  Leads to prolonged estrogen stimulation of the endometrium without progesterone counterbalance, causing irregular and heavy bleeding.

  Common in:

  Adolescents with immature hypothalamic-pituitary-ovarian axis.

  Perimenopausal women due to declining ovarian function.

  b. **Luteal Phase Defect**

  Insufficient progesterone production after ovulation.

  Causes irregular shedding of the endometrium, resulting in spotting or irregular bleeding.

c. Polycystic Ovary Syndrome (PCOS)
Chronic anovulation due to hyperandrogenism and insulin resistance.
Results in irregular, infrequent, or heavy bleeding.

d. Thyroid Dysfunction
Hypothyroidism or hyperthyroidism can disrupt the hypothalamic-pituitary-ovarian axis.
Hypothyroidism: Leads to prolonged, heavy bleeding.
Hyperthyroidism: Causes infrequent or light bleeding.

e. Hyperprolactinemia
Elevated prolactin levels interfere with ovulation.
Associated with menstrual irregularities and galactorrhea.

2. Structural and Organic Causes
Although structural causes are not classified as true DUB, they may present similarly. It is important to rule these out before diagnosing DUB.

a. Endometrial Polyps
Overgrowth of endometrial tissue causes intermenstrual bleeding.

b. Uterine Fibroids
Benign smooth muscle tumors can distort the uterine cavity and cause menorrhagia or irregular bleeding.

c. Adenomyosis
Endometrial tissue grows into the uterine muscle, leading to heavy and painful periods.

d. Endometrial Hyperplasia
Thickening of the uterine lining due to prolonged estrogen exposure without progesterone.
Can progress to endometrial cancer if untreated.

3. Systemic Causes

a. Coagulation Disorders
Bleeding disorders like von Willebrand disease or platelet dysfunction can lead to heavy menstrual bleeding.

b. Chronic Illness
Conditions like diabetes or liver disease affect hormonal balance and clotting factors, contributing to DUB.

c. Obesity
Excess adipose tissue produces estrogen, disrupting the hormonal balance and leading to heavy or irregular bleeding.

4. Medications
Certain drugs can interfere with normal coagulation or hormonal regulation.

a. **Contraceptives**

   Irregular bleeding is a common side effect of hormonal contraceptives, particularly with low-dose pills, intrauterine devices (IUDs), or after missing doses.

   b. **Anticoagulants**

   Medications like warfarin or aspirin can exacerbate menstrual bleeding.

   c. **Herbal Supplements**

   Certain herbs (e.g., ginseng or ginkgo biloba) may affect clotting or hormonal levels.

5. **Stress and Lifestyle Factors**

Psychological Stress: Disrupts the hypothalamic-pituitary-ovarian axis, leading to irregular ovulation.

Excessive Exercise: Reduces body fat and disrupts estrogen production.

Malnutrition or Eating Disorders: Affects hormonal production and menstrual regularity.

6. **Postmenopausal Hormonal Changes**

In postmenopausal women, unopposed estrogen therapy or estrogen-producing tumors can lead to abnormal bleeding.

7. **Idiopathic Causes**

In some cases, no definitive cause can be identified despite comprehensive evaluation. These cases are classified as **idiopathic DUB**.

Clinical Features

Abnormal Bleeding Patterns:

Types of Menstrual Disorders in Dysfunctional Uterine Bleeding (DUB)

Menorrhagia

Heavy or prolonged menstrual bleeding lasting more than 7 days or >80 mL blood loss per cycle.

Metrorrhagia

Irregular bleeding occurring between menstrual periods.

Menometrorrhagia

A combination of prolonged, heavy, and irregular bleeding.

Polymenorrhea

Frequent menstrual cycles occurring at intervals of less than 21 days.

Oligomenorrhea

Infrequent menstrual cycles with intervals greater than 35 days.

Hypomenorrhea

Light menstrual bleeding, with reduced flow or shorter duration.

Amenorrhea

Absence of menstruation for more than 3 months in women who previously had regular cycles.

Postmenopausal Bleeding

Vaginal bleeding occurring after menopause, which can sometimes overlap with DUB causes.

Polymenorrhea: Frequent periods (<21 days apart).

Associated Symptoms:

Fatigue due to anemia.

Pelvic discomfort in severe cases.

Complications

Anemia: Due to chronic blood loss.

Endometrial Hyperplasia: Prolonged unopposed estrogen stimulation.

Infertility: In cases of ovulatory dysfunction.

Psychological Impact: Stress and reduced quality of life.

Diagnosis

History and Physical Examination: To rule out structural causes.

Laboratory Tests:

Hormonal profiles (FSH, LH, TSH, Prolactin).

CBC for anemia evaluation.

Imaging:

Pelvic ultrasound to exclude fibroids or polyps.

Endometrial Biopsy: For women >35 years or with risk factors for endometrial cancer.

Management

Medical Treatment:

Hormonal Therapy: Combined oral contraceptives or progesterone.

NSAIDs: To reduce bleeding and pain.

Tranexamic Acid: For acute bleeding control.

Surgical Treatment:

Endometrial Ablation: For refractory cases.

Hysterectomy: In severe cases or when malignancy is suspected.

Lifestyle Modifications: Weight management, stress reduction.

Treatment of Underlying Conditions: Address thyroid dysfunction, PCOS, or other systemic issues.

Homeopathic Remedies for Dysfunctional Uterine Bleeding (DUB)

Homeopathy aims to address the root cause of DUB by considering the patient's unique symptoms and constitutional factors. Below are commonly used remedies:

1. **Sepia**

Indications:

Heavy bleeding with pelvic bearing-down sensation.

Irregular cycles with a tendency toward fatigue and irritability.

Other Symptoms: Yellowish vaginal discharge, aversion to family duties.

2. **Pulsatilla**

Indications:

Scanty or suppressed periods, often irregular.

Suitable for emotional individuals with weepy, changeable moods.

Other Symptoms: Relief in open air, craving for sympathy.

3. **Calcarea Carbonica**

Indications:

Profuse, prolonged bleeding with a tendency to gain weight.

Often used for individuals who are cold and sweaty, especially on the head.

Other Symptoms: Palpitations, fatigue, and sensitivity to exertion.

4. **Sabina**

Indications:

Bright red, clotted bleeding with cramping pain extending to the thighs.

Particularly useful for uterine hemorrhages and spotting.

Other Symptoms: Increased bleeding with slight movement.

5. **Phosphorus**

Indications:

Prolonged bleeding in tall, lean individuals with a tendency to anemia.

Bleeding worsens in the evening or after minor physical exertion.

Other Symptoms: Craving for cold food and drinks.

6. **Hamamelis**

Indications:

Dark, passive bleeding with soreness and heaviness in the pelvis.

Useful for venous congestion and varicose veins.

Other Symptoms: Weakness and throbbing pain.

7. **Trillium Pendulum**

Indications:

Gushing, bright red bleeding, often with faintness and weakness.

Associated with fibroids or other uterine conditions.

Other Symptoms: Pain in hips and back.

8. Ustilago

Indications:

Persistent spotting with dark, stringy clots.

Used for uterine conditions, including endometritis.

Other Symptoms: Tendency to low-grade fever.

9. Lachesis

Indications:

Profuse bleeding worsened by hot weather or tight clothing.

Often used in perimenopausal women.

Other Symptoms: Increased irritability and intolerance to heat.

10. Secale Cornutum

Indications:

Continuous, painless bleeding, often with burning sensation.

Suited for thin, feeble individuals with poor circulation.

Other Symptoms: Chilly yet desire for cold air.

Dysmenorrhea

Definition: Dysmenorrhea refers to the painful menstruation that typically occurs before or during the menstrual period. It is characterized by cramping pain in the lower abdomen or pelvis and is one of the most common gynecological conditions among women of reproductive age.

Types of Dysmenorrhea:

1. **Primary Dysmenorrhea:**
   - **Description**: It is menstrual pain that occurs without any underlying gynecological conditions. It usually starts within 6 months to a year after menarche (the first menstruation) and tends to improve with age or after childbirth.
   - **Cause**: The pain is caused by the release of prostaglandins, which induce uterine contractions.

2. **Secondary Dysmenorrhea:**
   - **Description**: It occurs due to underlying medical conditions like endometriosis, fibroids, pelvic inflammatory disease (PID), or adenomyosis. The pain typically starts later in life, often after the age of 30.
   - **Cause**: The pain is associated with pathological conditions such as fibroids or endometrial tissue growing outside the uterus (endometriosis).

Comparative Table: Primary vs. Secondary Dysmenorrhea

Feature	Primary Dysmenorrhea	Secondary Dysmenorrhea
Age of Onset	Usually begins within 6 months to 1 year after menarche.	Often starts after 30 years of age.
Duration of Pain	Pain lasts 1-3 days, typically during the first few days of menstruation.	Pain may last for longer and is not necessarily confined to menstruation.
Cause	Due to hormonal imbalances, particularly high prostaglandin levels.	Caused by underlying conditions such as fibroids, endometriosis, or pelvic infections.
Response to Treatment	Generally improves with age or after childbirth.	Requires treatment of the underlying condition.
Nature of Pain	Crampy, colicky pain in the lower abdomen.	Often more constant and can radiate to the lower back or thighs.

Feature	Primary Dysmenorrhea	Secondary Dysmenorrhea
Associated Symptoms	May have nausea, vomiting, and diarrhea.	Can have abnormal bleeding, pain during intercourse, or irregular menstrual cycles.

Causes of Dysmenorrhea:

- **Primary Dysmenorrhea:**
  o Increased prostaglandin production leading to stronger uterine contractions.
  o Lack of proper blood flow to the uterine muscles.
- **Secondary Dysmenorrhea:**
  o **Endometriosis**: Endometrial tissue growing outside the uterus causes inflammation and scarring.
  o **Uterine Fibroids**: Non-cancerous growths in the uterus that can cause pain.
  o **Adenomyosis**: Endometrial tissue embedded in the uterine wall.
  o **Pelvic Inflammatory Disease (PID)**: Infection of the female reproductive organs.
  o **Cervical Stenosis**: Narrowing of the cervix can restrict menstrual flow and increase uterine pressure.

Clinical Features of Dysmenorrhea:

- **Pain**: Cramping pain in the lower abdomen, which can radiate to the lower back and thighs.
- **Nausea and Vomiting**: Often seen in primary dysmenorrhea.
- **Headache**: Some individuals may experience tension headaches.
- **Fatigue**: Due to pain and discomfort.
- **Diarrhea or Constipation**: Some women experience gastrointestinal disturbances during menstruation.
- **Heavy Bleeding**: Especially in cases of secondary dysmenorrhea with conditions like fibroids.

Complications:

- **Chronic Pain**: If untreated, dysmenorrhea can lead to long-term chronic pelvic pain.
- **Impact on Quality of Life**: The pain can interfere with daily activities, work, and social life.
- **Infertility**: Conditions like endometriosis can affect fertility.
- **Anxiety and Depression**: Chronic pain can lead to psychological stress, including depression and anxiety.

Diagnosis:
1. **History and Physical Examination**: Detailed menstrual history and pelvic exam.
2. **Ultrasound**: To rule out fibroids, cysts, or other structural abnormalities.
3. **Laparoscopy**: A surgical procedure that may be performed if secondary dysmenorrhea is suspected, particularly for diagnosing endometriosis.
4. **Blood Tests**: To check for infections or hormonal imbalances.

Management in Modern Medicine:
1. **Pain Relief:**
   - **NSAIDs**: Non-steroidal anti-inflammatory drugs (e.g., ibuprofen) to reduce pain and inflammation.
   - **Antispasmodics**: Drugs like mefenamic acid that help relax the uterine muscles.
   - **Heat Therapy**: Application of heat to the abdomen to alleviate pain.
2. **Hormonal Therapy:**
   - **Oral Contraceptives**: Birth control pills reduce menstrual flow and suppress ovulation, reducing prostaglandin levels.
   - **IUD with Hormones**: Progestin-releasing IUDs can decrease menstrual bleeding and pain.
3. **Surgical Intervention:**
   - For secondary dysmenorrhea due to conditions like endometriosis or fibroids, surgery may be necessary to remove the cause (e.g., fibroid removal or laparoscopic surgery for endometriosis).
4. **Alternative Therapies:**
   - **Acupuncture**: Some women find relief through acupuncture treatments.
   - **Diet and Lifestyle Changes**: Increasing physical activity and consuming anti-inflammatory foods may help reduce symptoms.

Comparative Management in Modern Medicine vs Homeopathy:

Aspect	Modern Medicine	Homeopathic Treatment
Mechanism	Targets underlying biological mechanisms (e.g., prostaglandins).	Stimulates the body's self-healing response.
Treatment Approach	Symptomatic relief (NSAIDs, hormonal therapy).	Individualized remedies based on symptoms and constitution.
Duration of Treatment	Short-term for acute pain, long-term for chronic conditions.	Can be used for both acute and chronic management, often as long-term support.

Aspect	Modern Medicine	Homeopathic Treatment
Side Effects	Possible gastrointestinal issues with NSAIDs, hormonal side effects.	Minimal, though remedies may not work for everyone.
Effectiveness	High for immediate pain relief and management.	Effectiveness varies; often works well for mild cases or as adjunct therapy.

Homoeopathic management-

Homeopathic Remedy	Indications/Use	Effectiveness
Chamomilla	Intense pain with irritability, worse at night, and desire for warmth. Also for pain during labor or when the individual is in a highly sensitive or angry state.	Effective for severe pain with emotional sensitivity.
Magnesia Phosphorica	Spasmodic cramping pain, better with warmth or pressure, and worse with cold. Often used for painful, colicky cramps.	Highly effective for spasmodic and cramp-like pain.
Pulsatilla	Pain that is shifting in nature, relieved by crying or consolation, typically with a mild, weepy, or changeable mood.	Works well in individuals with changing symptoms and emotional sensitivity.
Belladonna	Sudden, intense, throbbing pain, often accompanied by fever, hot flashes, and sensitivity to light.	Effective for acute, intense pain with accompanying symptoms.
Cimicifuga	Deep, aching pain, especially associated with the lower back and pelvis, and feelings of stiffness. Used when there is pelvic congestion or heaviness.	Beneficial for deeper, aching pain or when there is associated muscle tension.

Homeopathic Remedy	Indications/Use	Effectiveness
Caulophyllum	Severe cramping and sharp pain, often with a sensation of the uterus being too large or heavy, typically in women with irregular menstrual cycles.	Effective for sharp, spasmodic pain, especially when irregular menstruation is present.
Nux Vomica	For pain with irritability, frustration, and sensitivity to stimuli. Pain can be worse in the morning or after overexertion.	Helpful for individuals with a stressful, overworked lifestyle.
Lachesis	Pain in the left side of the body, worse before menses, with a sensation of fullness or heaviness in the pelvis.	Used when menstrual pain is associated with emotional disturbances or left-sided pain.
Arsenicum Album	For burning pain with restlessness, anxiety, and a desire for warmth. Symptoms worsen at night.	Useful for burning, restless pain with emotional components.
Sepia	Dull, dragging pain in the lower abdomen with a feeling of exhaustion or irritability. Pain is worse with movement and better with rest.	Effective for women with hormonal imbalances or exhaustion during menstruation.
Kali Phosphoricum	For menstrual cramps associated with nervous tension, fatigue, or stress. Often used when there is emotional overwhelm.	Helpful for those who feel mentally exhausted and irritable.
Borax	For sharp, shooting pain during menstruation, often with a sense of coldness and fear. Can also be used for	Effective for those with intense, sharp pain during menses, particularly if anxiety or fear is present.

Homeopathic Remedy	Indications/Use	Effectiveness
	women who fear change or any major life transitions.	
Ignatia	For spasms or cramps that occur with emotional stress, particularly grief, disappointment, or frustration.	Ideal for women experiencing emotional upheavals that correlate with their menstrual cycle.
Aconite	Sudden onset of pain, typically after shock or fright. Pain is intense, sharp, and sudden.	Effective for acute, sudden pain that follows emotional trauma.
Murex Purpurea	For intense, shooting pain radiating down the legs, often with a bloated feeling in the abdomen or pelvic area.	Particularly useful when there is pelvic congestion or radiating pain.

Dyspareunia

Definition

Dyspareunia is persistent or recurrent pain during or after sexual intercourse. It can occur at the vaginal opening (superficial dyspareunia) or deep inside the pelvis (deep dyspareunia) and may have physical, psychological, or combined causes. It significantly impacts a person's quality of life, relationships, and mental health.

Types of Dyspareunia

Type	Characteristics
Superficial Dyspareunia	- Pain at the **vaginal entrance** or labia - **Causes:** Vaginal dryness, infections, vulvodynia, vaginismus
Deep Dyspareunia	- Pain felt **deep in the pelvis** during penetration - **Causes:** Endometriosis, fibroids, pelvic inflammatory disease (PID)
Primary Dyspareunia	- Present since the **first sexual experience** - Linked to anatomical issues, fear, vaginismus
Secondary Dyspareunia	- Develops **after a period of pain-free intercourse** - Often due to infections, surgeries, menopause
Situational Dyspareunia	- Occurs only in **specific conditions** (e.g., certain positions, with specific partners)

Causes and Risk Factors

Category	Causes
Physical Causes	- Vaginal infections (yeast infection, bacterial vaginosis) - Pelvic inflammatory disease (PID) - Endometriosis - Fibroids, ovarian cysts - Vaginal atrophy (due to menopause) - Tight hymen or insufficient lubrication
Psychological Causes	- Fear of pain or trauma - History of sexual abuse - Depression or anxiety

Hormonal Causes	- Estrogen deficiency (postmenopause, postpartum, breastfeeding) - Side effects of oral contraceptives
Neurological Causes	- Pudendal neuralgia (nerve pain in the pelvic area) - Vulvodynia (chronic vulvar pain)
Medical & Surgical History	- History of pelvic surgery or episiotomy - Radiation therapy (affecting vaginal elasticity)

Clinical Features

Category	Symptoms
Superficial Pain	- Burning or stinging at the vaginal entrance - Pain during **initial penetration**
Deep Pain	- **Pelvic pain** during deep thrusting - Worse in certain positions
Associated Symptoms	- Vaginal dryness - Post-coital bleeding - Lower abdominal pain
Psychological Symptoms	- Fear of intercourse - Emotional distress, depression, or avoidance of sex

Complications

Complication	Effects
Sexual Dysfunction	- Loss of sexual desire (low libido)
Infertility Issues	- Difficulty in conception due to avoidance of intercourse
Mental Health Impact	- Depression, anxiety, stress
Relationship Problems	- Emotional strain in marriage or partnerships

Diagnosis

Investigation	Findings
Clinical History	- Pain **onset, duration, and severity** - Menstrual, sexual, and medical history

Investigation	Findings
Pelvic Examination	- Assess for **vaginal infections, atrophy, or muscle tightness**
Swab Test	- **Vaginal discharge analysis** for infections
Ultrasound (Pelvic or Transvaginal USG)	- Identifies **fibroids, ovarian cysts, endometriosis**
MRI Pelvis	- **Detects deep pelvic pathologies** (e.g., adenomyosis, endometriosis)
Psychological Assessment	- Screens for **sexual trauma, relationship issues, anxiety**

Allopathic Drug Management

Category	Drugs and Dosage
Pain Relievers	- **Ibuprofen (400–600 mg PO every 6 hours as needed)** – Reduces pain
Hormonal Therapy	- **Topical estrogen cream (0.5g intravaginally once daily for 2 weeks, then twice weekly)** – For vaginal atrophy
Muscle Relaxants	- **Diazepam (2-5 mg PO at bedtime)** – Reduces pelvic muscle spasm
Topical Anesthetics	- **Lidocaine gel (5% applied before intercourse)** – Numbs the vaginal area
Antidepressants (If Psychological Factors Present)	- **Fluoxetine (20 mg/day PO)** – For depression and anxiety
Botox Injections	- **OnabotulinumtoxinA (50–100 units injected into vaginal muscles)** – For severe muscle spasms

Non-Pharmacological Management

- **Pelvic floor therapy** (Kegel exercises, vaginal dilators)
- Cognitive-behavioral therapy (CBT) for sexual anxiety
- Lubricants and vaginal moisturizers for dryness
- **Couples counseling** for emotional and relational support

Homeopathic Remedies for Dyspareunia

Remedy	Indications
Sepia	- Vaginal dryness, aversion to intercourse - Worse from pressure, better from warmth
Platina	- Severe vaginal tightness and pain - Hypersexual thoughts but fear of intercourse
Lachesis	- Deep pelvic pain, worsens before menstruation - Pain extending to thighs
Staphysagria	- Pain from past sexual trauma - Suppressed emotions, resentment
Ignatia Amara	- Pain with emotional distress, sadness, or grief
Causticum	- Pelvic muscle weakness, burning pain
Pulsatilla	- Timid, emotional women with fear of intimacy - Worse from warmth, better from open air
Hypericum	- Nerve pain in the vaginal region - Pain after surgery or injury

Comparative Table: Allopathy vs. Homeopathy

Aspect	Allopathy	Homeopathy
Approach	Pain relief, hormonal therapy, counseling	Treats both **physical and emotional** aspects
Mode of Action	Directly targets pain with medications	Stimulates self-healing
Side Effects	Hormonal therapy may cause bloating, weight gain	Minimal side effects, gentle action
Prognosis	Effective with therapy and medications	Supports **long-term healing**

Endometrial Cancer

Definition
Endometrial cancer is a malignant tumor that arises from the inner lining of the uterus (endometrium). It is the most common gynecological cancer and is often associated with prolonged estrogen exposure without progesterone opposition.

Types of Endometrial Cancer
Endometrial cancer is broadly classified into two types:

Type	Characteristics
Type I (Endometrioid Adenocarcinoma)	- Estrogen-dependent, associated with obesity and unopposed estrogen exposure. - Usually well-differentiated and has a better prognosis.
Type II (Non-Endometrioid Carcinoma)	- Estrogen-independent, often arises in atrophic endometrium. - Includes serous carcinoma, clear cell carcinoma, and carcinosarcoma. - More aggressive and has a worse prognosis.

Risk Factors

1. **Hormonal Factors**
   - Prolonged exposure to unopposed estrogen (HRT, anovulation, PCOS)
   - Tamoxifen therapy

2. **Metabolic Factors**
   - Obesity (increased peripheral estrogen conversion)
   - Diabetes

3. **Reproductive Factors**
   - Nulliparity (no childbirth history)
   - Early menarche, late menopause

4. **Genetic Factors**
   - Lynch syndrome (HNPCC)
   - Family history of endometrial, ovarian, or colorectal cancer

5. **Lifestyle Factors**
   - Sedentary lifestyle
   - High-fat diet

Etiology (Causes and Pathogenesis)
- **Estrogen stimulation** → Unopposed estrogen leads to endometrial hyperplasia → Malignant transformation.
- **Genetic mutations** (e.g., PTEN, PIK3CA, TP53 mutations) play a role in cancer development.
- **Chronic inflammation** and oxidative stress can contribute to carcinogenesis.

Clinical Features
- **Postmenopausal bleeding** (most common symptom)
- Abnormal uterine bleeding (in premenopausal women)
- Pelvic pain or pressure
- White or watery vaginal discharge
- Weight loss in advanced stages

Complications
- **Local spread**: Invades myometrium, cervix, vagina
- **Distant metastasis**: Lungs, liver, bones
- **Infertility** (in young patients)
- **Recurrence**: More common in high-grade tumors

Diagnosis

Investigation	Findings
Transvaginal Ultrasound (TVUS)	Thickened endometrium (>4 mm in postmenopausal women)
Endometrial Biopsy	Gold standard for diagnosis
Hysteroscopy with D&C	Direct visualization and biopsy
MRI/CT Scan	Staging and metastasis evaluation
CA-125 (Tumor Marker)	Elevated in advanced cases

Allopathic Management (Drugs & Doses)

Stage	Treatment Modality	Drugs and Dosage
Stage I (Localized, No Myometrial Invasion)	Total Abdominal Hysterectomy (TAH) + Bilateral Salpingo-Oophorectomy (BSO)	No chemotherapy needed
Stage II (Cervical Involvement)	Surgery + Adjuvant Radiation Therapy	External Beam Radiation (50 Gy)
Stage III (Pelvic Spread)	Surgery + Chemotherapy	**Paclitaxel (175 mg/m² IV)** + **Carboplatin (AUC 5–6 IV)** every 3 weeks
Stage IV (Distant Metastasis)	Palliative Chemotherapy	**Doxorubicin (60 mg/m² IV)** + **Cisplatin (50 mg/m² IV)** every 3 weeks

- **Hormonal Therapy**: In hormone receptor-positive tumors
    - Medroxyprogesterone acetate (200–400 mg/day PO)
    - Megestrol acetate (40–320 mg/day PO)

Homeopathic Remedies for Endometrial Cancer

Remedy	Indications
Conium Maculatum	Hard indurations in the uterus, slow-growing tumors, glandular swellings
Hydrastis Canadensis	Thick yellow vaginal discharge, weak digestion, cachexia
Carcinosin	Family history of cancer, perfectionist tendencies, history of suppressed grief
Kreosotum	Offensive, corrosive leucorrhea with itching, burning, and bleeding
Thuja Occidentalis	History of warts, sycotic constitution, excessive growth of tissues
Arsenicum Album	Weakness, burning pains, anxiety, marked restlessness
Phytolacca Decandra	Severe pain in pelvic region, weight loss, hard nodular masses
Sabina	Heavy, bright-red bleeding with clots, pain radiating to thighs

Comparative Table: Allopathy vs. Homeopathy

Aspect	Allopathy	Homeopathy
Approach	Surgery, chemotherapy, radiation	Holistic treatment based on symptom similarity
Mode of Action	Directly targets tumor cells	Stimulates body's self-healing response
Side Effects	Nausea, fatigue, hair loss, immunosuppression	Minimal side effects, gentle action
Prognosis	Effective for early-stage cancers	Supportive therapy, may slow progression

Secondary Spread and Its Clinical Manifestations

Site of Metastasis	Clinical Features
Pelvic and Para-aortic Lymph Nodes	Pelvic pain, lower limb edema (due to lymphatic obstruction), hydronephrosis (if ureters are compressed)
Lungs	Persistent cough, hemoptysis (coughing up blood), dyspnea (shortness of breath)
Liver	Hepatomegaly (enlarged liver), jaundice, right upper quadrant pain, weight loss
Bones	Bone pain (especially in the spine, pelvis, and long bones), pathological fractures
Peritoneum (Peritoneal Carcinomatosis)	Ascites (fluid accumulation in the abdomen), abdominal distension, bowel obstruction symptoms
Brain	Headache, seizures, altered mental status, focal neurological deficits (paralysis, vision changes)
Vagina	Vaginal nodules, recurrent bleeding, foul-smelling discharge

Metastatic spread is more common in **Type II** endometrial cancers (e.g., serous and clear cell carcinoma), which tend to be more aggressive.

Endometrial Polyp

Definition

An **endometrial polyp** is a benign, localized overgrowth of endometrial tissue projecting into the uterine cavity. These polyps consist of glands, stroma, and blood vessels and are attached to the uterine wall via a stalk (pedunculated) or a broad base (sessile).

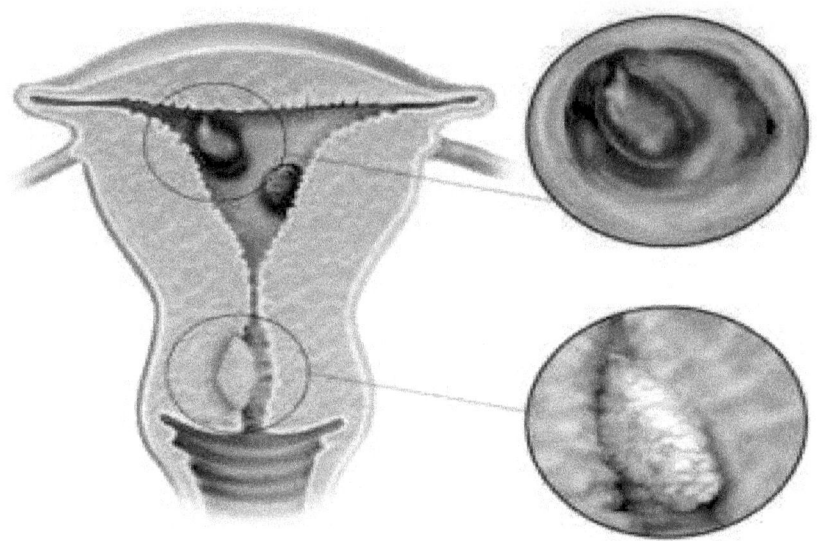

Types of Endometrial Polyps

1. **Functional Polyps**:
   - Responsive to hormonal changes in the menstrual cycle.
2. **Hyperplastic Polyps**:
   - Associated with excessive estrogen stimulation, often in postmenopausal women.
3. **Atrophic Polyps**:
   - Found in postmenopausal women; result from atrophy of endometrial tissue.
4. **Malignant Polyps**:
   - Rare but may undergo malignant transformation, especially in older women or those with risk factors like obesity or prolonged estrogen therapy.

Aetiology (Causes)

1. **Hormonal Imbalance**:
   - Excess estrogen or unopposed estrogen therapy.

2. **Chronic Inflammation:**
   - Long-standing endometritis or infections.

3. **Genetic Factors:**
   - Mutations in certain genes, e.g., PTEN or HMGI genes, may predispose individuals to polyp formation.

4. **Medications:**
   - Use of tamoxifen (a selective estrogen receptor modulator) can stimulate polyp growth.

5. **Other Risk Factors:**
   - Obesity, diabetes, hypertension, and polycystic ovarian syndrome (PCOS).

Clinical Features

1. **Symptoms:**
   - Abnormal uterine bleeding:
     - Intermenstrual bleeding.
     - Heavy or prolonged menstrual bleeding.
     - Postmenopausal bleeding.
   - Infertility or subfertility.
   - Pelvic pain or cramping (rare).

2. **Asymptomatic:**
   - Many polyps are found incidentally during investigations for other issues.

Complications

1. **Abnormal Uterine Bleeding:**
   - Persistent or severe bleeding leading to anemia.

2. **Infertility:**
   - Polyps can block the cervical canal or fallopian tube openings, interfering with fertilization or implantation.

3. **Recurrent Miscarriage:**
   - Polyps may disrupt the uterine lining, leading to pregnancy loss.

4. **Malignant Transformation:**
   - A rare complication, more common in postmenopausal women.

Diagnosis

1. **Transvaginal Ultrasound:**
   - Identifies echogenic masses in the uterine cavity.

2. **Saline Infusion Sonography (SIS):**
   - Enhances visualization of polyps by distending the uterine cavity with saline.

3. **Hysteroscopy:**
   - Direct visualization of polyps with the option for biopsy or removal.

4. **Endometrial Biopsy:**
   - Confirms the diagnosis and rules out malignancy.

5. **MRI or CT Scan:**
   - Rarely required but can help in complex cases.

Management

Modern Medical Management

1. **Medications:**
   - Progestins:
     - Used to shrink polyps and regulate menstrual bleeding.
   - GnRH Agonists:
     - Reduce estrogen levels and cause temporary regression of polyps.
   - Non-Steroidal Anti-Inflammatory Drugs (NSAIDs):
     - To manage associated pain or cramping.

2. **Follow-Up:**
   - Regular monitoring of small asymptomatic polyps, especially in premenopausal women.

Surgical Management

1. **Polypectomy:**
   - Hysteroscopic Polypectomy:
     - Gold standard for diagnosing and removing polyps.
     - Minimally invasive with faster recovery.
   - Polyps are removed using scissors, forceps, or electrosurgical techniques.

2. **Dilation and Curettage (D&C):**
   - Sometimes used alongside hysteroscopy to clear the uterine cavity.

3. **Hysterectomy:**
    o Recommended in cases of multiple recurrent polyps or suspicion of malignancy in postmenopausal women.

Post-Surgery Care:
- Regular follow-up to monitor recurrence.
- Treatment of underlying hormonal or metabolic imbalances.

Homeopathic Management

Comparison Between Modern Medicine and Homeopathy

Aspect	Modern Medicine	Homeopathy
Focus	Symptom management and mechanical removal of polyps.	Treats the root cause and considers the constitution.
Treatment Approach	Surgical (hysteroscopy, D&C), hormonal therapy.	Individualized remedies for the patient's symptoms.
Side Effects	Risks of surgery (infection, uterine perforation, recurrence).	Minimal to none if remedies are chosen correctly.
Recurrence Prevention	Depends on hormone regulation and periodic monitoring.	Prevented by holistic treatment of underlying causes.
Suitability	Effective for acute cases or large/malignant polyps.	Effective for chronic, recurrent, or mild polyps.

Remedy	Key Indications	Clinical Features	Modalities	Mental/Emotional Symptoms
Sabina	Polyps with profuse bleeding, clots, and pain radiating from the sacrum.	Bright red bleeding, often with clots. Severe uterine pain.	**Better:** Open air. **Worse:** Warm rooms.	**Irritable**, often feels as if they are ill.
Calcarea Carbonica	Obese, chilly patients with heavy menstrual flow and weakness.	Heavy periods, often with cramps, and a sense of fullness.	**Better:** Warmth. **Worse:** Cold, exertion.	**Anxious,** lacks confidence, fearful of illness.

Remedy	Key Indications	Clinical Features	Modalities	Mental/Emotional Symptoms
Thuja Occidentalis	Polyps with a history of genital infections or warts, irregular, foul-smelling discharge.	Thick, yellowish, or greenish discharge. Sometimes vaginal prolapse.	**Better:** Warmth. **Worse:** Dampness.	**Fearful**, low self-esteem, sensitive to cold.
Phosphorus	Bright red bleeding, weak, and anemic individuals with a tendency to hemorrhage.	Heavy bleeding with weakness, bright red, and profuse.	**Better:** Lying down, cool air. **Worse:** Heat.	**Anxious**, seeks reassurance, fears the future.
Ustilago	Polyps with dark, clotted bleeding, and uterine congestion.	Dark, clotted bleeding with a dragging sensation in the pelvis.	**Better:** Warmth. **Worse:** Rest.	**Restless**, often anxious and impatient.
Medorrhinum	Polyps with a history of chronic infections or inflammation, profuse bleeding.	Thick, acrid discharge, bleeding with pain in the pelvis.	**Better:** Evening. **Worse:** Damp weather.	**Restless**, anxious, irritable, and sensitive.
Sepia Officinalis	Polyps with bearing-down sensation, irregular bleeding, and pelvic heaviness.	Irregular menstrual bleeding, fatigue, and a bearing-down sensation.	**Better:** Activity. **Worse:** Rest.	**Indifferent**, exhausted, feels burdened.
Lachesis	Dark, offensive bleeding; sensitivity to touch and hormonal disturbances.	Dark, offensive bleeding, cramping pain. Tendency for varicose veins and hemorrhage.	**Better:** Free flow of discharge. **Worse:** Before menses.	**Jealous**, highly emotional, talkative.

Remedy	Key Indications	Clinical Features	Modalities	Mental/Emotional Symptoms
Hydrastis Canadensis	Chronic cervicitis or polyps with thick, yellowish discharge.	Thick, yellowish, or greenish discharge. Spotting between periods.	**Better:** Rest. **Worse:** Cold damp weather.	**Fatigued,** tends to be withdrawn and irritable.
Lilium Tigrinum	Polyps with pain and fullness, often with feelings of suffocation and pressure.	Uterine fullness, painful menstruation, and deep congestion.	**Better:** Pressure, hard pressure on the abdomen.	**Irritable,** restless, feels overwhelmed.

Endometriosis

Defination –

Presence of functioning endometrium other than the intrauterine cavity is called endometriosis.

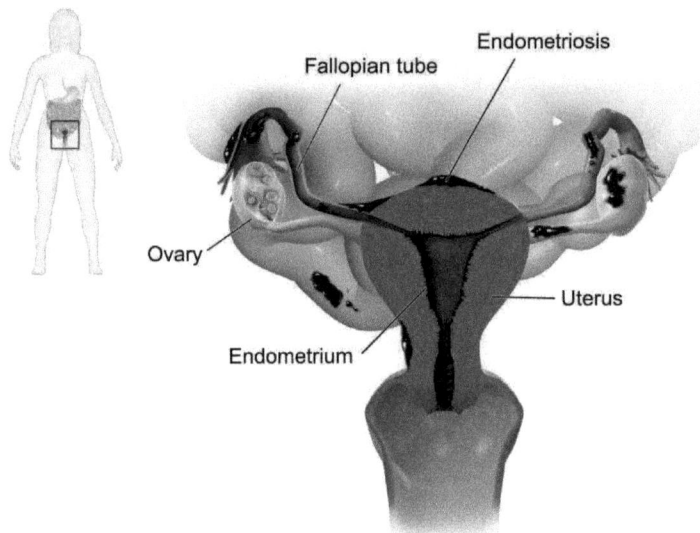

Aetiology-

The exact cause is unknown.
1. Sampson's theory of menstrual regurgitation and implantation (Metastatic theory)
   Retrograde menstruation

   Endometrial fragments are transported to peritoneal cavity through tubes
   Viable cells implant & grow
   Young girls with obstructive anomalies of genital tract often develop endometriosis.
2. Coelomic metaplasia theory:
   Original Coelomic membrane transforms into endometrial tissue.
   Explains endometriosis in ectopic sites.
3. Lymphatic & vascular metastasis theory:
   Lymphatic & hematogenous spread of endometrial cells
   Extensive communication of lymphatics between uterus, tubes,
   ovaries, pelvic & vaginal lymph nodes, kidneys & umbilicus.
   A. Genetic factors: risk is 7 times more if first degree relative has endometriosis.
4. Immunological factors: reduced clearance of endometrial cells due to decreased natural killer cell activity or decreased macrophage activity.

5. Inflammation: endometriosis maybe associated with subclinical peritoneal inflammation

1. Family history

If someone in your family has endometriosis, your risk for developing it is 7 to 10 times higher than those with no family history of the condition.

Endometriosis in immediate family members, such as your mother, grandmother, or sister, puts you at the highest risk for developing the condition. If you have distant relatives such as cousins who have it, this also increases your chances of being diagnosed.

Endometriosis can be passed down both maternally and paternally.

2. Menstrual cycle characteristics

The more exposure you have to menstruation, the higher the chance you have of developing endometriosis. Factors that increase your menstrual exposure and thus your risk include:
- Having 27 days or fewerTrusted Source between each period
- starting your first period before the age of 12 years
- experiencing periods that last seven days or longer each month

Pregnancy, which reduces the number of times you have periods, decreases risk. If you do have endometriosis and are able to become pregnant, your symptoms may fade during your pregnancy. It's common for symptoms to return after your baby is born.

3. Conditions that interfere with normal menstrual flow

One of the theories of causes associated with endometriosis is retrograde menstrual flow, or flow that moves backward. If you have a medical condition that increases, blocks, or redirects your menstrual flow, this could be a risk factor.

Conditions that can result in retrograde menstrual flow include:
- increased estrogen production
- uterine growths, like fibroids or polyps
- structural abnormality of your uterus, cervix, or vagina
- obstructions in your cervix or vagina
- asynchronous uterine contractions

4. Immune system disorders

Immune system disorders contribute to endometriosis risk. If your immune system is weak, it's less likely to recognize misplaced endometrial tissue. The scattered endometrial tissue is left to implant in the wrong places. This can lead to problems like lesions, inflammation, and scarring.

5. Abdominal surgery

Sometimes abdominal surgery like a caesarean delivery (commonly known as a C-section) or hysterectomy can misplace endometrial tissue.

If this misplaced tissue isn't destroyed by your immune system, it can lead to endometriosis. Review your surgical history with your doctor when discussing your endometriosis symptoms.

6. Age

Endometriosis involves uterine lining cells, so any woman or girl old enough to menstruate can develop the condition. In spite of this, endometriosis is most commonly diagnosed in women in their 20s and 30s.

Experts theorize this is the age at which women try to conceive, and for some, infertility is the main symptom of endometriosis. Women who don't have severe pain associated with menstruation might not seek assessment by their doctor until they're trying to get pregnant.

Reducing the risk

Until we better understand what leads to endometriosis, it's difficult to say how to prevent it.

You can probably reduce your risk by lowering the amount of estrogen in your system.

One of the functions of estrogen is to thicken your uterus lining, or endometrium. If your estrogen level is high, your endometrium will be thicker, which can cause heavy bleeding. If you have heavy menstrual bleeding, you're at risk for developing endometriosis.

Being in a healthy state balances hormones. To keep hormones such as estrogen at normal or lower levels, try these strategies:

- Exercise regularly.
- Eat whole foods and less processed foods.
- Consume less alcohol.
- Reduce your caffeine intake.
- Talk to your doctor about your birth control medication to see if there is a type you can switch to that contains less estrogen.

Pathophysiology-

Ovarian Endometriosis

Nodules implant in the lining of ovaries. When tissue around these areas hardens it can develop and proliferate into the fallopian tubes and bowels [4].

Deep Infiltrating Endometriosis

The nodules implant at least 5mm below the peritoneum [5]. Structures penetrated can include the uterosacral ligaments, bowel, bladder and ureters [4].

Peritoneal Endometriosis

The peritoneum is the lining of the abdomen. Peritoneal endometriosis occurs when endometrial cells travel to and implant in the peritoneal wall.

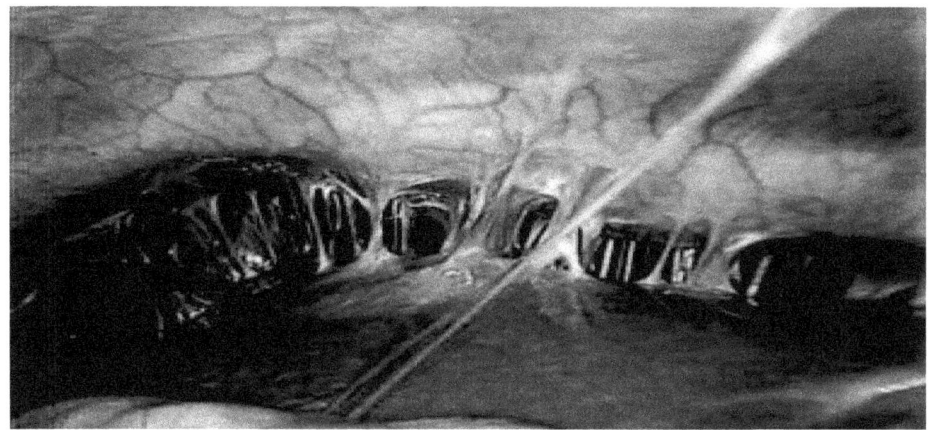

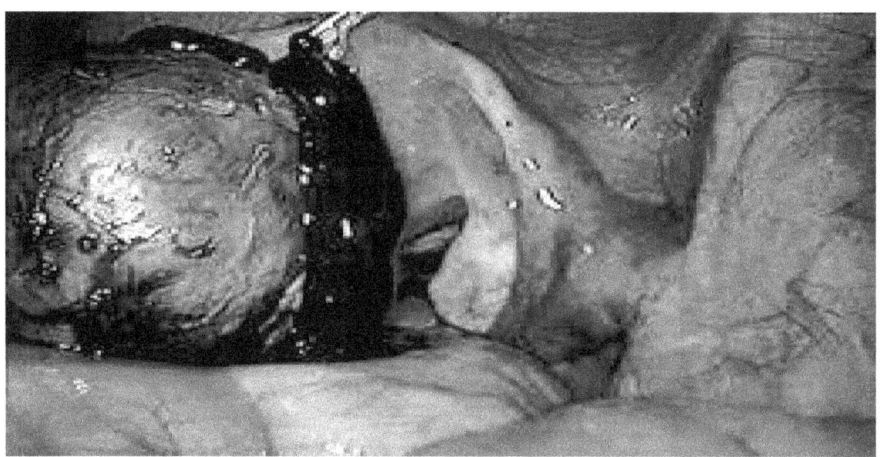

Fig. Chocolate Cyst, Ovarian Endometriosis

Sites Of Implantation -

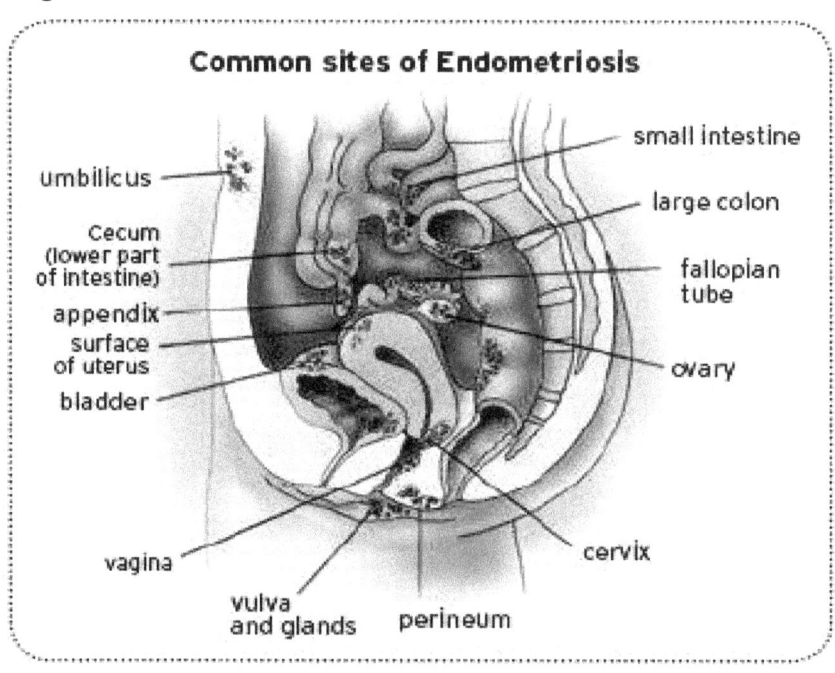

Sites of endometriosis-
- Pelvic
- Ovary
- Cul de sac
- Uterosacral LIGAMENTS
- Posterior surface of uterus
- Posterior broad ligament
- Rectovaginal septum
- Tubes and round ligament

Extrapelvic sites-

Intestines (rectosigmoid, cecum, terminal ilam, proximal colon, appendix)
- Lungs & thorax
- Urinary tract

Less common sites-
- Cervix
- Hernial sacs
- Umbilicus
- Laparotomy/episiotomy sites
- Tubal stumps after sterilization

Rarest-

Extremities

Clinical Features-

— MEMBRANOUS DYSMENORHEA; Painful periods. Pelvic pain and cramping may begin before and extend several days into a menstrual period. Also have lower back and abdominal pain.

— DYSPARENIA;Pain with intercourse. Pain during or after sex is common with endometriosis.

Dysuria Or Painfull Defication;

Pain with bowel movements or urination especially during a menstrual period.

Menorrhagea / Metrorrhagea;

Excessive bleeding. You may experience occasional heavy menstrual periods or bleeding between periods (intermenstrual bleeding). FOUL, FISHY ODOUR, MEMBRANOUS, THICK BLEED.

INFERTILITY; Sometimes endometriosis is first diagnosed in those seeking treatment for infertility. Ovarian endometriosis hampers ovulation, tubal endometriosis produces tubal adhesions and tubal blockage, cervical or vaginal lesions or adhesions produces obstruction for semen entry, and hence infertility.

Othersigns and symptoms;- Fatigue
- Diarrhea,
- Constipation,
- Bloating or nausea,
- Breast tenderness
- Painfull suture sites, specially during menstrual periods.

Signs-

On bimanual examination,
- A fixed, retroverted uterus
- Uterosacral ligament nodule
- General tenderness
- An enlarged, tender and boggy uterus is indicative of adenomyosis

Differential Diagnosis-

- Pelvic Inflammatory Disease: This can present with dyspareunia, pelvic pain and abnormal and/or heavy bleeding.
- Ectopic pregnancy. This can present with dyspareunia, pelvic pain and abnormal and/or heavy bleeding, and sometimes collECTION
- Fibroids: This can present with pelvic pain, long duration of menstrual bleeding, heavy menstrual bleeding, a feeling of a mass or bloating.
- Irritable Bowel Syndrome: abdominal pain, dyspareunia and bloating.

Investigations-

The gold standard in the diagnosis of endometriosis is laparoscopy. It is particularly effective at differentiating between endometriosis and chronic infection.

findings include:
- Chocolate cyst
- Adhesions
- Peritoneal deposits

A pelvic ultrasound scan can also help determine the severity of endometriosis and o ught to be undertaken before any surgery. A skilled operator can demonstrate "kissing ovaries" - where bilateral endometrioma are adherent together. Pelvic mobility can be demonstrated, including any involvement of bowel.

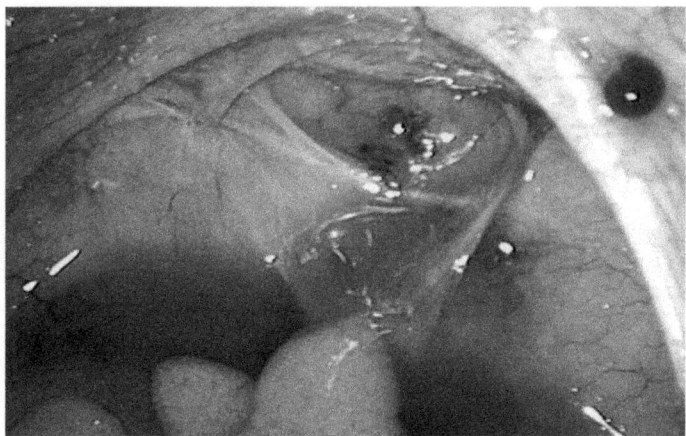

fig. Signs of endometriosis in POD in laparoscopy.

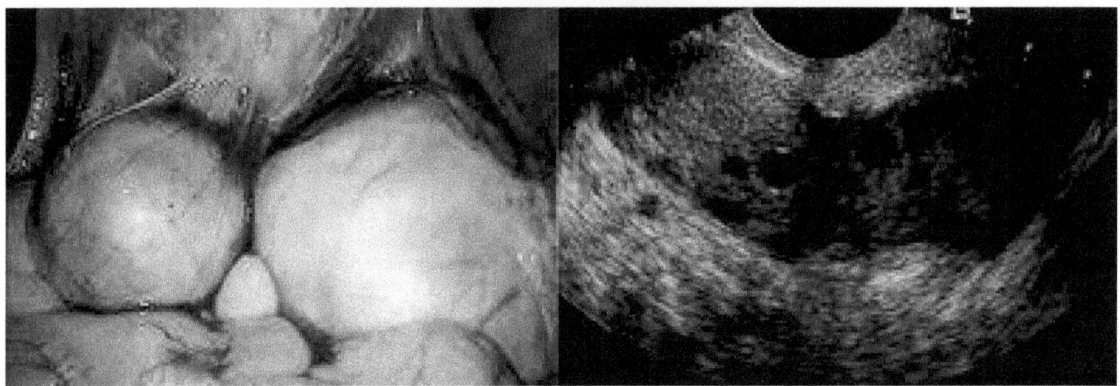

Fig. kissing overies in laparoscopy and in USG

Management:

The treatment is based on the individual requirements of each patient. If the patient is asymptomatic, no treatment is needed.

Analgesics-

Pain can be managed through analgesia or NSAIDs.

Ovulation Supressing Hormones-

Suppressing ovulation for 8-12 months can cause atrophy of the endometriosis lesions and therefore a reduction in symptoms.

A low dose combined oral contraceptive pill or norethisterone can be used. Injected hormones or intrauterine devices such as the Mirena coil can also be used. The Mirena has the benefit of containing a low dose of hormone.

Surgery-

The surgical option is used if the endometriosis symptoms seriously affect the patient's
-Excision, fulguration and laser ablation aim to completely remove the ectopic endometrial tissue in the peritoneum, uterine muscle and pouch of Douglas to reduce pain.

Hysterectomy-

When complaints relapses or intolerable or leads to severe anaemia ultimate management may be a hysterectomy and oferectomy.

followed by [HRT],hormone replacement until the age of the menopause.

Drugs In Management-

1. **Pain Management**
   - **NSAIDs (Non-Steroidal Anti-Inflammatory Drugs)**: Medications like **Ibuprofen** and **Naproxen** help reduce inflammation and relieve pain by inhibiting prostaglandin production.
   - **Benefits**: Effective for mild to moderate pain relief.
   - **Side Effects**: Stomach irritation, ulcers, and kidney issues with long-term use.

2. **Hormonal Therapy**

These treatments suppress estrogen and ovulation, reducing endometrial tissue growth and pain.

  a. **Combined Oral Contraceptives (COCs)**
   - **Examples**: Ethinyl estradiol + Progestin.
   - **Mechanism**: Suppresses ovulation, reduces menstrual flow, and prevents endometrial tissue growth.
   - **Benefits**: Reduces pain and prevents disease progression.
   - **Side Effects**: Nausea, breast tenderness, risk of blood clots.

  b. **Progestins**
   - **Examples**: Norethindrone, Dienogest, Medroxyprogesterone.
   - **Mechanism**: Thins the endometrial lining and suppresses estrogen levels.
   - **Benefits**: Effective pain relief and suppression of menstrual bleeding.
   - **Side Effects**: Weight gain, mood changes, irregular bleeding.

  c. **GnRH Agonists**
   - **Examples**: Leuprolide, Goserelin.
   - **Mechanism**: Induces temporary menopause by shutting down estrogen production.
   - **Benefits**: Significantly reduces endometriosis growth and pain.
   - **Side Effects**: Hot flashes, bone loss, vaginal dryness.

  d. **GnRH Antagonists**
   - **Examples**: Elagolix, Relugolix.
   - **Mechanism**: Directly blocks GnRH receptors, reducing estrogen levels.
   - **Benefits**: Fast-acting, effective for pain relief.
   - **Side Effects**: Headaches, nausea, osteoporosis risk.

  e. **Aromatase Inhibitors**
   - **Examples**: Letrozole, Anastrozole.

- **Mechanism**: Blocks estrogen production in peripheral tissues.
- **Benefits**: Used in severe or treatment-resistant cases.
- **Side Effects**: Joint pain, hot flashes, bone loss.

3. **Surgical Management**
   - **Laparoscopy**: A minimally invasive procedure that removes or ablates endometrial implants, improving pain and fertility.
   - **Hysterectomy**: A last-resort option involving the removal of the uterus (sometimes ovaries), offering permanent relief in severe cases.
   - **Risks**: Surgery-related complications, recurrence of endometriosis, and hormonal imbalances if ovaries are removed

4. **Emerging Therapies (Experimental)**
   - **Immune Modulators**: Target immune system dysfunction linked to endometriosis.
   - **Anti-angiogenic Drugs**: Aim to block new blood vessel formation in endometrial lesions, potentially preventing disease progression.

Homoeopathic Management-

For Severe Dysmenorrhea

1. Cimicifuga/ Actea Racemosa/ Xynthophyllum -For Endometriosis with Painful Periods

Significant medicine for endometriosis with painful periods are Xanthoxylum and Cimicifuga. Xanthoxylum is best suited when periods are very painful, with excruciating pain in the pelvis, back, thighs and legs. The menses are profuse and exhausting Cimicifuga is another useful of medicine for endometriosis with pain during periods. It is indicated in case of severe, bearing down pain in the lower abdomen, uterine region, and the lower back during periods. It is also prescribed for darting pain in the pelvis from hip to hip More the menstrual flow, mere the pain. Sharp electricity like pains may appear in various parts of the body as a reflex from uterine ovarian irritation in such cases where Cimicifuga will prove one of the best medicines for endometriosis .

2. SABINA, SEPIA, and PULSATILLA - For Endometriosis with Pelvic Pain

Sabina, Sepia and Pulsatilla are noted to be the best on the long list of medicines for endometriosis with pelvic pain. Homeopathic medicine Sabina is indicated when colicky or Labour-like pains appear in the pelvis. Marked pains in the small of the back and from sacrum and pubis are also behaved in such cases The menses are profuse, panly fluid and pan allotted. Sepia is another of the reliable medicines for endometriosis indicated in case of marked bearing down pains in the pelvis Mca prescribed Sepa may also complain of gripping, stitching, cutting pain in the pelvis. Pulsatilla is the most effective among medicines for endometriosis for pelvic pain during periods, attended with chills, restlessness and tossing in bed

3. Sepia and Platina - For Pain during Intercourse (dyspareunia)

Sepia and Platina are top grade medicines for endometriosis with dyspareunia Both work as best prescriptions in case of women who complain of marked pain during intercourse. Buming and soreness is also present. The genitals are sensitive to touch In fact, women prescribed Sepia usually have a low sex drive while those needing Platina have an increased sexual desite.

For Rectal Complaints Due To Endometriosis-

4. Nux Vomica, Ammonium Mur and Lachesis -

Nux Vomica. Ammonium Mur and Lacheüs are helpful medicine for endometriosis with rectal symptoms Nux Vomica is prescribed when pain in the rectum appears during periods. Ineffectual urging for stool may accompany rectum pain. The stool in unsatinfa…: endometriosis with a bleeding rectum during menses. The bleeding is usually accompanied by pain in the rectum

For Dysuria -

5. Sepia and Natrum Mur - For Endometriosis with Urinary Troubles

Beneficial medicines for endometriosis with urinary complaints are Sepia and Natrum Mur. Sepia is considered the most useful among medicines for endometriosis where it is accompanied by urinary urgency and frequency. A bearing down sensation in the pubic region may be felt. Pain while passing urine from endometriosis lesions also indicates use of Sepia. Pain in the bladder of aching (dull) and burning nature during menses also points to the use of Sepia. Natrum Mur is one of the most effective medicines for endometriosis which is mainly prescribed when bleeding from the urinary bladder appears simultaneously with the menses.

MERC SOL- MILK IN BREAST INSTEAD OF MENSES. PAINFULL BREASTS AS IF ULCERATED DURING EVERY MENSES.

MERC COR-BLOODY DYSENTRY WITH SEVERE RECTAL AND BLADDER TENESMUS, NOT RELIVED EVEN AFTER STOOLS

SILICEA-Constipation before ,during,after menses

PLUMBUM-String like pulling sensation around nevel

THALPSI BURSA-Alternate menses are profuse,continue until next menses start with constant colic and clots.

Cholera like symptoms during menses-ammonium carb,bovista,veritum alb.

AMMONIUM CARB-Yawning and thigh pains during menses with offensive,acrid,decomposed menstruations.

APIS-Rt.sided chocolate cyst with severe stinging pains

AURUM MET-Menstrual excess of uterine hypertrophy,foul mouth breath in girls at puberity.

MAG.CARB- Severe dysmenorrhea with cutting labour like abdominal pais and backache. ACRID,DARK,PITCH LIKE MENSES, DIFFICULT TO WASH. Night time menses with every 3 wks diarrhea with severe tenesmus.

LACHESIS- LT.SIDED chocolate cyst ,but all complaints relived with menstrual flow.

CROCUS SATIVUS- Dysmenorrhea, metrorrhagea with DARK,STRINGY, BLACK menstrual discharges. HANGING DOWN IN LONG STRINGS FROM BLOODY SURFACE.

Headache before, during and after menses.

USTILAGO- Dysmenorrhea where pains radiating from back to loin and womb.NAUSEA, FLATULENCE AROUND MENSES RELIEVED AFTER EATING.Frequent,profuse urination during menses.

VIBRINUM OPULUS-Black ,stringy clots ,continued upto next menses.VICARIOUS MENSTRUATION FROM LUNGS,BOWELS at climacteric age .

TRILLIUM-Dark ,clotted,profuse ,EVERY 2 wk. MENSES,LONG LASTING. Sensation as if small of back bone brocken into SMALL PIECES.

XANTHOXYLUM- NEURALGIC DYSMENORRHEA esp. lt ovarian region. Dark,stringy profuse menses lasting upto 2 wks with SEVERE NEURALGIC PAINS ALONG GENITAL CRUCIAL NERVE,radiating toward knees.NO POSITION GIVES RELIEF IN PAIN. Headache during menses with desire to tight it with band.

Symptom	Homeopathic Remedy	Indications	Potency & Dosage
Severe Pelvic Pain	Belladonna	Sudden, intense pelvic pain, heat, and throbbing sensations	30C or 200C, 2–3 times daily
Cramping & Dysmenorrhea	Magnesia Phosphorica	Severe cramping, relieved by warmth and pressure	6X or 30C, every few hours as needed
Heavy Menstrual Bleeding (Menorrhagia)	Sabina	Profuse bleeding with clots, pain extending to thighs	30C or 200C, once or twice daily
Dark, Scanty, or Clotted Menses	Lachesis	Blackish, clotted flow with left-sided ovarian pain	30C or 200C, once daily

Symptom	Homeopathic Remedy	Indications	Potency & Dosage
Irritability & Emotional Symptoms	Sepia	Depression, mood swings, aversion to loved ones	30C or 200C, once daily
Endometriosis with Digestive Issues (Bloating, Constipation)	Nux Vomica	Indigestion, bloating, constipation, worsened by stress	30C, 2–3 times daily
Fatigue & Weakness	Kali Phosphoricum	Chronic fatigue, mental exhaustion, low energy	6X, 3–4 times daily
Lower Back Pain	Calcarea Carbonica	Aching pain in lower back, worsens before menstruation	30C, once daily
Sharp Ovarian Pain (Right-Sided)	Lycopodium	Right ovarian pain, bloating, gas, digestive issues	30C, once or twice daily
Sharp Ovarian Pain (Left-Sided)	Pulsatilla	Left-sided ovarian pain, irregular cycles, weepiness	30C, once or twice daily
Suppressed or Irregular Menses	Apis Mellifica	Swollen ovaries, suppressed periods, stinging pain	30C, once daily

Fibroid Uterus

Defination- also known as uterine fibroids or leiomyomas, are non-cancerous growths that develop in or on the uterus. The exact cause of fibroids is not fully understood, but several factors are thought to contribute to their development.

Aetiology-

1. Hormonal Factors: Estrogen and progesterone, the hormones that regulate the menstrual cycle, are believed to promote the growth of fibroids. Fibroids tend to shrink after menopause due to a decrease in hormone levels.
2. Genetic Factors: A family history of fibroids increases the likelihood of developing them. Certain genetic mutations are also linked to fibroid growth.
3. Growth Factors: Substances that help the body maintain tissues, such as insulin-like growth factors, may affect fibroid development.
4. Extracellular Matrix (ECM): ECM, the material that helps cells stick together, is increased in fibroids, making them more fibrous. ECM also stores growth factors that may cause fibroids to grow.
5. Other Factors:
— Obesity: Higher body fat can lead to increased estrogen levels, which may promote fibroid growth.
— Diet: A diet high in red meat and low in green vegetables, fruit, and dairy may be linked to an increased risk of fibroids.
— Early Menstruation: Starting menstruation at an early age is associated with a higher risk of developing fibroids.
— Vitamin D Deficiency: Low levels of vitamin D are associated with an increased risk of fibroids.
— Lifestyle Factors: Alcohol consumption, particularly beer, has been linked to an increased risk of fibroid.

Risk factors of fibroids:

1. Inflammatory Factors:

Chronic inflammation in the body may contribute to the development of fibroids. Some studies suggest that inflammatory processes within the uterus could stimulate fibroid growth.

2. Pregnancy:

Pregnancy increases the production of estrogen and progesterone, which can cause fibroids that were already present to grow more rapidly.

3. **Environmental Factors:**

Exposure to environmental toxins, such as certain chemicals in plastics (e.g., bisphenol A, or BPA), may influence the development of fibroids. These chemicals can mimic estrogen in the body, potentially leading to fibroid gr

4. **Race and Ethnicity:**

African-American women are more likely to develop fibroids and tend to experience them at a younger age and with more severe symptoms compared to women of other ethnicities. The reasons for this disparity are not fully understood but may involve a combination of genetic, environmental, and lifestyle factors.

5. **Age:**

The likelihood of developing fibroids increases as women age, particularly during the reproductive years (30s and 40s). However, they tend to shrink after menopause when hormone levels decrease.

6. **Menstrual Cycle Characteristics:**

Longer and heavier menstrual cycles are sometimes associated with a higher risk of fibroids. This may be linked to the higher cumulative exposure to estrogen over time.

7. **Reproductive History:**

Women who have never given birth (nulliparity) may have a higher risk of developing fibroids. Conversely, women who have had more pregnancies are at a lower risk, possibly due to changes in hormone levels during pregnancy.

8. **Stress:**

While research is still ongoing, chronic stress has been suggested as a potential risk factor for fibroid development. Stress can affect hormone levels, which may influence fibroid growth.

Types-

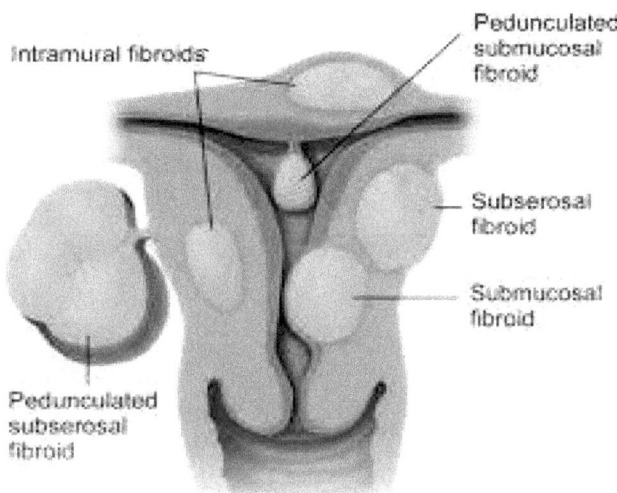

According to sites where they present-
Uterine [Pedunculated or Non-pedunculate]
Cervical[Pedunculated or Non-pedunculate]
According to layer of uterus they accupied-
SUBMUCOSAL-lies inside the uterine cavity
INTRAMURAL- lies within the myometrium
SUBSEROSAL-lies outside of uterus

Clinical Features -

Symptoms may vary depending on the size, number, and location of the fibroids.

1. **Menstrual Symptoms:**
   — Heavy Menstrual Bleeding (Menorrhagia): One of the most common symptoms of fibroids is heavy or prolonged menstrual bleeding. This can lead to anaemia and fatigue.
   — Menstrual Clotting: Passing large blood clots during menstruation can be a sign of fibroids.
   — Prolonged Menstrual Periods: Periods that last longer than seven days can be associated with fibroids.
   — Dysmenorrhea: Spasmodic dysmenorrhea
   — DUB

2. **Pelvic Pain and Pressure:**
   — Pelvic Pain or Pressure: Fibroids can cause a sensation of heaviness or pressure in the pelvis.
   — Sensation of something live moving inside the abdomen.
   — Lower Back Pain: If fibroids press on nerves or muscles in the lower back, they can cause chronic back pain.
   — Abdominal Swelling: Larger fibroids can cause noticeable swelling or distension in the abdomen, making a woman look pregnant.

3. **Bladder and Bowel Symptoms due to pressure-**
   — Frequent Urination: Fibroids can press on the bladder, leading to a frequent need to urinate or difficulty emptying the bladder completely.
   — Urinary Incontinence: In some cases, the pressure on the bladder may cause a loss of bladder control.
   — Constipation: Fibroids that press on the rectum can cause constipation or difficulty with bowel movements.
   — Painful Bowel Movements: Pressure on the rectum or surrounding structures may lead to discomfort or pain during bowel movements.

4. **Reproductive and Sexual Health Symptoms:**
   — Infertility: Although not common, fibroids can interfere with fertility by blocking the fallopian tubes or distorting the shape of the uterus, making it difficult for an embryo to implant.
   — Recurrent Miscarriages: Fibroids, particularly submucosal ones that grow inside the uterine cavity, can increase the risk of miscarriages.
   — Pain During Intercourse (Dyspareunia): Fibroids, especially those located near the cervix or along the uterus, can cause pain during sexual intercourse.

5. **Pregnancy Complications:[Effect of fibroid on pregnancy]**
   — Preterm Birth: Fibroids can increase the risk of preterm labour or delivery.
   — Abnormal presentations of faetus : The presence of fibroids can affect the baby's position in the uterus, leading to breech /transverse/oblique presentation.
   — Placent: In rare cases, fibroids may increase the risk of the placenta detaching from the uterine wall before delivery.

6. **Anaemia**

Iron-Deficiency Anaemia: Due to heavy menstrual bleeding, some women with fibroids may develop anaemia, leading to symptoms such as fatigue, weakness, dizziness, and shortness of breath.

7. **General Symptoms**
   — Fatigue: This can result from anaemia or the physical toll of carrying larger fibroids.
   — Emotional and Psychological Impact*: Chronic pain, heavy bleeding, and fertility issues can affect a woman's mental health, leading to stress, anxiety, or depression.

Risk factors-

1. Hormonal Factors: Estrogen and progesterone, the hormones that regulate the menstrual cycle, are believed to promote the growth of fibroids. Fibroids tend to shrink after menopause due to a decrease in hormone levels.
2. Genetic Factors: A family history of fibroids increases the likelihood of developing them. Certain genetic mutations are also linked to fibroid growth.
3. Growth Factors: Substances that help the body maintain tissues, such as insulin-like growth factors, may affect fibroid development.
4. Extracellular Matrix (ECM): ECM, the material that helps cells stick together, is increased in fibroids, making them more fibrous. ECM also stores growth factors that may cause fibroids to grow.
5. ther Factors:
   — Obesity: Higher body fat can lead to increased estrogen levels, which may promote fibroid growth.

- Diet: A diet high in red meat and low in green vegetables, fruit, and dairy may be linked to an increased risk of fibroids.
- Early Menstruation: Starting menstruation at an early age is associated with a higher risk of developing fibroids.
- Vitamin D Deficiency: Low levels of vitamin D are associated with an increased risk of fibroids.
- Lifestyle Factors: Alcohol consumption, particularly beer, has been linked to an increased risk of fibroids.

Additional factors and insights into the causes and risk factors of fibroids:

1. Inflammatory Factors:

Chronic inflammation in the body may contribute to the development of fibroids. Some studies suggest that inflammatory processes within the uterus could stimulate fibroid growth.

2. Pregnancy:

Pregnancy increases the production of estrogen and progesterone, which can cause fibroids that were already present to grow more rapidly.

3. Environmental Factors:

Exposure to environmental toxins, such as certain chemicals in plastics (e.g., bisphenol A, or BPA), may influence the development of fibroids. These chemicals can mimic estrogen in the body, potentially leading to fibroid growth.

4. Race and Ethnicity:

African-American women are more likely to develop fibroids and tend to experience them at a younger age and with more severe symptoms compared to women of other ethnicities. The reasons for this disparity are not fully understood but may involve a combination of genetic, environmental, and lifestyle factors.

5. Age:

The likelihood of developing fibroids increases as women age, particularly during the reproductive years (30s and 40s). However, they tend to shrink after menopause when hormone levels decrease.

6. Menstrual Cycle Characteristics:

Longer and heavier menstrual cycles are sometimes associated with a higher risk of fibroids. This may be linked to the higher cumulative exposure to estrogen over time.

7. **Reproductive History:**

Women who have never given birth (nulliparity) may have a higher risk of developing fibroids. Conversely, women who have had more pregnancies are at a lower risk, possibly due to changes in hormone levels during pregnancy.

8. **Stress:**

While research is still ongoing, chronic stress has been suggested as a potential risk factor for fibroid development. Stress can affect hormone levels, which may influence fibroid growth.

9. **Endocrine**

clinical features of fibroids:

1. **Menstrual Symptoms:**
   — Heavy Menstrual Bleeding (Menorrhagia): One of the most common symptoms of fibroids is heavy or prolonged menstrual bleeding. This can lead to anaemia and fatigue.
   — Menstrual Clotting: Passing large blood clots during menstruation can be a sign of fibroids.
   — Prolonged Menstrual Periods: Periods that last longer than seven days can be associated with fibroids.

2. **Pelvic Pain and Pressure:**
   — Pelvic Pain or Pressure: Fibroids can cause a sensation of heaviness or pressure in the pelvis. This can be due to the fibroids pressing on surrounding organs.
   — Lower Back Pain: If fibroids press on nerves or muscles in the lower back, they can cause chronic back pain.
   — Abdominal Swelling: Larger fibroids can cause noticeable swelling or distension in the abdomen, making a woman look pregnant.

3. **Bladder and Bowel Symptoms:**
   — Frequent Urination: Fibroids can press on the bladder, leading to a frequent need to urinate or difficulty emptying the bladder completely.
   — Urinary Incontinence: In some cases, the pressure on the bladder may cause a loss of bladder control.
   — Constipation: Fibroids that press on the rectum can cause constipation or difficulty with bowel movements.
   — Painful Bowel Movements: Pressure on the rectum or surrounding structures may lead to discomfort or pain during bowel movements.

4. **Reproductive and Sexual Health Symptoms:**
   — Infertility: Although not common, fibroids can interfere with fertility by blocking the fallopian tubes or distorting the shape of the uterus, making it difficult for an embryo to implant.
   — Recurrent Miscarriages: Fibroids, particularly submucosal ones that grow inside the uterine cavity, can increase the risk of miscarriages.
   — Pain During Intercourse (Dyspareunia): Fibroids, especially those located near the cervix or along the uterus, can cause pain during sexual intercourse.

5. **Pregnancy Complications:**
   — Preterm Birth: Fibroids can increase the risk of preterm labour or delivery.
   — Breech Birth: The presence of fibroids can affect the baby's position in the uterus, leading to breech presentation.
   — Placental Abruption: In rare cases, fibroids may increase the risk of the placenta detaching from the uterine wall before delivery.

6. **Anaemia:**
   — Iron-Deficiency Anaemia: Due to heavy menstrual bleeding, some women with fibroids may develop anaemia, leading to symptoms such as fatigue, weakness, dizziness, and shortness of breath.

7. **General Symptoms:**
   — Fatigue: This can result from anaemia or the physical toll of carrying larger fibroids.
   — Emotional and Psychological Impact: Chronic pain, heavy bleeding, and fertility issues can affect a woman's mental health, leading to stress, anxiety, or depression.

8. **Asymptomatic Fibroids:**
   — No Symptoms: Many women with fibroids have no symptoms at all and only discover the fibroids during a routine pelvic exam or imaging study for another condition.

9. **Rare Complications:**
   — Torsion of Pedunculated Fibroids: A fibroid on a stalk (pedunculated) can twist, cutting off its blood supply, which may cause severe, sudden pelvic pain and require emergency treatment.
   — Degeneration: If a fibroid outgrows its blood supply, it may degenerate and cause acute pain, fever, and elevated white blood cell counts.

The severity and combination of symptoms can vary widely, and some women may need treatment to manage their symptoms, while others may only require monitoring. If you need more details on any of these symptoms or are interested in treatment options, feel free to ask!

Here are some of the potential effects of fibroids on pregnancy:

1. **Increased Risk of Miscarriage:**
   — Early Pregnancy Loss: Fibroids, particularly submucosal ones that distort the uterine cavity, can increase the risk of miscarriage. They may interfere with the implantation of the embryo or disrupt the growing placenta, leading to early pregnancy loss.
   — Recurrent Miscarriages: Women with large or multiple fibroids may have a higher risk of recurrent miscarriages.

2. **Preterm Labour and Delivery:**
   — Preterm Labour: Fibroids, especially large ones, can increase the risk of preterm labour by causing uterine irritability or reducing the space available for the growing baby.
   — Preterm Delivery: If the fibroids lead to complications such as bleeding or placental issues, early delivery may be necessary to protect the health of both mother and baby.

3. **Placental Abruption:**
   — Placental Abruption*: Fibroids can increase the risk of placental abruption, where the placenta partially or completely detaches from the uterine wall before delivery. This is a serious condition that can lead to heavy bleeding and may compromise the baby's oxygen supply.

4. **Fetal Growth Restriction (IUGR):**
   — Intrauterine Growth Restriction (IUGR): Large fibroids can restrict the space available in the uterus, limiting the baby's growth. This can result in IUGR, where the baby is smaller than expected for gestational age.

5. **Breech or Abnormal Fetal Position:**
   — Abnormal Fetal Presentation: Fibroids can affect the baby's position in the uterus, leading to abnormal presentations, such as breech (bottom-first) or transverse (sideways) positions. This can complicate labour and increase the likelihood of a caesarean delivery.

6. **Labour Complications:**
   — Prolonged Labour: Fibroids, particularly those located in the lower part of the uterus or near the cervix, can obstruct the birth canal, leading to prolonged or obstructed labour.
   — Caesarean Section: Due to complications such as obstructed labour, abnormal fetal position, or placental issues, women with fibroids are more likely to require a caesarean section (C-section) for delivery.

7. **Postpartum Haemorrhage:**
   — Excessive Bleeding After Delivery: Fibroids can increase the risk of postpartum haemorrhage, which is heavy bleeding after childbirth. This can occur because fibroids may interfere with the uterus's ability to contract effectively after delivery, leading to increased blood loss.

8. **Placenta Previa:**
   — Placenta Previa: In some cases, fibroids may cause the placenta to implant lower in the uterus, covering the cervix (placenta previa). This condition can lead to complications such as bleeding during pregnancy and may require a C-section delivery.

9. **Increased Risk of Uterine Rupture:**
   — Uterine Rupture: Although rare, very large fibroids or those deeply embedded in the uterine wall can increase the risk of uterine rupture during pregnancy or labour. This is a serious complication that requires emergency medical intervention.

10. **Pre-eclampsia:**
    — Pre-eclampsia: Some studies suggest that women with fibroids may have a slightly increased risk of developing pre-eclampsia, a condition characterized by high blood pressure and damage to organs such as the liver and kidneys.

11. **Pregnancy-Related Pain:**
    — Fibroid Degeneration: During pregnancy, fibroids may outgrow their blood supply and undergo degeneration, causing severe pain. This is known as "red degeneration" and can lead to localized…

key effects of pregnancy on fibroids:

1. **Fibroid Growth:**
   — Hormonal Stimulation: During pregnancy, the levels of estrogen and progesterone increase significantly. Since fibroids are hormone-sensitive, they may grow in response to these elevated hormone levels. However, not all fibroids enlarge during pregnancy; some may remain stable in size or even shrink.
   — First-Trimester Growth: Fibroids are more likely to grow during the first trimester when hormone levels rise rapidly. After the first trimester, growth may slow down or stabilize.

2. **Fibroid Degeneration:**
   — Red Degeneration: As fibroids grow, they may outstrip their blood supply, leading to a process called red degeneration (also known as carneous degeneration). This results in the breakdown of fibroid tissue, which can cause severe pain, fever, and

sometimes bleeding. Red degeneration is more common during the second and third trimesters.
— Acute Pain: The degeneration of fibroids can lead to acute abdominal pain, which may require hospitalization for pain management. However, this condition usually resolves on its own with supportive care.

3. **Changes in Symptoms:**
   — Increased Pressure and Discomfort: As the uterus expands during pregnancy, fibroids may cause increased pressure on surrounding organs, leading to symptoms such as urinary frequency, constipation, and pelvic discomfort.
   — Shifting Position: The growing uterus may push fibroids into different positions, potentially reducing or increasing their impact on pregnancy-related symptoms.

4. **Impact on Fibroid Location:**
   — Migration of Fibroids: As the uterus enlarges, fibroids may change their position. For example, a fibroid that was initially located near the cervix may be pushed upward as the uterus grows, reducing the risk of obstructing the birth canal.
   — Increased Contact with Placenta: In some cases, fibroids may come into closer contact with the placenta, potentially affecting placental function and leading to complications like placental abruption or restricted fetal growth.

5. **Fibroid Size After Delivery:**
   — Postpartum Shrinkage: After childbirth, fibroids typically shrink as hormone levels decrease. Many women find that their fibroid-related symptoms improve significantly after delivery.
   — Long-Term Changes: While some fibroids may shrink after pregnancy, others may remain the same size or even grow larger over time. In some cases, new fibroids may develop after pregnancy.

6. **Impact on Uterine Function:**
   — Altered Uterine Contractions: Fibroids may interfere with the normal contractions of the uterus during pregnancy and labour. This can lead to challenges in labour progression and may increase the likelihood of requiring medical interventions such as induction or C-section.

7. **Postpartum Complications:**
   — Postpartum Haemorrhage: Fibroids can increase the risk of postpartum haemorrhage due to their impact on uterine contractions and the ability of the uterus to contract effectively after delivery. This can lead to excessive bleeding and may require medical intervention to manage.

8. **Reduced Symptoms:**
   — Symptom Relief: In some cases, pregnancy-related changes in blood flow and hormone levels may reduce fibroid symptoms. Some women find that their fibroids become less symptomatic during pregnancy, especially if the fibroids are small.

9. **Risk of Recurrence:**
   — Potential for New Fibroid Growth: While pregnancy may lead to shrinkage of existing fibroids, the hormonal changes associated with pregnancy can also stimulate the development of new fibroids. This means that women who have fibroids during one pregnancy may develop additional fibroids in subsequent pregnancies.

10. **Breastfeeding and Fibroid Changes:**
    — Lactation-Related Hormonal Effects: Breastfeeding can suppress estrogen levels due to the production of prolactin, which may contribute to the continued shrinkage of fibroids postpartum. Women who breastfeed may experience a slower return of fibroid-related symptoms compared to those who do not breastfeed.

In summary, pregnancy can lead to various changes in fibroids, ranging from growth and degeneration to shifts in symptoms and location. While some women may experience an increase in fibroid-related discomfort during pregnancy, others may find that their symptoms improve. Postpartum, many fibroids shrink, and symptoms often lessen. Regular monitoring during pregnancy and postpartum care are important for managing the potential effects of fibroids.

Primary Methods Used To Diagnose Fibroids:

1. **Clinical Evaluation:**
   — Medical History: A thorough medical history is taken, focusing on symptoms such as heavy menstrual bleeding, pelvic pain or pressure, frequent urination, constipation, and reproductive issues. A history of family members with fibroids may also be relevant.
   — Physical Examination: During a pelvic exam, the doctor may palpate (feel) the uterus through the abdomen to check for an enlarged or irregularly shaped uterus, which could indicate the presence of fibroids.

2. **Imaging Studies:**
   — Ultrasound: The most common and non-invasive imaging test used to diagnose fibroids. It can be performed transabdominally (through the abdomen) or transvaginally (through the vagina). Ultrasound provides images of the uterus and can help identify the size, number, and location of fibroids.
   — Magnetic Resonance Imaging (MRI): MRI provides a more detailed image of fibroids than ultrasound. It's particularly useful for mapping fibroids in women who

are considering surgery or other treatments. MRI can distinguish between different types of fibroids and other conditions like adenomyosis.
- Hysterosonography (Sonohysterography): This is a special type of ultrasound where sterile saline is injected into the uterine cavity to provide a clearer view of the endometrial lining. It's particularly useful for detecting submucosal fibroids, which may distort the uterine cavity.
- Hysterosalpingography (HSG): An X-ray procedure where contrast dye is injected into the uterus and fallopian tubes. This test can show abnormalities in the uterine cavity, including fibroids, and is often used in fertility evaluations.

3. **Hysteroscopy*:**
- Direct Visualization: A hysteroscopy involves inserting a thin, lighted telescope (hysteroscope) through the cervix into the uterus. This allows for direct visualization of the inside of the uterine cavity. It's especially useful for diagnosing submucosal fibroids and can also be used to remove small fibroids.

4. **Laparoscopy:**
- Minimally Invasive Surgery: Laparoscopy involves inserting a small camera through a small incision in the abdomen to visualize the outside of the uterus. This technique can be used to diagnose and sometimes treat fibroids, especially if they are causing pelvic pain or fertility issues.

5. **Laboratory Tests:**
- Complete Blood Count (CBC): For women with heavy menstrual bleeding, a CBC is often ordered to check for anemia (low red blood cell count), which is a common complication of fibroids.
- Hormonal Tests: These may be conducted to rule out other causes of abnormal bleeding, such as thyroid disorders or hormonal imbalances.
- Endometrial Biopsy: In cases where abnormal bleeding is a concern, especially in women over 40, an endometrial biopsy may be performed to rule out other conditions, such as endometrial hyperplasia or cancer. This involves taking a small sample of the uterine lining for examination.

6. **Other Diagnostic Procedures:**
- Pap Smear: While not specifically used to diagnose fibroids, a Pap smear may be part of the overall evaluation to rule out other causes of abnormal bleeding or pelvic pain.
- Biopsy of Fibroid: Though rare, a biopsy might be performed if there's concern about malignancy, particularly if the fibroid has unusual features on imaging.

7. **Differential Diagnosis:**
   — Ruling Out Other Conditions: The diagnosis of fibroids also involves ruling out other conditions that may cause similar symptoms, such as ovarian cysts, adenomyosis, endometriosis, or malignancies. This is done through a combination of the above diagnostic methods and clinical judgment.

Once diagnosed, the specific characteristics of the fibroids—such as size, number, and location—will guide treatment decisions. The choice of diagnostic tool depends on the patient's symptoms, age, reproductive plans, and overall health.

The Main Strategies For Managing Fibroids:

1. **Watchful Waiting (Conservative Management):**
   — Asymptomatic Fibroids: If fibroids are not causing symptoms, or if symptoms are mild and manageable, watchful waiting may be the best approach. This involves regular monitoring with pelvic exams and ultrasounds to track the size and growth of the fibroids.
   — Post-Menopausal Women: Fibroids often shrink after menopause due to a decrease in hormone levels. In post-menopausal women, conservative management is often preferred unless the fibroids are causing significant symptoms.

2. **Medical Management:**
   — Hormonal Therapies:
   — Gonadotropin-Releasing Hormone (GnRH) Agonists: These medications, such as leuprolide, reduce estrogen and progesterone levels, leading to temporary shrinkage of fibroids. They are often used preoperatively to reduce fibroid size or to manage symptoms. However, long-term use is limited due to side effects like bone loss.
   — Progestin-Only Therapies: Progestin-only pills, intrauterine devices (IUDs), or injections (like Depo-Provera) can help control heavy menstrual bleeding associated with fibroids. The levonorgestrel-releasing IUD (e.g., Mirena) is particularly effective.
   — Combined Oral Contraceptives: Birth control pills that contain estrogen and progestin can help regulate menstrual cycles and reduce heavy bleeding, but they may not shrink fibroids.
   — Selective Progesterone Receptor Modulators (SPRMs): Medications like ulipristal acetate can shrink fibroids and control bleeding. However, use may be restricted due to concerns about liver safety.
   — Non-Hormonal Therapies:
   — Nonsteroidal Anti-Inflammatory Drugs (NSAIDs): NSAIDs like ibuprofen can help manage pain related to fibroids but do not reduce bleeding or shrink the fibroids.

- Tranexamic Acid: An antifibrinolytic medication that reduces heavy menstrual bleeding by stabilizing blood clots. It is taken during menstruation and does not affect fibroid size.
- Iron Supplements: For women with anemia due to heavy bleeding, iron supplements can help manage symptoms of anemia.

3. **Minimally Invasive Procedures:**
   - Uterine Artery Embolization (UAE): This procedure involves blocking the blood supply to the fibroids, causing them to shrink. It is effective for reducing symptoms and can be a good option for women who want to avoid surgery. However, it may not be suitable for women who wish to become pregnant in the future.
   - Magnetic Resonance-Guided Focused Ultrasound (MRgFUS): This non-invasive treatment uses focused ultrasound waves to heat and destroy fibroid tissue. It is performed under MRI guidance and is an option for women with certain types of fibroids.
   - Endometrial Ablation: This procedure destroys the lining of the uterus to reduce menstrual bleeding. It is generally not recommended for women who wish to maintain fertility and is most effective for small submucosal fibroids.

4. **Surgical Management:**
   - Myomectomy: Surgical removal of fibroids while preserving the uterus. Myomectomy can be performed via different approaches depending on the size, number, and location of the fibroids:
   - Hysteroscopic Myomectomy: For submucosal fibroids, this procedure is done through the vagina and cervix using a hysteroscope.
   - Laparoscopic Myomectomy: A minimally invasive approach where fibroids are removed through small incisions in the abdomen.
   - Abdominal Myomectomy: An open surgery that involves a larger incision in the abdomen. It is typically used for larger or more numerous fibroids.
   - Postoperative Considerations: Women who undergo myomectomy may need to wait several months before attempting pregnancy. There is also a risk of fibroid recurrence.
   - Hysterectomy: The definitive treatment for fibroids, involving the removal of the uterus. Hysterectomy completely eliminates fibroids and their associated symptoms. It is considered in women who do not wish to preserve fertility or when other treatments have failed. There are different types of hysterectomy:
   - Total Hysterectomy: Removal of the uterus and cervix.
   - Subtotal (Partial) Hysterectomy: Removal of the uterus while leaving the cervix intact.

— Hysterectomy with Oophorectomy: Removal of the ovaries along with the uterus, often considered in cases where ovarian conditions or risks are present.
— *Considerations*: Hysterectomy is a major surgery with longer recovery time but offers a permanent solution. It is recommended for women with severe symptoms who do not wish to preserve fertility.

5. **Fertility Considerations:**
— Fertility-Sparing Treatments: For women who wish to maintain fertility, myomectomy is the preferred surgical option. Minimally invasive procedures like UAE and MRgFUS may have limited effects on fertility, and careful consideration should be given to the choice of treatment.
— Fertility Evaluation: Women with fibroids who are experiencing difficulty conceiving may need additional fertility evaluation and treatment, such as IVF, depending on the impact of the fibroids.

6. **Lifestyle and Supportive Measures:**
— Diet and Exercise: While not directly proven to shrink fibroids, maintaining a healthy diet and regular exercise can help manage symptoms and improve overall health.
— Stress Management: Chronic stress can exacerbate symptoms, so stress-reduction techniques such as yoga, meditation, and counselling may be beneficial.

7. **Alternative and Complementary Therapies:**
— Herbal Remedies and Supplements: Some women explore herbal supplements and natural remedies for fibroid management. However, the safety and effectiveness of these treatments are not well-established, and it's important to discuss them with a healthcare provider.
— Acupuncture: Some studies suggest that acupuncture may help relieve symptoms associated with fibroids, though evidence is limited.

8. **Follow-Up and Monitoring:**
— Regular Check-Ups: For women undergoing conservative management or after treatment, regular follow-up with pelvic exams and imaging is important to monitor fibroid growth or recurrence.
— Symptom Tracking: Keeping a record of symptoms can help guide treatment decisions and assess the effectiveness of interventions.

Conclusion:

Management of fibroids is highly individualized, taking into account the patient's symptoms, reproductive goals, and person

9. **Rare Complications*:**
   — Torsion of Pedunculated Fibroids: A fibroid on a stalk (pedunculated) can twist, cutting off its blood supply, which may cause severe, sudden pelvic pain and require emergency treatment.
   — Degeneration: If a fibroid outgrows its blood supply, it may degenerate and cause acute pain, fever, and elevated white blood cell counts.

Remedy	Key Indications	Menstrual Symptoms	Pain Characteristics	Other Notable Symptoms
Calcarea Carbonica	Large, soft fibroids; obesity; sluggish metabolism	Heavy, prolonged periods with **clots**	**Dull, aching pain** in pelvis	Weakness, cold intolerance, sweating, craving eggs
Thuja Occidentalis	Fibroids with abnormal growths; left-sided affections	Scanty, irregular, or delayed periods	**Cutting, darting pains** in uterus	Warts, cysts, oily skin, history of vaccination issues
Sepia Officinalis	Uterine prolapse; bearing-down sensation	**Scanty, irregular, or suppressed periods**	Heaviness, dragging pain, relieved by exercise	Irritability, aversion to family, cold hands/feet
Phosphorus	Fibroids with excessive bleeding and weakness	**Bright red bleeding, lasts long**	**Burning, stitching pain** in uterus	Thirsty, loves cold drinks, nervous exhaustion
Lachesis	Left-sided fibroids; intolerance to tight clothing	Dark, offensive bleeding, worsens with menopause	**Congested, pulsating pain** in pelvis	Jealous, talkative, feels suffocated
Ustilago Maydis	Fibroids with **severe hemorrhage**	**Dark, stringy clots, continuous bleeding**	**Cramps, soreness** in uterus	Weakness, dizziness, history of miscarriages

Sabina	Fibroids with **excessive, gushing bleeding**	Bright red blood, worse from movement	**Violent, throbbing pain**, extends to thighs	Worse from warm rooms, history of abortions
Trillium Pendulum	Fibroids with **profuse bleeding and weakness**	Bright red bleeding, **fainting tendency**	**Severe backache**, improves with tight bandages	Exhaustion, cold extremities
Belladonna	Acute inflammation of fibroids; sudden onset	**Bright red, hot bleeding**, sudden onset	**Sharp, throbbing pain**, sudden	High fever, flushed face, sensitive to light
Conium Maculatum	Fibroids with slow, gradual growth; right-sided issues	Suppressed, delayed, or scanty periods	**Stitching pain**, aggravated by touch	Dizziness, weakness, sensation of fullness in abdomen
Bovista	Fibroids with **fibrocystic changes**	**Heavy bleeding, with clots**	**Cramps, distension** in abdomen	Indigestion, swelling of glands, intolerance to milk
Aconitum Napellus	Fibroids with acute pain, sudden onset of symptoms	**Short, early periods** with **heaviness**	**Burning, sharp pain**, sudden and intense	Anxiety, fear, restlessness, worsened by cold air
Hydrastis Canadensis	Fibroids with **chronic uterine infections**	**Mucous discharge**, excessive bleeding	**Dragging pain**, with a feeling of fullness	Loss of appetite, thin, yellowish discharge
Cimicifuga Racemosa	Fibroids with **nervousness and menstrual irregularities**	**Painful, irregular menses**	**Cramps** extending to the back and thighs	Exhaustion, restlessness, sensitivity to touch and pressure

Silicea	Fibroids with **chronic, chronic inflammation**	**Delayed periods, scanty bleeding**	**Sharp, cutting pain** during periods	Weak nails, excessive perspiration, sensitivity to cold
Magnesia Phosphorica	Fibroids with **cramping pain and bloating**	Painful, spasmodic periods	**Cramp-like, colicky pain**, improved by warmth	Better from warmth, nervous tension, muscular weakness
Natrum Muriaticum	Fibroids with **emotional disturbances** and stress	**Irregular menses**, worsened by emotional stress	**Stitching pain**, aggravated by exertion	Thirsty, withdrawal from others, grief, headaches

Genital Prolapse

Defination:- The herniation of the pelvic organ through the vagina is called genital prolapsed.

Types:-
- Cystocele
- Rectocele
- Enterocele
- Urethrocele
- Uterine prolapse
- Vault prolapsed

I] CYSTOCELE

Descent of urinary bladder with anterior vaginal wall below the cervix.

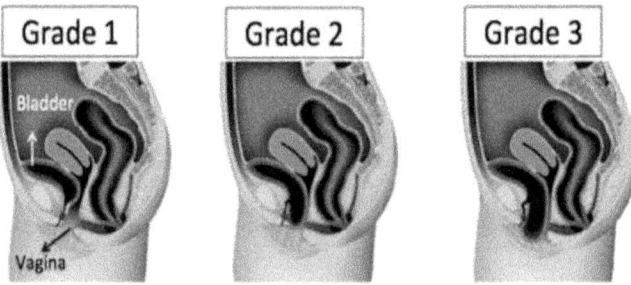

II] RECTOCELE

Descent of rectum with posterior wall of vagina.

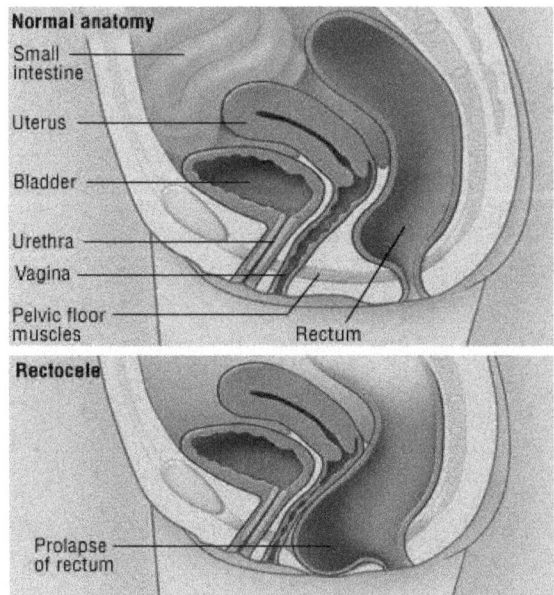

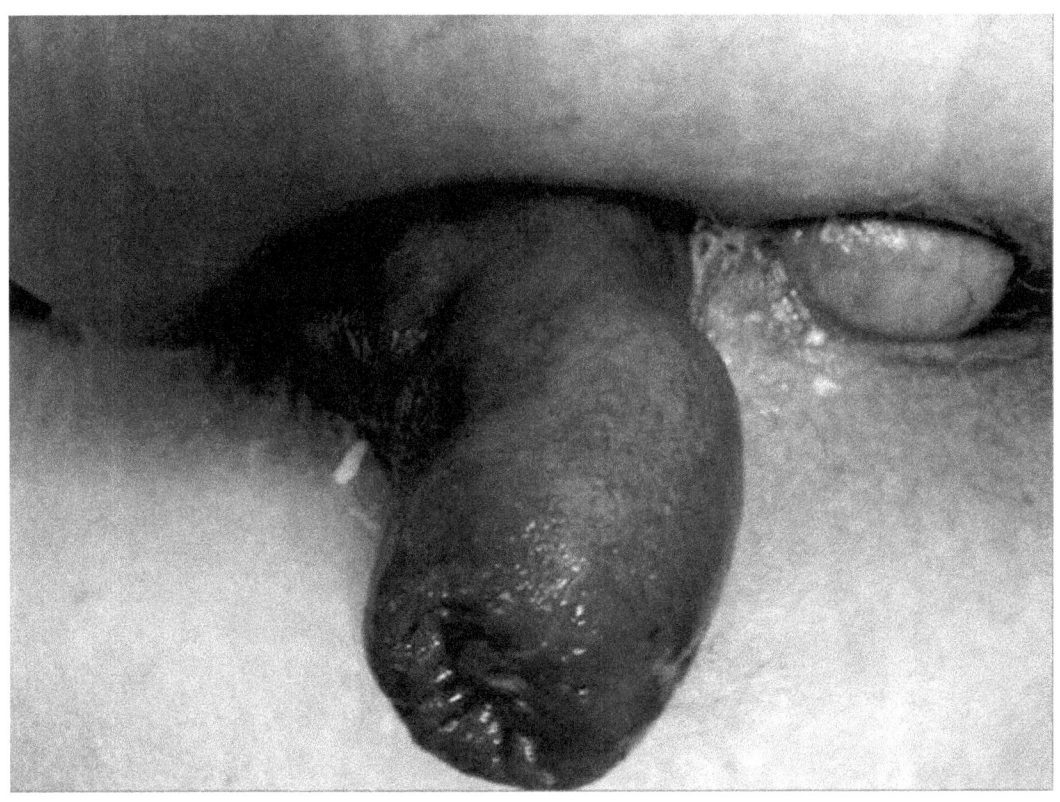

III] URETROCELE
Descent of urethra with lower part of anterior vaginal wall.

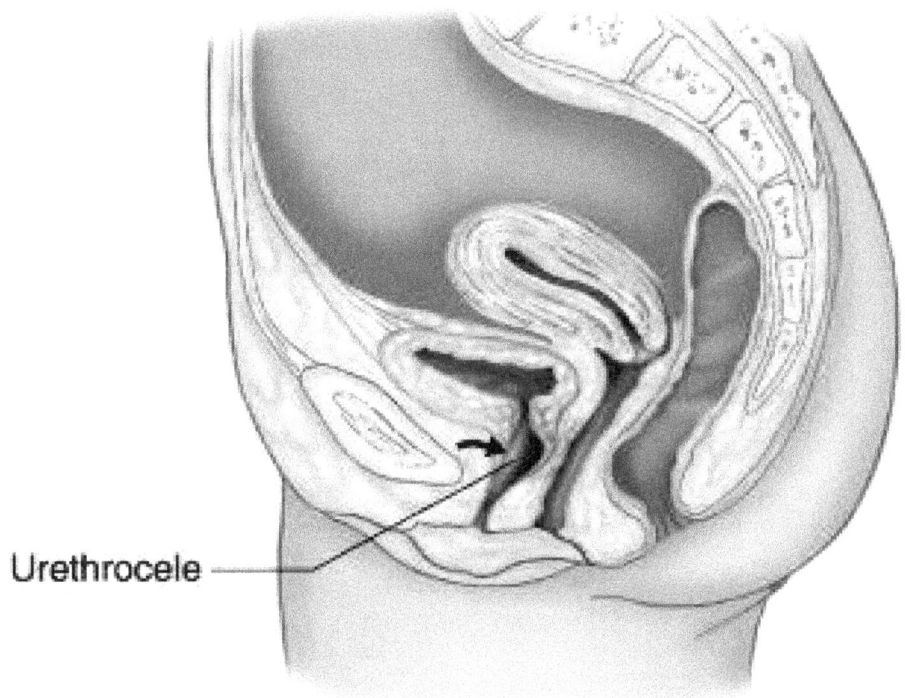

IV] ENTEROCELE

Descent of pouch of Douglus with posterior vaginal wall and containts like loop of intestines or omentum.

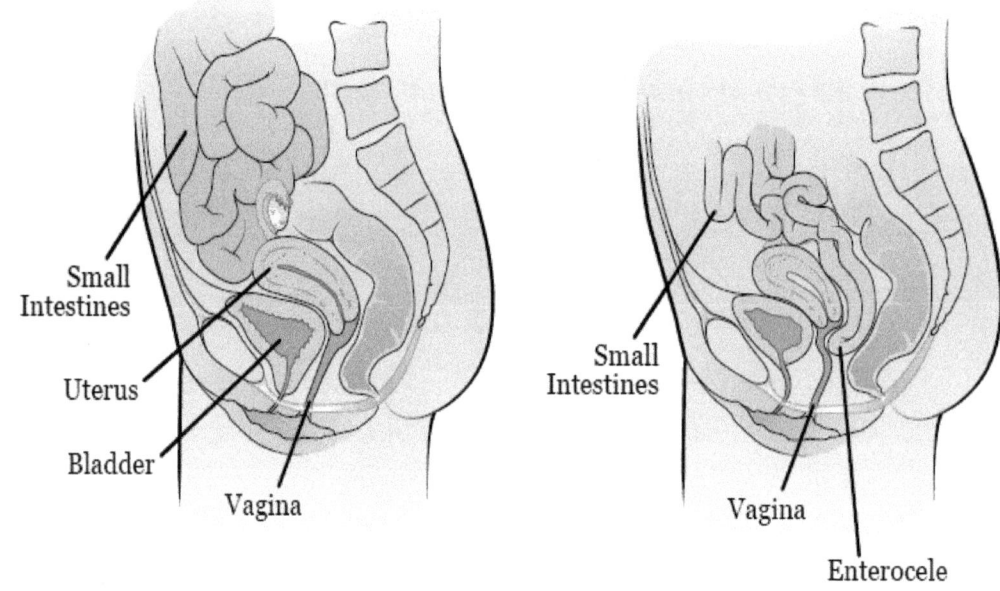

V] UTERINE PROLAPSE

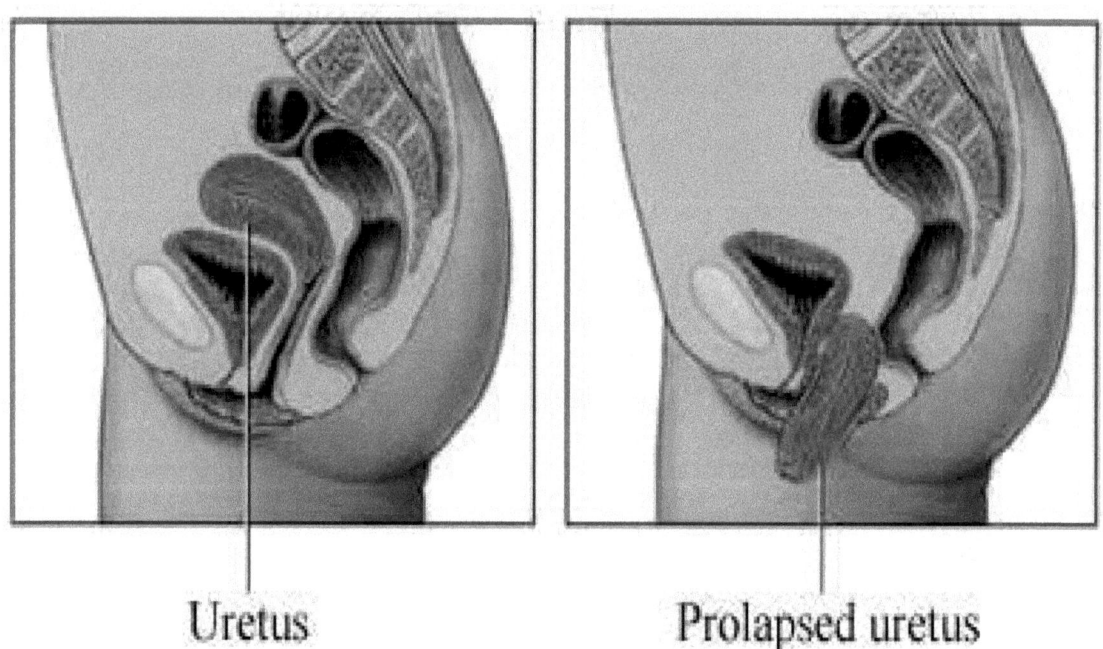

Descent of uterus through vagina.
Vagino –uterine prolapse, primarily vaginal prolapsed drags down the uterus.
Utero-vaginal prolapsed, primary uterine prolapse causes invertion of vagina.

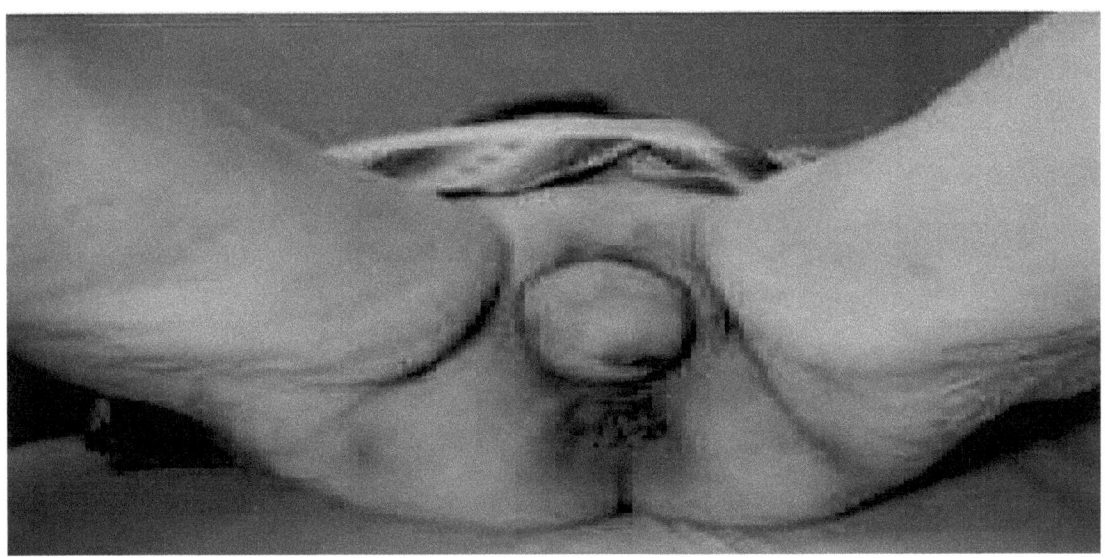

Fig. "COMPLETE PROCEDENTIA

VI] VAULT PROLAPSE

Prolapse of vaginal flora along with enterocele and uterovaginal prolapse.

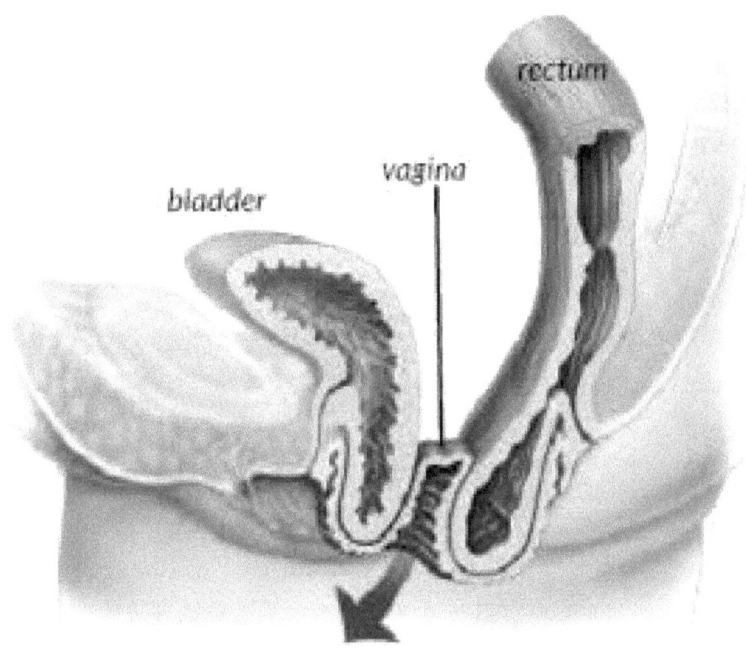

Degrees Of Prolapse :-

-Ist or Mild degree: Herniating part descents down from its normal position below the level of cervix.

— II nd or Moderate degree : Herniating part descents down upto vaginal introitus.

— IIIrd or Severe degree : Herniating part descends outside the vaginal introitus.

Complete Procedentia- It is the IVth degree uterine prolapse also called as complete uterine prolapse where wholw uterus descends outside the vagina and vagina is almost completely inverted.

Aetiology :-

I] Failure of pelvic supports

II] Raised intra abdominal pressure

I] Failure of pelvic supports-

- Congenital causes-
— -weakness of pelvic muscles and ligaments
— spina bifida occulta
— postmenopausal nulliparous women
- Aquired causes-

childbirth:

— stretching, tearing of pelvic fascia and widenind of vaginal canal.
— perineal trauma
— dammage to pelvic floor due to recurrent abortions and recurrent deliveries.
— early bear down
— excessive fundal pressure
— delivery without emptying of bladder and rectum
— poor puerperal management.

atrophy:

— after menopause
— undernutrition

postsurgical causes:

— subtotal hysterectomy
— vaginal hysterectomy
— abdominal subtotal/ total hysterectomy

II] Raised intra-abdominal pressure-

- Chronic cough
- Chronic constipation
- Chronic dysentery
- Lifting heavy weight
- Obesity
- Fibroid uterus or pelvic tumours.

Pathophysiology:

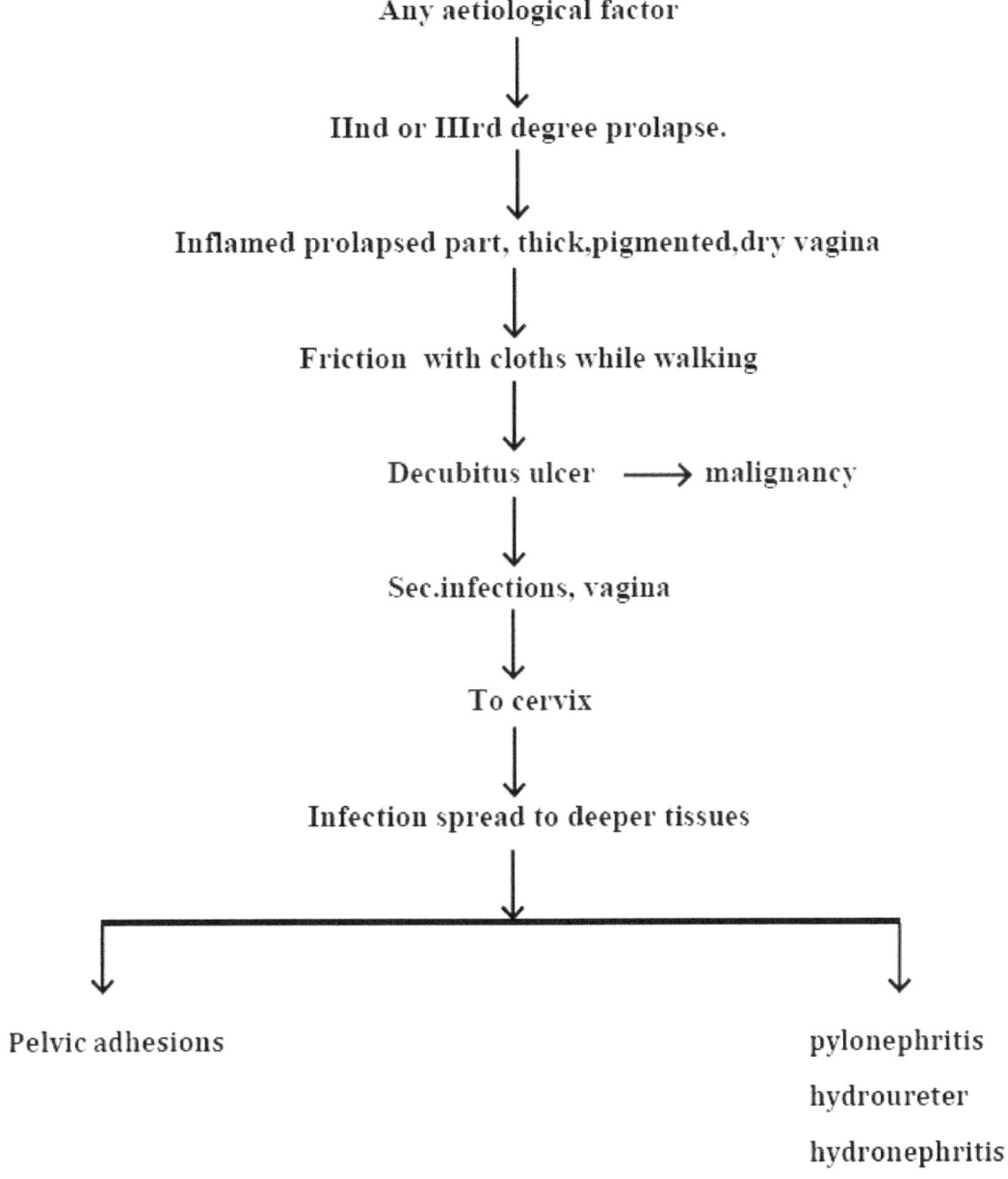

Clinical Features:-

Uterine Prolapse-

— Bearing down sensation as if something is falling down from the vagina, aggravated esp. after prolonged standing and straining.
— Backache with localized tenderness. Sacral or lumbosacral due to overstretching of ligaments.

- White P/V discharges, due to vaginitis. It becomes blood stained in decubitus ulcers, yellowish-greenish in mixed type of bacterial infections.
- Feeling of loss of vaginal tightness in sexual intercourse, Fluor seminitis.
- P/V bleeding after sexual intercourse in decubitus ulcers.
- Rarely, menstrual abnormalities like menorrhagia, metrorrhagia.

Additional Symptoms In Cystocele –
- Frequent micturation
- Cystitis, burning micturation, recurrent UTI
- Required straining for emptying of bladder
- Stress incontinence.
- Involuntary passage of urine while laughing, coughing.

Additional Symptoms In Rectocele-
- Constipation
- Difficult emptying of bowel, pt.want to bend backwards for emptying.
- SIGNS :-
- Anaemia
- Lax abdomen
- P/V Exam-Descent of cervix, or herniating part through vagina while straining or coughing.
- Bulging of ant.vaginal wall in cystocele and bulging of posterior vaginal wall in rectocele.

Prevention:
- Good puerpural management.
- Avoid early bear down during labour.
- Smooth 2nd stage conduction of labour.
- Early diagnosis and management of chronic cough, chronic constipation, chronic diarrhea, obesity.
- Avoid over weight lifting or aggrassive jim work, esp sudden after delivery or abortion.
- Proper spacing between two pregnancies with proper contraception so that good ligamental and pelvic flour strength recovery.
- Proper repair of vaginal vault after vaginal or abdominal hysterectomy

Curative Management:-
- Physiotherapy, pelvic floor exercises to strengthen the muscles and ligaments in I st grade prolapsed.
- Curative management for causative factors like cough, constipation, obesity.

- Pessary management in I st grade or in pregnancy with prolapsed uterus.
- Packing with cotton filled with glycerine in case of friction ulcers.

Surgical Management:-

Applicable in II nd and III rd grade or in complications like decubitous ulcers or malignancy.

- Anterior colporrhaphy: For correction of cystourethrocele
- Paravaginal repair: For correction of cystourethrocele
- Posterior compartment defects-
- Posterior colporrhaphy: For correction of rectocele and deficient perineum
- Enterocele repair: For correction of enterocele
- Apical prolapsed:
— vaginal hysterectomy, for repair of uterovaginal prolapsed
— Sacrospinous ligament fixation/ Abdominal sacrocolpopexy, for vaginal vault prolapsed.
- Fothergill's operation/ Monchester's operation:
In uterine prolapse with preservation of uterus
- Ward mayo's operation:
Vaginal hysterectomy with pelvic floor repair for complete procedentia.
- Le fort's operation:
For old ladies with atrophied uterus.

1. **Modern (Allopathic) Drug Management**

Treatment	Details
Hormone Replacement Therapy (HRT)	**Estrogen creams (Premarin, Estradiol), Vaginal Rings (Estring)** – Strengthens pelvic tissues and improves vaginal tone. Side effects: Breast tenderness, nausea, increased clotting risk.
Pain Relief (NSAIDs & Analgesics)	**Ibuprofen, Diclofenac, Paracetamol** – Reduces pain and discomfort associated with prolapse. Side effects: Gastric irritation, nausea.
Pessary Insertion	**Silicone or rubber pessary** – Supports the prolapsed organs, commonly used in mild to moderate cases. Side effects: Vaginal irritation, increased risk of infection.
Antibiotics (If Infection Occurs)	**Amoxicillin, Metronidazole, Clindamycin** – Treats infections due to ulceration or pessary use. Side effects: Nausea, diarrhea, allergic reactions.

Treatment	Details
Pelvic Floor Rehabilitation	**Kegel exercises, Physical therapy** – Strengthens pelvic muscles and prevents worsening of prolapse. No side effects.
Surgical Management (Severe Cases)	**Colporrhaphy (Vaginal Repair), Hysterectomy, Mesh Repair** – Used when conservative treatments fail. Risks: Post-surgical infection, bleeding, pain.

2. Homeopathic Therapeutic Management

Symptom	Homeopathic Remedy & Details
General Pelvic Weakness & Prolapse	**Sepia** – Best remedy for uterine prolapse, heaviness, bearing-down sensation (30C or 200C, once daily).
Prolapse with Lower Back Pain & Fatigue	**Lilium Tigrinum** – Used when there is dragging pain in the pelvis and pressure in the perineum (30C, 2-3 times daily).
Bladder Weakness & Stress Incontinence	**Staphysagria** – Helps with prolapse associated with urinary leakage and weakness (30C, 2 times daily).
Prolapse Worsened by Standing or Walking	**Podophyllum** – For heaviness in the uterus and rectum, worsens with movement (30C, 2 times daily).
Uterine Prolapse with Constipation	**Murex** – Helps when there is a sensation of pressure in the uterus along with constipation (30C, once daily).
Vaginal Pain & Sensation of Internal Pressure	**Helonias Dioica** – Used when there is a dragging sensation, exhaustion, and weak pelvic muscles (30C, 2-3 times daily).
Prolapse with Vaginal Irritation or Infection	**Kreosotum** – Helps relieve vaginal burning, itching, and irritation due to prolapse (30C, 2 times daily).
Swelling & Pelvic Congestion	**Pulsatilla** – For swelling, fullness, and varicose veins in the vaginal region (30C, once or twice daily).

1. SEPIA- A topmost remedy for prolapsed uterus around menopausal age group in ladies with h/o recurrent abortions, recurrent deliveries, prolonged hormonal management for all type of menstrual irregularities and with characteristic symptoms of menopausal syndrome. Digust of sex, indifference to loved ones, lothing of life.Constant sense of bear down when kneeling or in squatting position.sense as if something is coming down from the vagina and sits cross leg to prevent it.agrravation of complaints on thinking of them, CONSOLATION, in kneeling position. Prolapse in asthmatic women feeling better when dancing and when busy.

2. LIL.TIG.- Prolapse in ladies which are always hurried and worried,always busy and accupied. The cause of prolapse is laxed pelvic ligaments and subinvolution of uterus ,retroversion of uterus. constant bearing down sensation and hold the private parts to prevent that. HOT, EXCESSIVE SEXUAL DESIRE, INTENSE CRAVING OF MEAT.Keep accupied herself to suppress sexual desire.due to mobile retroversion, cystocele and rectocele also have characteristic rectal and urinary symptoms.Costant desire to pass urine, stool with sense of fullness, requires great straining but passes only little urine and stool at a time with ball like sensation inside. HOT, SCANTY AND OFFENSSIVE DISCHARGES like urine, stool, menses. Menstrual flow only in movements,stops in resting position.

3. MUREX- Another excellent remedy for uterine prolapsed at climacteric age ladies. Constant beardown sensation, sits cross leged to prevent it. INTENSE SEXUAL DESIRE WITH VIOLENT EXCITEMENT IN SEXUAL ORGANS,aggravated by slightest touch. Menses heavy, clotted with right sided abdominal pains ref to lt.sided breast. Leucorrhea alternate with mentles .

4. NAT.MUR –Excellent remedy for cystocele in climacteric age fastidious, irritable, hot, hysterical, extrememly emotional lady.

Frequent desire to pass urine,long strains but passes few drops with sense of lot of urine remains behind.involuntary passing of urine while laughing,coughing, sneezing.SHE CANT PASS URINE IN PRESENSE OF OTHERS. All type of menstrual irregularities with thyroid disorders.Headace before menses,consolation aggravation.Sunstroke, sunrise to sunset aggravation of complaints.

5. CAN.INDICA- Excellent remedy for a prolapsed in lady with many wonderfull imaginations and hallucinations, constantly theorizing but with great forgetfulness esp .about words while talking . SENSE OF BALL IN RECTUM, SOMETHING MOVING IN ABDOMEN.Dribbling urine even after great straining.

6. LAPPA ART.-Excelllent remedy for prolapsed with constant soreness of pelvis and backache. Aggravation while walking and standing with dragging down sensations at genitals.

7. FRAXINUM AMERICANA- Prolapse due to huge uterine tumours,fibroids or pelvic tumours.

Huge enlarged uterus with heavy feeling in pelvic region with constant backache.

8. ARNICA-Remady for rectocele with ribbon like soft stool with prolonged straining. Sore, lame .brushed feeling at genitals, rectum relieved after worm water application. Excellent remedy for prolapsed genitals following blunt instrumental injuries during labour like forceps,ventose delivery or due to prolonged and excessive fundal pressure .

9. CAUSTICUM- Remedy for vault prolapse following surgery. She can pass stool only in standing position. Passes urine in dribbling when want to pass but involuntary passage of urine while laughing and coughing.

VAULT PROLAPSE

GENITAL PROLAPSE

PESSARY MANAGEMENT

Genital Tuberculosis

Definition
Genital tuberculosis (GTB) in females refers to the infection of the female reproductive tract by *Mycobacterium tuberculosis*. It is typically secondary to primary tuberculosis in other parts of the body, most commonly the lungs, and spreads via hematogenous, lymphatic, or direct routes. It is an important cause of infertility, pelvic pain, and menstrual irregularities.

Aetiology

1. **Causative Organism**
   - *Mycobacterium tuberculosis* (MTB), an acid-fast bacillus.
   - Rarely, atypical mycobacteria may be involved.

2. **Primary Focus**
   - Most cases result from the reactivation of dormant bacilli from primary foci, usually in the lungs or lymph nodes.

3. **Modes of Spread**
   - Hematogenous: From primary pulmonary TB, the most common route.
   - Lymphatic Spread: From infected mesenteric or para-aortic lymph nodes.
   - Direct Spread: From the peritoneum or adjacent organs such as the intestines.

4. **Risk Factors**
   - Immunosuppression (e.g., HIV infection).
   - Malnutrition.
   - Close contact with TB patients.
   - History of pulmonary TB.

Clinical Features
The presentation is often subtle and non-specific, leading to delayed diagnosis.

1. **General Symptoms**
   - Low-grade fever, night sweats.
   - Weight loss.
   - Fatigue.

2. **Gynecological Symptoms**
   - Infertility: The most common presentation, seen in 40–80% of cases.
   - Menstrual Disturbances:
     - Amenorrhea or oligomenorrhea due to endometrial involvement.

- Menorrhagia or intermenstrual bleeding in rare cases.
    - Pelvic Pain: Chronic lower abdominal or pelvic pain.
    - Vaginal Discharge: Purulent or blood-stained discharge in advanced cases.
3. **Physical Examination**
    - Adnexal masses or tenderness.
    - Irregular, fixed, or bulky uterus due to pelvic adhesions.

Complications

1. **Infertility**
    - Due to tubal obstruction, endometrial scarring, or pelvic adhesions.
2. **Pelvic Inflammatory Disease (PID)**
    - Chronic infection leading to adhesions and hydrosalpinx or pyosalpinx.
3. **Ectopic Pregnancy**
    - Secondary to tubal damage.
4. **Asherman's Syndrome**
    - Uterine synechiae (adhesions) caused by endometrial scarring.
5. **Generalized Peritonitis**
    - Due to ruptured tubercular abscesses.
6. **Systemic Spread**
    - Dissemination to distant organs such as the liver, kidney, or bones.

Diagnosis

Diagnosing genital TB is challenging and often requires a combination of clinical suspicion, imaging, microbiology, histopathology, and molecular techniques.

1. **Clinical History and Examination**
    - Infertility, chronic pelvic pain, or menstrual irregularities in a patient with a history of TB should raise suspicion.
2. **Laboratory Investigations**
    - Blood Tests: Elevated ESR, positive Mantoux test.
    - Sputum Examination: For suspected coexisting pulmonary TB.
3. **Imaging**
    - Ultrasound (USG): May reveal tubo-ovarian masses, endometrial thickening, or calcifications.
    - Hysterosalpingography (HSG): "Beaded appearance" of fallopian tubes or rigid tubal outlines.
    - MRI/CT Scan: For detailed pelvic assessment.

4. **Microbiological and Histopathological Tests**
   - Endometrial Biopsy: Presence of caseating granulomas.
   - Acid-Fast Bacilli (AFB) Staining: Direct smear of samples like endometrial tissue or fluid.
   - Mycobacterial Culture: Gold standard but time-consuming.
5. **Molecular Diagnostics**
   - GeneXpert MTB/RIF: Rapid detection of MTB and rifampicin resistance.
   - PCR: Highly sensitive for detecting MTB DNA.
6. **Laparoscopy**
   - Diagnostic laparoscopy shows tubercles, adhesions, hydrosalpinx, or frozen pelvis.

Management

Management of genital TB includes antitubercular therapy (ATT), surgical intervention for complications, and addressing infertility.

1. **Medical Management**
   - Antitubercular Therapy (ATT):
     - Standard 6-month regimen:

Intensive Phase (2 months): Isoniazid, Rifampicin, Pyrazinamide, and Ethambutol (HRZE).

Continuation Phase (4 months): Isoniazid and Rifampicin (HR).
   - Duration may be extended in severe cases.

Supportive Therapy:
   - Nutritional supplementation.
   - Management of anemia and immunosuppression.

2. **Surgical Management**
   - Indications: Tubo-ovarian abscess, ruptured mass, or severe adhesions.
   - Procedures:
     - Adhesiolysis.
     - Salpingectomy or salpingo-oophorectomy.

3. **Infertility Treatment**
   - Assisted reproductive technologies (ART), such as IVF, may be considered after completion of ATT if tubal damage or uterine scarring persists.

   Anti-Tubercular Treatment (ATT) for Genital Tuberculosis (GTB)

ATT in Non-Pregnant Women with Genital Tuberculosis

Principles of Treatment

1. Focus on complete eradication of *Mycobacterium tuberculosis*.

2. Prevent progression of disease and preserve fertility.
3. Address drug resistance if present.

Standard ATT Regimen

1. **Intensive Phase (2 months)**
   - Four first-line drugs: Isoniazid (H), Rifampicin (R), Pyrazinamide (Z), and Ethambutol (E) (HRZE).
   - These drugs target active and dormant bacilli.
2. **Continuation Phase (4 months)**
   - Two drugs: Isoniazid (H) and Rifampicin (R) (HR).

Monitoring and Adjustments

1. **Baseline Investigations:**
   - Liver function tests (LFTs), renal function tests, and complete blood count.
   - Visual acuity testing (for ethambutol).
2. **During Treatment:**
   - Monthly LFTs to monitor for hepatotoxicity.
   - Monitor adherence and manage side effects like gastrointestinal upset or peripheral neuropathy.
3. **Adjunct Therapy:**
   - Pyridoxine (Vitamin B6): 10–25 mg daily to prevent isoniazid-induced peripheral neuropathy.
   - Nutritional support to enhance immunity.
4. **For Drug-Resistant GTB (MDR-TB):**
   - Use second-line drugs (e.g., fluoroquinolones, bedaquiline) under expert guidance.

ATT in Pregnant Women with Genital Tuberculosis

Special Considerations

1. Safety of the fetus is a priority, so only drugs with proven safety are used.
2. Treatment is initiated as soon as GTB is diagnosed because untreated TB poses significant risks to both the mother and fetus, including miscarriage, preterm birth, and low birth weight.

Standard ATT Regimen for Pregnancy

1. **Intensive Phase (2 months)**
   - Isoniazid (H), Rifampicin (R), Pyrazinamide (Z), and Ethambutol (E) (HRZE).
   - All these drugs are considered safe in pregnancy and effective for treating GTB.

2. **Continuation Phase (4 months)**
   o **Isoniazid (H)** and **Rifampicin (R) (HR)**.

Drugs to Avoid in Pregnancy

- **Streptomycin** and other aminoglycosides: Risk of fetal ototoxicity.
- **Fluoroquinolones** (e.g., Levofloxacin): Potential fetal cartilage damage.
- **Second-line injectables** (e.g., Kanamycin, Capreomycin): Not recommended.

Monitoring and Safety in Pregnancy

1. **Maternal Monitoring:**
   o Regular LFTs to monitor for hepatotoxicity.
   o Symptoms of anemia, gastrointestinal upset, and neuropathy should be addressed.
   o Vitamin B6 supplementation (pyridoxine) to prevent neuropathy.

2. **Fetal Monitoring:**
   o Ultrasounds to assess fetal growth and detect any abnormalities.
   o Supplement maternal nutrition to prevent intrauterine growth restriction (IUGR).

Risks of Untreated GTB in Pregnancy

- Increased maternal complications: severe pelvic pain, systemic spread, or peritonitis.
- Fetal risks: miscarriage, preterm labor, low birth weight, and congenital TB.

Comparison of ATT in Pregnant vs. Non-Pregnant Women with GTB

Aspect	Non-Pregnant Women	Pregnant Women
Drug Regimen	HRZE (intensive) + HR (continuation)	HRZE (intensive) + HR (continuation)
Excluded Drugs	Fluoroquinolones for drug resistance if needed.	Streptomycin, fluoroquinolones, kanamycin.
Monitoring	Focus on organ function and adherence.	Additional fetal monitoring and maternal care.
Adjunct Therapy	Pyridoxine, nutritional support.	Pyridoxine, folic acid, and Vitamin K.
Outcomes	Good with early diagnosis; infertility remains a challenge.	Reduced maternal and fetal risks with early treatment.

Homeopathic Remedy	Indications
1. Tuberculinum	Tuberculinum is a constitutional remedy for individuals with a **family history of tuberculosis** or those who are **predisposed to tuberculosis infections**. It is often prescribed when there is **chronic cough**, **night sweats**, and **fatigue**, along with **marked emaciation**. This remedy helps strengthen the **immune system** and assists in fighting off **latent tuberculosis**. It is suitable for **recurrent infections** and **weakness** during the disease.
2. Bacillinum	Bacillinum is used for patients suffering from **tuberculosis** and those with a history of **chronic respiratory infections**. It is often indicated when there is a **chronic cough**, **low-grade fever**, **night sweats**, and **fatigue**. This remedy is helpful for **tubercular lesions** in the genital region, **painful menstruation**, and **uterine involvement**. It supports the body in overcoming latent infections and improving **immune function**.
3. Kali Carbonicum	Kali Carbonicum is suitable when there are chronic symptoms, weakness, and sweats, especially night sweats. It is helpful in cases of tubercular endometritis and tubercular pelvic inflammation, with stitching pain in the lower abdomen. This remedy is useful when the patient feels exhausted and experiences emotional breakdowns with poor stamina. It is also beneficial for dryness in the genital tract and abnormal uterine bleeding.
4. Silicea	Silicea is used when there is **chronic, sluggish healing** of tubercular lesions in the genital region, with **suppuration** or **abscess formation**. It is beneficial for individuals who have **a history of infections** and suffer from **frequent colds**, **low immunity**, and **weak tissues**. Silicea helps in expelling **toxins** and is useful for **post-inflammatory scarring** in the genital tract.
5. Calcarea Carbonica	Calcarea Carbonica is indicated for those suffering from chronic conditions, weakness, and low energy due to tuberculosis. Women who experience recurrent infections with genital tuberculosis that leads to uterine prolapse, heavy bleeding, and loss of appetite may benefit from this remedy. It

	strengthens the immune system and helps with fatigue, cold intolerance, and emotional instability.
6. Natrum Muriaticum	Natrum Muriaticum is useful when there are **chronic uterine infections** with **painless tubercular lesions**, **irregular menstrual cycles**, and **dryness** in the genital region. This remedy is indicated when the patient experiences **emotional withdrawal**, **grief**, or **depression** due to long-term health issues. It is helpful for **immune system support** and promotes **healing** in tubercular cases of the **reproductive system**.
7. Lycopodium	Lycopodium is beneficial when there is **weakness**, **abdominal bloating**, and **digestive problems** along with **chronic pelvic pain** from genital tuberculosis. It helps with **chronic infections**, **bladder irritability**, and **irregular menstruation**. Lycopodium is often indicated for those with a **history of emotional or mental stress** and **self-doubt**, which may exacerbate physical ailments like **tuberculosis**.
8. Phosphorus	Phosphorus is indicated when there are **chronic infections**, **weakness**, and **emaciation** due to tuberculosis. This remedy is helpful for those with **pulmonary involvement** and **genital TB**, especially when there are **burning sensations** in the genital region. Phosphorus is beneficial for **patients with a tendency to excessive sweating**, **delirium**, and **sensitivity to cold**.
9. Arsencium Album	Arsencium Album is useful for weak, exhausted patients with genital tuberculosis. It is indicated when there is marked emaciation, chronic exhaustion, burning sensations in the pelvis, and sensitivity to cold air. This remedy also helps with diarrhea, frequent urination, and restlessness in tubercular cases. It is beneficial for tubercular abscesses that do not heal easily.
10. Mercurius Solubilis	Mercurius Solubilis is prescribed when there are foul-smelling discharges, inflammation, and swelling in the pelvic area due to genital tuberculosis. It helps with night sweats, excessive salivation, and stinging pains in the genital region. This remedy is effective when tubercular lesions cause ulceration and abscesses and is often helpful in resolving tubercular infections in the uterus and cervix.

Management Strategy

1. **Acute Phase**
   - Remedies targeting active inflammation, abscesses, or discharge.
   - For example: Silicea, Mercurius Solubilis.

2. **Chronic Phase**
   - Focus on constitutional and miasmatic treatment.
   - For example: Tuberculinum, Calcarea Phosphorica, Bacillinum.

3. **Supportive Therapy**
   - Boost immunity and improve general health with remedies like Phosphorus or Arsenicum Album.

4. **Infertility Management**
   - Remedies to address scarring, adhesions, and hormonal imbalances.
   - For example: Sepia, Pulsatilla, Kali Carbonicum.

5. **Adjunct Measures**
   - Encourage proper nutrition with iron, vitamins, and a high-protein diet.
   - Promote rest, hygiene, and stress management.

Role of Miasmatic Treatment

- **Tubercular Miasm**: Most cases of GTB require remedies that address tubercular miasm (e.g., *Tuberculinum* or *Bacillinum*).
- **Other Miasms**: In cases with secondary complications (e.g., syphilitic scarring), additional remedies may be chosen.

Harmone Replacement Thearapy...

Hormone replacement therapy (HRT) is a treatment that can help ease some of the symptoms associated with menopause—the point in time when a person's menstrual cycle has stopped for 12 straight months and permanently ends.

During the transition into menopause, the body gradually makes less of the hormones.estrogen and progesterone, causing bothersome symptoms like night sweats, hot flashes, and vaginal dryness.

Risks may include an increased chance of developing serious conditions like breast cancer and heart disease in certain people.

Types of Hormone Replacement Therapy-

Hormone replacement therapy is made with either one or two types of hormones:
- **Estrogen only**, which helps reduce night sweats, hot flashes, vaginal dryness, and urinary discomfort, in addition to bone loss that's associated with aging, and is recommended for people who have had their uterus removed (hysterectomy)
- **Estrogen with added progesterone**, which helps protect against the risk of endometrial cancer in people who still have a uterus

Systemic Hormone Therapy-

Systemic therapies allow the hormones—whether estrogen alone or with added progesterone—to circulate throughout the body via the bloodstream. This method impacts the vasomotor symptoms (night sweats and hot flashes) of menopause.

Systemic HRT is provided in the following ways:
- **Pill formulas** that are taken orally (by mouth)
- **Topical formulas** that absorb through the skin via a patch, gel, or spray
- Transdermal implants.
- **Vaginal rings** that are inserted into the vagina every few months 5

Low-Dose Vaginal Products-

Low-dose vaginal therapies release smaller amounts of hormones to the affected area through placement into the vagina.

Because they work locally instead of systemically, these products are typically used to just treat menopause symptoms that affect the vagina or urinary tract, such as vaginal dryness. They do this by helping to thicken vaginal tissues and boost moisture.

Low-dose HRT is available in the form of a vaginal cream, ring, or tablet. They most often contain estrogen alone.

Advantages of HRT-

For many healthy adults who are experiencing moderate or severe menopausal symptoms, there are benefits to using hormone replacement therapy that may override potential risks of this treatment.

Medical experts note that the benefits of HRT can include:
- Relief from moderate to severe hot flashes
- Relief from vaginal dryness and discomfort
- Prevention of bone loss (osteoporosis) and bone fractures
- Protection against colorectal cancer

Risks of Hormone Replacement Therapy-

— higher risk of breast cancer,

— heart disease

— stroke,

— blood clots,

— urinary incontinence,

— gallbladder disease,

— dementia.

Risks may be more likely in people who

- Begin HRT at age 60 or older
- Begin HRT more than 10 years after the start of menopause
- Have a personal or family history of conditions like cancer and heart disease
- Taking harmones for more than 5 yrs

Hormone replacement therapy is not recommended for people who:

- May be pregnant
- Have issues with abnormal vaginal bleeding
- Have a family or personal history of breast cancer
- Have a personal history of heart disease, stroke, blood clots, or liver disease
- Have a family history of gallbladder disease
- Are allergic to estrogen or progesterone

Adverse effects-
- Irregular bleeding or spotting
- Breast tenderness
- Headaches
- Bloating
- Nausea and vomiting
- Hair loss
- Vaginal yeast infection

Hysterectomy

Defination-

A hysterectomy is a surgical procedure that completely or partially removes a person's uterus. The uterus, also known as the womb, is where a fetus grows during pregnancy. The uterine lining also produces menstrual blood.

A person who has a hysterectomy will no longer have menstrual periods or become pregnant.

TYPES According To Parts Removed-

- **Partial (supracervical) hysterectomy:** During a partial hysterectomy, a surgeon only removes the upper portion of the uterus.
- **Total hysterectomy:** Surgeons use this procedure to remove both the uterus and cervix.
- **Radical hysterectomy:** During this procedure, a surgeon removes the womb, cervix, and upper part of the vagina. They may also remove the ovaries, fallopian tubes, and surrounding lymph nodes.
- **Total hysterectomy with bilateral salpingo-oophorectomy:** This type involves the removal of one or both of a person's ovaries and fallopian tubes. A surgeon can perform a salpingo-oophorectomy during a hysterectomy.

TYPES According To Route Of Surgery-

- **Vaginal hysterectomy:** This method involves removing the uterus through the vagina, which does not require any external incisions and leaves no visible scarring. The American College of Obstetricians and Gynecologists recommend vaginal hysterectomies whenever possible.
- **Abdominal hysterectomy:** A surgeon removes the uterus through a small incision below the bellybutton. This type of hysterectomy has a longer recovery periodTrusted Source than a vaginal hysterectomy.
- **Laparoscopic-assisted hysterectomy:** A surgeon inserts an instrument called a laparoscope (a long, thin tube with a light and high resolution camera on the end) through a small incision in the bellybutton. Once they locate the uterus with the laparoscope, they will cut it into small pieces, which they will remove through two or three additional incisions in the abdomen.

Type-Wise Detailed Indications for Hysterectomy.

1. Total Hysterectomy (Removal of Uterus and Cervix)

Benign Conditions:
Uterine Fibroids: When symptomatic with heavy bleeding, pain, or pressure.

Adenomyosis: Severe pain and heavy bleeding not responding to other treatments.

Endometriosis: Severe cases causing chronic pelvic pain or organ damage.

Chronic Abnormal Uterine Bleeding: Not responsive to hormonal or other therapies.

Malignant Conditions:

Endometrial Cancer: Early-stage cases.

Cervical Cancer: When confined to the uterus and cervix.

Other Conditions:

Uterine rupture.

Unmanageable postpartum hemorrhage.

2. Subtotal (Supracervical) Hysterectomy (Removal of Uterus, Cervix Intact)

Benign Conditions:

Uterine fibroids, adenomyosis, or abnormal uterine bleeding where cervical preservation is preferred.

When the cervix is healthy, and there's a desire to preserve sexual function or pelvic floor support.

Other Considerations:

Often chosen for younger patients without cervical disease.

3. Radical Hysterectomy (Removal of Uterus, Cervix, Upper Vagina, and Surrounding Tissues)/ Wertheim,s Hysterectomy

Cervical Cancer:

Stage IA2, IB1, or early-stage II.

Endometrial Cancer:

Advanced or recurrent cases.

Vaginal Cancer:

When originating from or invading adjacent tissues.

4. Total Hysterectomy with Bilateral Salpingo-Oophorectomy (Removal of Uterus, Cervix, Ovaries, and Fallopian Tubes)

Ovarian or Fallopian Tube Cancer:

Preventive or therapeutic removal.

Severe Endometriosis:

When ovarian involvement leads to pain or cysts.

BRCA Mutation or High-Risk Patients:

Prophylactic removal to prevent cancer.

Pelvic Inflammatory Disease:

Severe, recurrent cases causing tubo-ovarian abscess.

5. Vaginal Hysterectomy (Removal via Vaginal Approach)

Uterine Prolapse:

When the uterus descends into the vaginal canal.

Pelvic Organ Prolapse:

Includes bladder or rectal prolapse with uterine descent.

Non-Malignant Conditions:

Small fibroids or benign growths.

6. Laparoscopic/Robotic-Assisted Hysterectomy

Minimally Invasive Approach for Any Indication:

Uterine fibroids, adenomyosis, endometriosis, or abnormal bleeding.

Preferred when faster recovery and less postoperative pain are desired.

Early-Stage Cancers:

Endometrial or cervical cancer.

Special Indications Based on Conditions

Obstetric Indications:

Ruptured Uterus: During or after delivery.

Placenta Accreta/Increta/Percreta: Unmanageable bleeding after delivery.

Trauma:

Severe uterine injury due to accidents or surgery.

Pelvic Pain:Severe chronic pain unresponsive to other treatments caused by conditions like fibroids, endometriosis, or adhesions

Contraindications

1. Severe uncontrolled medical conditions (e.g., cardiovascular disease).
2. Active pelvic infection.
3. Desire for future fertility (if alternatives exist).
4. High surgical risk due to obesity or coagulopathy.

Preoperative Care-

- stop taking blood-thinning medication and aspirin a week before the procedure
- avoid smoking a few days before the procedure
- avoid eating and drinking several hours before the procedure
- pack an overnight bag in case a doctor recommends an extended hospital stay
- arrange transportation to and from the hospital
- Counseling on expectations, recovery, and risks.
- Ensure no active infections.
- Anemia correction (if present).
- Fasting 6-8 hours before surgery.
- Before the procedure, people should also inform their doctor if they:

are currently taking any prescription or over-the-counter medications, vitamins, or supplements know or suspect that they are pregnant

have breathing problems, such as asthma or sleep apnea

have an allergy to any medications or anesthetics

Postoperative Care

- Immediate Postoperative:
- Monitor vitals and bleeding.
- Pain management with medications.
- Early ambulation to prevent deep vein thrombosis (DVT).
- Hospital Stay:
- 1-3 days (varies with the type of procedure).
- Recovery:
- Full recovery in 6-8 weeks for abdominal hysterectomy.
- 2-4 weeks for minimally invasive methods.
- Instructions:
- Keep the surgical site clean and dry.
- Report any signs of infection (fever, redness, or foul discharge).
- should avoid the following activities for 4–6 weeks after surgery:
- lifting heavy objects
- pushing or pulling objects
- swimming
- using tampons
- douching
- sexual intercourse

Complications-

Immediate complications-

- pain
- scarring
- vaginal bleeding or spotting
- constipation
- difficulty urinating
- digestive issues
- damage to blood vessels, nerves, or surrounding organs
- delayed healing
- localised haematomas

Remote complicatons-

- following symptoms of menopauseTrusted Source if they undergo the removal of their ovaries:

hot flashes, vaginal dryness, changes in libido, difficulty sleeping

mood changes ,symptoms of depression or anxiety

- Fistula [VVF/RVF]
- Vault prolapse
- Vaginal prolapse
- Urine incontinence
- Chronic pains at suture site
- Chronic backache
- Infertility

Type Of Anaesthetia-

Preferable is Spinal /Epidural

In contraindicated conditions for spinal, general anaesthetia

In vaginal hysterectomy additional local anesthetia sos

Comparison of Anesthesia Types

Anesthesia Type	Advantages	Disadvantages
General Anesthesia	Complete unconsciousness, muscle relaxation, and control of airway.	Longer recovery, risk of nausea/vomiting, and potential respiratory depression.
Spinal Anesthesia	Better postoperative pain control, faster recovery, and fewer systemic risks.	Risk of hypotension, spinal headache, or incomplete block.
Epidural Anesthesia	Adjustable dose, longer duration of anesthesia, and less systemic impact.	Slower onset, potential for incomplete anesthesia, and catheter-related risks.
Local Anesthesia + Sedation	Minimally invasive, minimal systemic effects, and faster discharge.	Limited to minor surgeries or highly selected cases.

Special Considerations

- Patient Factors:
  o Cardiac, pulmonary, or metabolic conditions may favor regional anesthesia to avoid the risks of GA.
- Surgical Complexity:
  o Extensive surgeries (e.g., radical hysterectomy) require GA.
  - Surgeon's Preference:
  o Some surgeons prefer GA for better control during laparoscopic and robotic-assisted procedures.
- Patient Preference:
  o Patients may choose based on their comfort with being conscious during the surgery.

Comparitive Points-

Factor	Abdominal Hysterectomy (AH)	Vaginal Hysterectomy (VH)
Surgical Approach	Incision in the abdomen	Through the vagina
Anesthesia	General	General/spinal/epidural
Duration	2–3 hours	1–2 hours
Recovery	6–8 weeks	2–4 weeks
Postoperative Pain	Higher due to abdominal incision	Lower since no external incision
Scarring	Visible abdominal scar	No external scars
Hospital Stay	4–7 days	1–3 days
Complications	Higher risk of wound infection and hernia	Lower, but vaginal cuff issues possible
Bleeding	More intraoperative blood loss	Less blood loss
Suitability for Obesity	More challenging	Better option for obese patients
Costs	Higher due to extended hospital stay	Lower costs
Intra-abdominal Visibility	Better visibility for associated conditions	Limited visibility
Pelvic Adhesions	Easier to manage severe adhesions	Challenging if adhesions are extensive

Factor	Abdominal Hysterectomy (AH)	Vaginal Hysterectomy (VH)
Surgeon Expertise	General surgical skills	Requires specific expertise in vaginal surgery
Risk of Organ Injury	Higher (e.g., bowel or bladder injury)	Lower but still possible
Indications	Used for large fibroids, cancer, or adhesions	Used for prolapse, small fibroids, or accessible uterus
Operative Field Access	Allows better access to ovaries and tubes	Limited access to upper abdominal organs
Uterine Size	Suitable for large uterus	Best for smaller uterus
Risk of Postoperative Hernia	Higher due to abdominal incision	Minimal risk
Cosmetic Results	Visible scar on the abdomen	No visible scars
Postoperative Recovery Activities	Delayed, with restrictions on lifting for weeks	Quicker return to activities
Risk of Adhesion Formation	Higher due to abdominal entry	Lower risk
Associated Surgeries	Easier to combine with other abdominal procedures (e.g., appendectomy)	Limited compatibility
Future Pelvic Stability	May weaken abdominal wall	May preserve pelvic floor stability
Position During Surgery	Supine (lying on the back)	Lithotomy (legs in stirrups)

Factor	Open Abdominal Hysterectomy (AH)	Laparoscopic Hysterectomy (LH)
Surgical Approach	Large incision in the abdominal wall	Small keyhole incisions with laparoscopic tools
Incision Type	Horizontal or vertical incision (6–8 inches long)	Multiple small incisions (0.5–1 cm each)
Anesthesia	General anesthesia	General anesthesia

Factor	Open Abdominal Hysterectomy (AH)	Laparoscopic Hysterectomy (LH)
Surgical Duration	2–3 hours	1.5–2 hours
Recovery Time	6–8 weeks	2–4 weeks
Hospital Stay	Longer (4–7 days)	Shorter (1–2 days)
Postoperative Pain	More pain due to large incision	Less pain due to smaller incisions
Scarring	Visible, larger scar on the abdomen	Minimal scars, often cosmetically better
Bleeding	More blood loss during surgery	Less blood loss
Risk of Infection	Higher due to larger wound and exposure	Lower due to minimally invasive technique
Complications	Higher risk of wound dehiscence or hernia	Lower overall risk of wound-related issues
Cosmetic Outcome	Larger scar	Minimal visible scarring
Recovery Activities	Limited mobility and restrictions on lifting	Faster return to daily activities
Suitability for Complex Cases	Better for large fibroids, malignancies, or severe adhesions	Less suitable for extremely large uterus or complex pelvic conditions
Visibility of Surgical Field	Direct visualization	Relies on camera and laparoscopic view
Risk of Adhesions	Higher risk of postoperative adhesions	Lower risk due to reduced tissue handling
Cost	Typically lower (equipment costs are less)	Higher due to specialized equipment and expertise
Postoperative Hernia Risk	Higher risk due to large abdominal incision	Minimal risk
Learning Curve for Surgeons	Straightforward, well-established	Requires advanced laparoscopic expertise
Indications	Preferred for complex or large cases	Suitable for smaller uterus and routine hysterectomies

Factor	Open Abdominal Hysterectomy (AH)	Laparoscopic Hysterectomy (LH)
Blood Loss Management	May require transfusion in some cases	Less need for transfusion
Patient Comfort	More discomfort due to larger incision	Less discomfort and faster recovery
Hospital Stay Cost	Higher due to longer recovery	Lower due to early discharge
Pelvic Floor Impact	May weaken the abdominal wall	Minimally affects pelvic floor stability
Associated Procedures	Easier to combine with other open surgeries (e.g., bowel resection)	Suitable for certain minimally invasive procedures (e.g., oophorectomy)

Homoeopathic Management-

Homeopathic Remedies for Supportive Care

1. **Pre-Surgery Support:**
   - **Arnica montana**: To reduce surgical shock and bleeding.

2. **Post-Surgery Recovery:**
   - **Staphysagria**: For pain and healing of incisions.
   - **Calendula officinalis**: To promote wound healing and prevent infection.
   - **Bellis perennis**: For deep abdominal tissue healing.

3. **Emotional Support:**
   - **Ignatia amara**: For grief or emotional disturbances related to hysterectomy.
   - **Sepia officinalis**: For hormonal imbalance and associated mood changes.

4. **Chronic Pain or Fatigue:**
   - Hypericum perforatum: For nerve pain.
   - **Phosphoric acid**: For post-surgical fatigue and weakness.

Infertility

DEFINATION :- Infertility or Sterility means inability to conceive after 1 year of sexual life without use of any contraception.
Infertility - Failure to conceive
Sterility' :- Absolute state of inability to conceive.

TYPES :-

I] Primary :- Conception never occurs.
II] Secondary :- Conception has failed to occur after a period of fertility, that means there is h/o previous conception.

AETIOLOGY :-

1] Physiological - Before puberty
- During pregnancy
- After menopause
- Sometimes during lactation

2] Pathological - Faulty male factors
- Faulty female factors.
- Combined effect of both.

The causes behind them will be —
- Systemic
- Immunological
- Psychological
- Coitus difficulty
- Endocrinal
- Genital defects

Male Infertility :

Systemic causes :
- Age above 45 yrs
- Alcoholism
- Constant heat exposure
- Obesity
- Fatiqué
- Diabetes.

Psychological causes:
-Nervousness about sex
-Depression
-Fatigue

Endocrinopathy : -
-Hypothyroidism
-Pituitary dysfunction
-Diabetes

Immunological :
-Orchitis, vas.deferance obstruction, Heavy smoking,
fall on testis, may cause autoimmuno antibodies formation
against own sperms.

Coitus Difficulty :
-Fear
-Too few of many frequent sexual intercourse.
-Painful coitus e.g; in phimosis & hydrocele.

Genital Defects :
-Intersex
-Klinefelter's Syndrome
-Undescended' testes
-Hypogenidism
-Testicular damage after small pox, mumps, varicocele, hydrocele,
-Increased scrotal temp.
-Postoperative or post illness [monococccal, tubercular, mycoplasma inf]

FEMALE INFERTILITY-

Systemic Causes –
-Age > 35 yrs.
-Obesity
-Severe anaemia
-Diabetes
-Recurrent urinary tract infections
-TORCH infections

Psychological –
-Fear of sex
-Marital dyshormoney..

-Vaginismus.

Endocrinal :

-Thyroid disorders

-Hypogonadism

-Meteoropathic bleeding

-POOD

Immunological factors -

-Accumulated autoantibodies in. cervical mucus against speams .

-ABO incompatibility

Genital factors :

-Cervix –

-Estrogen, Thick cervical mucus,

- Cervicitis after pyogenic, tubercular, gonococcal infection

Ca Cervix

- Polyp

-Vaginal :-

-Narrow vag.introitus

-Vaginismus

-Vaginitis

-Vaginal introitus or stenosis

-Escape of semen ofter coitus [Flour seminitis]

Uterine

-Fibromyoma

-Fibromyosis

-Uterine hypoplasia

-Tubercular endometritis

-Endometriosis

Tubal :-

 -Long tubes

 - Tubal adhesion

 - Pyogenic, gonococcal, tuberculous   Salpingitis.

- Ovarian :-

-Anovulatory cycles in responds to

-Hyperprolactinaemia,

-Hypothyroidism

Investigations :

When to do
Women age < 25 yrs, infertile even after 2 yrs.
  Women age ~ 25-35 yrs ,after 1 yr.
  Women age > 35 yas after 6 mts of infertility

Seven Steps Of Investigations :-
Step 1 :- Clinical Evaluation of Both life Partners
Step 2 :- Semen Analysis of Husband
Step 3 :- Dilatation and Curettage [THEURAPEUTIC D AND C]
Step 4 :- Tubal patency test or HSG [Hystosalphingography]
Step 5 :- Ovulation Tests
Step 6 :- Test for cervical factors.
Step 7 :- Laparoscopy:
Step 7b :- Chromosomal analysis of both partners.

STEP I : EVALUATION OF BOTH PARTNERS

Evaluation of wife;-
-H/O irregular menses,PAINLESS SCANTY MENSES.
- H/o leucorrhoea
-Marital dyshormony
-Abortion
- Difficulties in sexual intercourse
-Systemic diseases
-Genital checkup.
-Chronic Use of contraceptive pills or any medicine.
-Stressfull occupation
-Family history of infertility and menopause,premature ovarian
-Failure
-Uterine or ovarian history

GENERAL EXAMINATION-
-S/O PCOD
-Obesity
-p/v exam, vaginal infections,transverse septum,elongated vagina

Evaluation of Husband :-
-HIO Sexual dysfunction
-Dietary habits
-Addiction..

-Systemic diseases
-Coitus frequency
-Genital checkup.
-Heat exposue,
-Radiation exposue
-Tight wearing of cloths.
-Prematuare ejaculation.
 GENERAL EXAM- look for
-Hypospadiasis
-small gonads
-varicocele

II] SEMEN ANALYSIS:- SEMINOGRAM / SPERMIOGRAM

-Should done after 3 days of sexual abstinence.
-After 2hrs. Of collection of liquefaction.
-Diagnosis for Aspermia [unability to produce semen],
-Azoospermia [total absence of sperms in semen],
-Oligospermia [sperm concentration below 20million/ml of semen],
-Teratospermia [increased percentage of abnormal morphology of sperms with defective head, neck or tail]
-Asthenospermia [less than 40% motility of sperms]
-Asthenozoospermia [100% immotile sperms]
-Hypospermia [low semen volume <1ml]
-Hyperspermia [high sperm volume >5ml]
-Leucospermia [leucocytes more than 1lakh/ml]
-Hyperviscous semen [homogenous semen with persistant viscocity which will not change by time]
-Hypoviscous semen [semen without homogenous consistency

SEMEN ANALYSIS

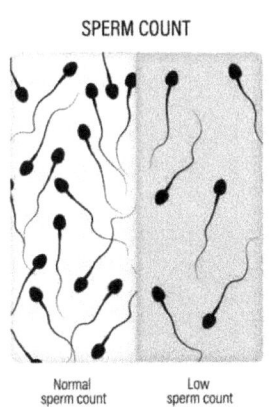
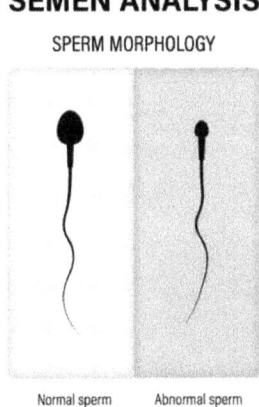
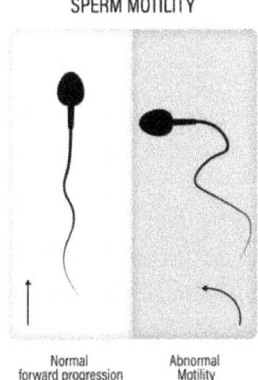

NORMAL SPERM COUNT:
@ Per ejaculation: 40 millions or more
Per ml : 20 millions/ml
Lowest normal count: 15 millions/ml

III] DILATATION AND CURRATAGE:[20%]

If pregnancy fails to occur within 6 months after treating the causes in 1st two investigations ,call for diagnostic/ theuraputic D& C.

-It should be done in secretory phase of menses that is around 22nd day of menstrual cycle. The collected endometrium then sended for histopathological studies.

-It gives diagnosis of infertility causes regarding endometrium.e.g; endometrial hypoplasia,hyperplasia,tuberculosis,abnormal or poor secretory functions of endometrium,harmomal deficiencies,endometritis,pyometritis.

-Endometrial tuberculosis is the commonest uterine cause for infertility.

IV] TUBAL PATENCY TEST- [30%]

-Six months after D & C if pregnancy not occurs.

-Within a week following end of menses

-Helpful in diagnosis of site of block,

-TB salpingitis

-Mycoplasma,Clamedial,Gonococcal infections are the most common causes for obstructive salphingitis.

-congenital anomelies of uterus and follipian tubes like septed uterus,unicorniated uterus,long tubes,tortuous tubes,narrowing of tubal lumen,etc.

It is a lab procedure where the radio opaque die get injected in uterus through a vaginal probe ,allow it to spread spontaneously and then xrays are taken at regular intervals.

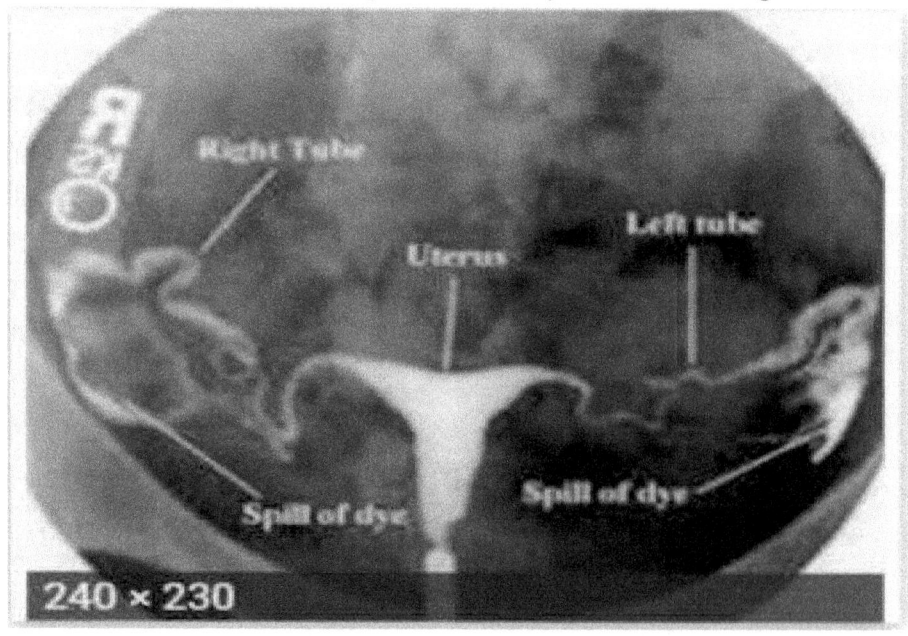

V] OVULATION TEST – [40 %]

-6 months after HSG

BBT - Mouth femp. de corded in 3-4 cycles

Sudden drop of temp. by 0 5° F on day of Ovulation followed by sustained rise of 1 degree F temp.

In anovulatory cycles, no RISE IN BODY TEMP. is seen.

CYCLIC USG, from 10th day of menses to observe follicular growth ,ovulation pattern and endometrial development of individual.

-Follicular growth to 18- 25 mm & rupture follicle with coprpus luteal production is seen.

-No growth ,or no rupture but only cyst formation will show ovuln failure !

-it also gaves d diagnosis of anovulatory cycles,follicular growth failures,endometrial hyperplasia, PCOD.

-corpus luteum insufficiency causing deficient progesterone which is important for maintainance of pregnancy.

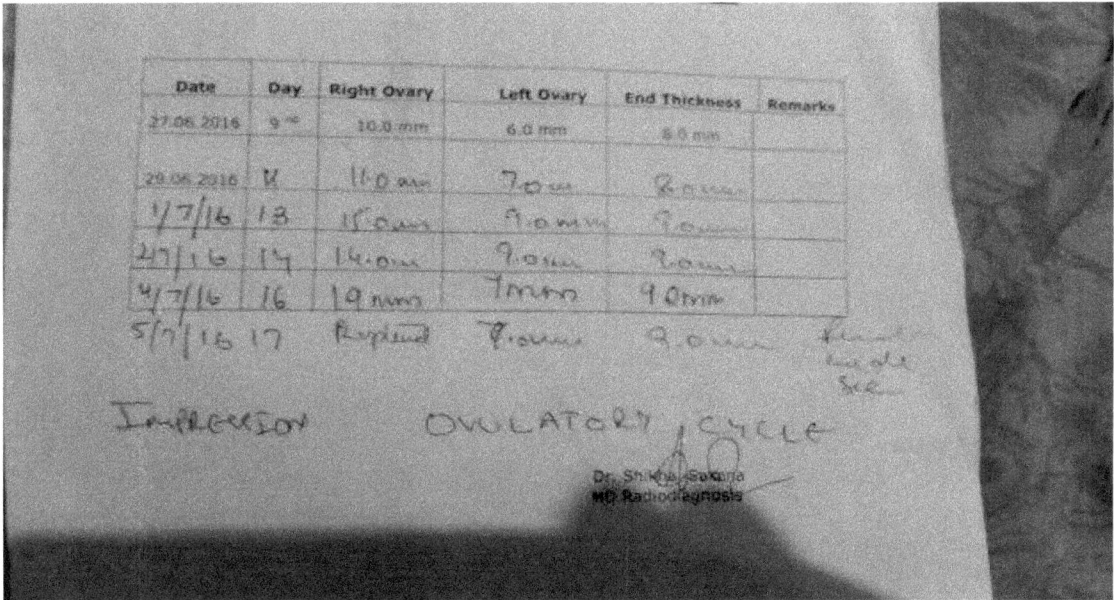

-Poor follicular growth indicates FSH deficiency.

-Cystic formation without ovulation shows LH deficiency.

-Poor endometrial growth which must be more than 7mm at secretary phase,will indicates endometrial hypoplasia with aestrogen and progesterone deficiency.

-multiple small follicles at single menstrual cycle will indicate PCOD.

-Another signs and symptoms in PCOD are,

-SECONDARY AMENNORRHEA

-Obesity with moon face or oedematous face.

-ACANTHOSIS NIGRICANS; is a skin disorder with velvety,light brown or blackish pigmentation over nape of nake,armpits,groins and under breast due to insulin intorence with raised level of insulin and hyperglycemia.

-Hirsutism; due to increased testesteron level leading to abnormal ,excessive facial hear growth.

-PIMPLES;due to increased secretary functions of sebascious glands.

Relative levels of AMH-ANTI MULLERIAN HARMONE ,rules out various ovarian causes of infertility.

-normal level of AMH -1.5 TO 5

-Less than normal level indicates PREMATURE OVARIAN FAILURE,i.e, ovary is unable to produce follicles before the age.

-Higher than normal AMH indicates PCOD.

- Management with deficient harmones will correct the faulty ovulation.
- Inj.HMG is resenmbance with FSH ,so advice for follicular growth,started fronm 2nd day sos with 75mg dose…may required to150 mg dose.
- Inj. HCG,resemblance like LH ,ADVICABLE IN 2000IU/5000IU/10000IU for induction of ovulation.
- In endometrial hypoplasia implantation of fertilized ovum occurs,to overcome it progesterone pills required.
- Tab. Glyciphase 500 mg is the management for PCOD induced hyperglycemia.
- Another advice is dietory manangement and exrcises to overcome Obesity.

IV] CERVICAL FACTOR TEST OR Fern test : [10%]

-Palm leaf like appearance of Cx mucus on slide after doying due to oestrogen effect.

-It starts on 5th to 0th day, completely absent by . 22nd day of cycle.

 -Max. 24-48 hours before ovulation

-Presence of fearning by 22nd day of cycle indicates anovulatory cycles

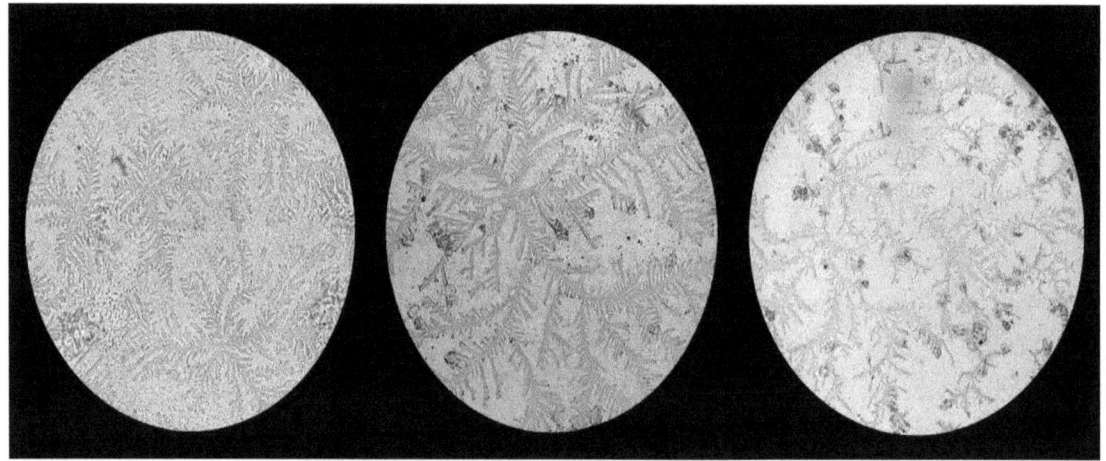

MULLER,S TEST /PCT TEST i.e, postcoital test-
-It is an outdated test for autoantibodies detection in cervivcal mucus.
-semen sample from vagina get collected after 36hrs of sexual intercourse
And tested for active sperms.
-If less than 10% active sperms exists in sample it denotes autoantibodies presence .

VII] LAPAROSCOPIC DYE TEST-

-If all above steps results NORMAL
-HSG have any abnormal findings.
Preparation -
1st 10 days sexual abstinence .
-Daily or alternate intercourse on 11th to 18 day of next month menstrual cycle. ie; around ovulation period
-Avoid exertion, stress following 20th day to
avoid hormonal imbalance.
It is always associated with therapeutic as well as diagnostic laparoscopy,find the cause and treat it.
Mostly done with hysteroscopy
Laparoscopic dye test rule out tubal patency,blockages,site of blockages.
Hysteroscopy will rule out congenital uterine and tubal anomelies like septed uterus,uni or bicornuated uterus,long tubes, fibroids, ASHERMAN,S SYNDROME.

MANAGEMENT :-
-**Treat The cause**

FEMALE INFERTILITY

-**If systemic causes : -**
> DIET AND EXERCISE
-modification plan in obesity.
-Reduction of wt.
-Early *diagno*sis and treatment of sy*s*temic diseas*es.*e.g, Hypertension, Diabetes , hyperlipidemia.
 -Control over smoking, alcoholism and stress .

- **If psychological causes :**
- Pooper sexual education.
- Removal of fear.
 - *Anti*depressan*t* & consol" therap*y*
 - Advice' for outdoor holidays.
- yoga, pranaym, meditation for mentle relaxation and to come over mentle stress.

-If Endocrinal causes:-

Hormonal investigates & corresponding treatment

-Diabetes control

- *Hormonal therapy* for menstrual regularization.

In Genital defects /Obstructions:-

-*Medicinal* & Surgical management to relieve *the obstuctions* e.g, *TB*, *Undes*cended testis

Hydrocele,

-vaginal or cervical *stenosis* - D&C.

* Medical Treatment –

If Anovulation Or Oligoovul" :

-Clomiphene citrate or resemblance medicinal thereapy for artificial follicular development and ovulation induction.

e.g; Tab. Clofert/ Rejun / Fertyl super 50 or 100mg-3rd day onward of M.C for further 5 days.

-Vit E 400 mg H S x mt

–inj. Hmg - In FSH deficiency, 75 or 150mg /day from 7th day sos.

-HCG - For' ovulation 2000/5000 /10000 units

-Corticosteroid therapy in resistant cases.

-Bromocreptin in hyperprolactenamia.

-Antibiotics,AKT,antiviral therapy IN INFECTIVE CAUSES.

-Clomifene citrate hyperstimulates ovaries so avoid in pcod.

-Another drug in management is, LETROVAL

2.5 OR 5 mg …fronm 2nd day to 6th day of m.c.

-Surgical Treatment :

- Widening of vagined introitius

For relieve tight hymenal ring , Vaginismus .

-Correction of Retroversion -To avoid recurrent abortions

-Myomectomy ,If presence of submucous fibromyoma

-D and C followed by Cu T insertion for 3 months,if Asherman's syndrome..

-Metroplasty : in congenital uterine anomelies like double , arcuate or septed uterus .

-Tuboplasty : To remove the tubal block ,adhesions,post tubectomy.

-Neosalphingostomy,in reversal of posttubectomy.

-Cervical ligation :

-To avoid midterm abortion,in cervical incompetence

-Conservative surgery in Pelvic endometriosis

MALE INFERTILITY

Impotency & Frigidity –

-Alternate day coitus advice to improve desire:

-loving care of wife should improve

-Nervousness, Tecnique of sexual act educated.

-Klinefeltes's Syndrome : Oral testesteron

-Hypothalamic- Pituitary dysfunction – Hormonal assay followed by corresponding supportive therapy.

-Diabetes mellitus – EaRly detection N management.

-Antidepressants ,anti hypertensives to tranquillars.

-Harmonal management with FSH, to increase sperm production, LH increases testesteron production.

-Scrotal USG done transrectal to conclude blockages in vas deference or epididymis.

IUI [INTRAUTEINE INSEMINATION];-

-AIH [ARTIFICIAL INSEMINATION OF HUSBAND]

When HUSBAND"S sperm count is normal but have erectiile dysfunction, or in oligospermia, semen sample is collected in lab,chemical wash given to separate out dead, poor quality sperms, only good, progressive sperms get collected in syring which gets inserted in wifes uterus through vagina on d day ovulation.

-Surgical treatment for obstructive azoospermia

-AID:- [Artificial Insemination of DONOR]:

If husband is totally sterile or azospermic, donar having same blood group of husband is selected and donors semen sample is used for IUI.

Single IUI:

-When follicle size reaches to 18 to 20 mm size.

-Preovulatary

Double IUI:

Twice IUI in single cycle

1st IUI 12 hrs before ovulation

2nd IUI 36 hrs. later 1st IUI

- IN OBSTRUCTIVE AZOSPERMIA SOME OTHER SPERM RETRIEVAL PROCEDURES are required to collect the sperms rather than ejaculation.
- Other sites of collection are vas deference ,epididymis,testis
- MESA:MICROSERGICAL EPIDIDYMAL SPERM ASPIRATION
- dissection of epididymis and collection of sample from tubules.
- PESA:PERCUTANEOUS EPIDIDYMAL SPERM ASPIRATION.
- TESE: TESTICULAR SPERM EXTRACTION

— TESA: TESTICULAR SPERM ASPIRATION

— Intracytoplasmic sperm injections

-GIFT - Gamete Intra fallipian Transfer. Also called as IVF-InVitroFertilization or TESTTUBE BABY.

Here the artificially ripen follicles of wife and lab collected sperms of husband met together under microscope in lab,allow them to develop in embryo in lab itself and then pushed inside the uterus and allowed to implant.

When natural conception is impossible it is adviced.

-ZIFT: Zygote intrafollipian transfer,fertized egg allow to develop in zygote in lab,and then transfer inside the uterus via vagina for further development.

SURROGATE MOTHERSHIP:-

When wife have good follicles to fertilise but anable to grow the faetus inside her womb, IVF followed by implantation of embryo in other womens uterus until delivery is allowed,is called surrogate mothership.

Adoption :- when no other choice remain

HSG

Semen analysis

D & C

HYSTEROSCOPY

DIAGNOSTIC LAPAROSCOPY WITH OVARIAN DRILLING IN PCOD

IUI

IVF in hindi

SPERM RETRIEVAL PROCEDIURES

PCOD

S/O OVULATION

Leucorrhea

Definition:
- **Leucorrhea** refers to the **abnormal vaginal discharge**, typically **white or yellowish**, which may vary in consistency (thin, watery, or thick) and is often a symptom of an underlying gynecological condition.
- It is important to differentiate **physiological leucorrhea** (which is a normal, natural discharge) from **pathological leucorrhea** (which is associated with diseases or infections).

Aetiology (Causes):
The causes of leucorrhea can be broadly classified into **physiological** and **pathological**.

1. **Physiological Causes:**
   - **Hormonal changes**: Leucorrhea can be caused by **increased estrogen levels** during different stages of the menstrual cycle, especially during ovulation, pregnancy, or puberty.
   - **Pregnancy**: During pregnancy, there is an increase in **cervical mucus** due to hormonal changes.
   - **Ovulation**: In the middle of the menstrual cycle (around ovulation), the cervix produces more mucus to facilitate the passage of sperm, leading to a clear or white discharge.
   - **Post-menstrual phase**: After menstruation, a slight increase in vaginal discharge may occur as the body prepares for ovulation.

2. **Pathological Causes:**
   - Infections:
     - **Bacterial vaginosis (BV)**: An imbalance of normal vaginal flora, leading to a thin, milky, or gray discharge with a foul odor.
     - **Candidiasis (yeast infection)**: Characterized by thick, white, cottage cheese-like discharge, usually with itching and irritation.
     - **Trichomoniasis**: A parasitic infection that leads to greenish or frothy discharge, often with a strong odor.
     - **Sexually transmitted infections (STIs)**: Such as **gonorrhea** and **chlamydia**, both of which may lead to yellowish or greenish discharge.
   - **Cervicitis**: Inflammation of the cervix due to infections, trauma, or irritation.
   - **Pelvic inflammatory disease (PID)**: Infections of the upper reproductive tract, such as **salpingitis** (inflammation of the fallopian tubes), which can lead to purulent discharge.

- **Tumors**: Benign or malignant tumors of the uterus or cervix may lead to abnormal vaginal discharge.
- **Foreign body**: Presence of a foreign body such as a retained tampon or contraceptive device can cause vaginal discharge.
- **Diabetes**: Uncontrolled diabetes can predispose women to yeast infections, leading to thick, white discharge.

3. **Other Causes:**
   - **Allergic reactions**: Irritation or allergic response to soaps, perfumes, douches, or other chemicals.
   - **Menopause**: Atrophic vaginitis or thinning of the vaginal walls due to reduced estrogen production in post-menopausal women can cause vaginal dryness and increased discharge.
   - **Poor hygiene**: Poor genital hygiene or the use of tight clothing may alter the pH of the vagina and promote infections.

Types of Leucorrhea:

Leucorrhea is classified based on its **color, consistency**, and **associated symptoms**:

1. **Physiological Leucorrhea:**
   - Typically **clear to milky** in appearance.
   - **Non-irritating**, without associated symptoms like itching or pain.
   - Occurs in **normal conditions** such as pregnancy, puberty, menstruation, and ovulation.

2. **Pathological Leucorrhea:**
   - **Yellowish/greenish** discharge, often with a foul odor, indicating infection (e.g., bacterial vaginosis, gonorrhea, trichomoniasis).
   - **Thick and cheesy** discharge, which is characteristic of **candidiasis**.
   - Watery discharge may indicate a viral infection, such as human papillomavirus (HPV) or herpes simplex virus (HSV).
   - **Purulent** discharge can be associated with **pelvic inflammatory disease (PID)** or cervical infection.

Clinical Features:

The clinical presentation of leucorrhea depends on its underlying cause:

1. **Physiological Features:**
   - **Clear to milky discharge** that may increase at certain times of the menstrual cycle (such as during ovulation or pregnancy).
   - **Non-irritating**, without itching, burning, or redness.

2. **Pathological Features:**
   - **Itching**: Vaginal or vulvar itching is common with **fungal infections** (e.g., candidiasis) or **trichomoniasis**.
   - Burning sensation: Especially when urinating, which is common in urinary tract infections (UTIs) or gonorrhea.
   - **Odor**: Foul-smelling discharge, especially with bacterial infections such as **bacterial vaginosis**.
   - **Abdominal pain or discomfort**: Pain during intercourse or lower abdominal pain could indicate underlying conditions like **PID** or **cervicitis**.
   - Bleeding or spotting: Associated with cervical cancer, polycystic ovary syndrome (PCOS), or cervical polyps.
   - **Painful intercourse (dyspareunia)**: Often observed in infections or inflammatory conditions.

Complications of Leucorrhea:

If left untreated, leucorrhea may lead to several complications:
- **Chronic infection**: Persistent infections such as **candidiasis** or **trichomoniasis** can cause recurrent symptoms.
- **Pelvic inflammatory disease (PID)**: Untreated infections, such as those caused by **gonorrhea** or **chlamydia**, can ascend to the uterus, fallopian tubes, and ovaries, leading to PID, which may result in infertility.
- **Cervical cancer**: Abnormal discharge associated with **cervical cancer** can progress to more severe stages if not diagnosed and treated early.
- **Infertility**: Recurrent infections that cause inflammation or scarring in the reproductive organs can lead to difficulties in conceiving.
- **Sepsis**: In rare cases, untreated infections in the reproductive organs can lead to systemic infections or sepsis.

Diagnosis of Leucorrhea:

The diagnosis of leucorrhea involves a **comprehensive assessment**, including a detailed **history, physical examination**, and relevant **laboratory investigations**.

1. **History:**
   - Onset, **duration**, and **characteristics** (color, consistency, odor) of the discharge.
   - Associated symptoms such as **pain, itching, bleeding**, or **odor**.
   - **Menstrual history**, sexual activity, use of contraceptives, and any history of **STIs**.

2. **Physical Examination:**
   - **Pelvic examination** to assess the **vagina, cervix, vulva**, and **uterus** for signs of infection, inflammation, or tumors.

- **Speculum examination** to obtain a sample of the discharge for microscopic analysis.

3. **Laboratory Investigations:**
   - **Microscopic examination** of the vaginal discharge to identify the presence of **bacteria**, **yeast**, or **trichomonads**.
   - Culture to isolate specific pathogens (e.g., gonorrhea, chlamydia, group B streptococcus).
   - Pap smear to screen for cervical cancer and precancerous lesions.
   - **Urine culture** if urinary tract infection is suspected.
   - **Ultrasound** or **CT scan** to evaluate for underlying structural causes, such as **fibroids**, **ovarian cysts**, or **pelvic masses**.

Management of Leucorrhea:

1. **Conservative Management (For Physiological Leucorrhea):**
   - **Maintaining hygiene**: Regular washing of the vaginal area with lukewarm water. Avoid the use of harsh soaps or douches.
   - **Menstrual hygiene**: Regular change of sanitary pads or tampons.
   - **Dietary changes**: Ensure adequate hydration and a balanced diet to prevent infections.

2. **Pharmacological Treatment (For Pathological Leucorrhea):**
   - **Antibiotics** for bacterial infections such as **bacterial vaginosis** or **gonorrhea**.
   - Antifungal treatment for candidiasis, often in the form of oral or topical antifungals (e.g., fluconazole or clotrimazole).
   - Antiprotozoal agents for trichomoniasis, such as metronidazole.
   - Hormonal therapy for conditions such as menopausal atrophic vaginitis or hormonal imbalances (e.g., estrogen therapy).
   - Analgesics for pain relief associated with pelvic inflammatory disease or cervicitis.
   - Surgical treatment for underlying conditions like cervical polyps, fibroids, or cervical cancer.

3. **Lifestyle and Home Remedies:**
   - **Probiotics**: Oral probiotics can help maintain vaginal flora and prevent recurrent infections.
   - **Diet**: Increase intake of **yogurt**, **garlic**, and **vitamin C** to support immune health.
   - **Hydration**: Drinking plenty of water helps flush out toxins and supports vaginal health.

Here is a table summarizing the differentiating points between **Physiological Leucorrhea** and **Pathological Leucorrhea**:

Characteristic	Physiological Leucorrhea	Pathological Leucorrhea
Cause	Normal physiological processes like hormonal changes, menstruation, pregnancy, ovulation, or puberty.	Caused by infections, inflammations, tumors, or other pathological conditions.
Color	White or milky discharge, may appear clear.	Can be yellow, green, thick, cheesy, or even bloody.
Consistency	Thin or slightly thick, non-viscous.	Thick, sticky, or frothy, depending on the cause (e.g., cottage cheese-like with candidiasis).
Odor	No significant odor or a mild, non-offensive odor.	Foul, fishy, or unpleasant odor, depending on the underlying infection (e.g., bacterial vaginosis, trichomoniasis).
Associated Symptoms	No itching, burning, or pain; no other discomfort.	May be associated with itching, burning, pain during urination, abdominal pain, or fever.
Duration	Normal, intermittent, and temporary, fluctuating with the menstrual cycle.	Persistent, lasting for days to weeks, often worsening with time.
Accompanying Conditions	No underlying infection or disease.	Often associated with infections (e.g., bacterial vaginosis, yeast infection, STIs), or other gynecological conditions (e.g., PID, cervical cancer).
Vaginal pH	Normal vaginal pH (4.5 to 5.5).	May show an altered vaginal pH, usually more alkaline (e.g., bacterial vaginosis with pH > 4.5).
Discharge Volume	Mild to moderate, varies with the menstrual cycle (especially around ovulation).	Often excessive or profuse discharge, may require frequent pad changes.
Response to Treatment	No treatment required; resolves naturally.	Requires medical treatment (antibiotics, antifungals, or other appropriate therapies).

Characteristic	Physiological Leucorrhea	Pathological Leucorrhea
Systemic Symptoms	No systemic symptoms; remains localized.	May present with systemic symptoms like fever, fatigue, and general discomfort.

Here's a table comparing **Candidal Vaginitis**, **Trichomonal Vaginitis**, and **Gonorrheal Vaginitis** based on various key characteristics of leucorrhea:

Characteristic	Candidal Vaginitis	Trichomonal Vaginitis	Gonorrheal Vaginitis
Causative Organism	Candida albicans (fungus/yeast)	**Trichomonas vaginalis** (protozoan parasite)	Neisseria gonorrhoeae (bacteria)
Color of Discharge	White, thick, curd-like (cottage cheese appearance)	Yellow-green, frothy, often with a fishy odor	Yellow or green, purulent (pus-like) discharge
Consistency	Thick, clumpy, or cottage cheese-like	Frothy, bubbly, and thin	Watery to purulent, sometimes thick
Odor	Mild or no odor, may have a slight yeast smell	Foul, fishy odor	Strong, foul odor
Itching	Intense itching and irritation, especially around the vulva	Itching, vulvar irritation, and discomfort during urination	May have some irritation or discomfort, but less intense than candidiasis
Associated Symptoms	Redness, swelling, pain during urination and intercourse	Painful urination, burning sensation, discomfort during sex	Painful urination, pelvic pain, vaginal bleeding, lower abdominal pain
Vaginal pH	Acidic, usually < 4.5	Slightly alkaline, around 5 to 6	Alkaline, usually > 4.5
Microscopic Findings	Buds, pseudohyphae of Candida, spores	Motile **trichomonads** (pear-shaped protozoa)	Gram-negative **diplococci** (Neisseria gonorrhoeae)

Characteristic	Candidal Vaginitis	Trichomonal Vaginitis	Gonorrheal Vaginitis
Common Risk Factors	Antibiotic use, diabetes, pregnancy, tight clothing	Multiple sexual partners, lack of condom use, poor hygiene	Unprotected sex, multiple sexual partners, lack of condom use
Diagnosis	Wet mount showing yeast cells or culture on agar	Wet mount showing motile trichomonads, or culture	Gram stain, culture, or nucleic acid amplification test (NAAT)
Treatment	**Antifungal treatment** (e.g., fluconazole, clotrimazole)	Antiprotozoal treatment (e.g., metronidazole)	**Antibiotic treatment** (e.g., ceftriaxone, azithromycin)
Complications	Chronic infections, recurrent episodes, spread to partner	Pelvic inflammatory disease (PID), infertility, increased susceptibility to HIV	Pelvic inflammatory disease (PID), infertility, complications in pregnancy, increased risk of HIV
Sexual Transmission	Not sexually transmitted but may recur with sexual contact	Primarily sexually transmitted	Primarily sexually transmitted

Key Differentiating Points:

- **Candidal Vaginitis** is caused by a **fungal infection** and presents with thick, **white, cottage cheese-like** discharge, accompanied by itching and vulvar redness.
- **Trichomonal Vaginitis** is caused by a **protozoan parasite** and results in frothy, yellow-green discharge, along with a **foul, fishy odor** and **vulvar irritation.**
- Gonorrheal Vaginitis is caused by a bacterial infection and presents with a yellow-green, purulent discharge, often accompanied by painful urination, pelvic pain, and abdominal discomfort.

Homoeopathic Management-

1. **Calcarea Carbonica**
   - Indications:
     - Leucorrhea with thick, milky, white discharge.

- Weakness and profuse perspiration.
- Often indicated in women with low vitality, especially during puberty or menopause.
- Coldness, chilly sensations, and profuse sweating.
- Symptoms may worsen in **warm weather** or after eating.
- Clinical Features:
  - White, creamy or curd-like discharge.
  - May be accompanied by **itching** or **irritation**.
  - Backache or pelvic pain.
  - Tendency to sweat excessively.
- **Management**: This remedy is especially useful in cases where the discharge is thick and white, and when the patient feels **cold** or **chilly**.

2. **Sepia**
   - Indications:
     - Leucorrhea associated with **hormonal changes** (e.g., pregnancy, menopause, or during menstruation).
     - **Greenish-yellow** discharge that is often **watery**, **thin**, or **frothy**.
     - The patient may feel irritable, depressed, and have a disconnected feeling.
     - Symptoms tend to worsen with **mental stress**, **heat**, or **during menstruation**.
   - Clinical Features:
     - Profuse, yellowish, or greenish discharge.
     - Accompanied by vaginal itching, and sometimes offensive odor.
     - Women feel better in the open air and worse with heat or during menstruation.
     - Often accompanied by a feeling of heaviness in the pelvic region.
   - **Management**: Sepia is effective in treating **hormonal** imbalances and is especially useful for **menopausal women** or those with **mood disturbances** due to hormonal fluctuations.

3. **Pulsatilla**
   - Indications:
     - Leucorrhea that is **yellow, thick, or creamy** and may be accompanied by **itching**.
     - Often indicated for women who are **changeable**, **sensitive**, and have a tendency to feel **weepy** or **emotionally unstable**.
     - Leucorrhea may be associated with **irregular periods** or **delayed menstruation**.
   - Clinical Features:
     - Yellowish or creamy discharge, typically thin or watery.

- o The discharge may be more pronounced in the morning and associated with itching or burning sensations.
- o The patient tends to feel better in cool air and may have emotional instability or mood swings.
- o Often worse from heat or in the evening.
- **Management**: Pulsatilla works well for those who have **emotional symptoms** and fluctuating symptoms, particularly for **young women** and those with **irregular cycles**.

4. **Borax**
   - Indications:
     - o Leucorrhea with a **stringy, jelly-like** discharge that is **offensive** and may be **yellow** or **green**.
     - o **Strong, acrid odor** to the discharge.
     - o Often seen in cases of chronic vaginal infections or after childbirth.
     - o Menstrual irregularities, along with itching and burning sensations.
   - Clinical Features:
     - o **Offensive** yellow or green discharge.
     - o The discharge may be **thick** and **sticky**, often with a **stringy** consistency.
     - o **Itching** and **irritation** of the vagina.
     - o The patient may feel **anxious** or **restless**.
   - **Management**: Borax is used when the discharge is **offensive**, **thick**, and **stringy**, particularly in chronic infections.

5. **Natrum Muriaticum**
   - Indications:
     - o Leucorrhea with **thick, white**, sometimes **milky discharge**.
     - o Associated with emotional issues, such as grief or suppressing emotions.
     - o Typically indicated when the patient experiences a **lack of warmth** or **moodiness**, often after emotional stress or **depression**.
     - o The discharge can be worse during **menstruation**.
   - Clinical Features:
     - o Thick, white, or milky discharge.
     - o The patient may have a history of emotional trauma or grief.
     - o Symptoms worsen from warmth and during menstruation.
     - o The patient is usually reserved, withdrawn, and has a tendency to suppress emotions.
   - **Management**: Natrum Muriaticum is useful for treating leucorrhea that is accompanied by **emotional suppression**, especially in women who have had **emotional trauma**.

6. **Thuja Occidentalis**
    - Indications:
        - Leucorrhea with offensive, greenish, or yellowish discharge.
        - Associated with chronic vaginal infections or wart-like growths.
        - Often used in cases of HPV (human papillomavirus) infections or wart formations in the genital area.
        - The discharge can be thick, fetid, and sometimes accompanied by itching or burning.
    - Clinical Features:
        - **Offensive**, often **greenish** or **yellow** discharge.
        - Painful urination, itching, and a feeling of burning.
        - May be associated with the formation of **warts** or **growths** around the vagina or cervix.
        - Worse in warmth or after intercourse.
    - **Management**: Thuja is useful in **chronic vaginal infections** and cases with **genital warts** or **HPV** infections.

7. **Mercurius Solubilis**
    - Indications:
        - Profuse, yellowish, offensive discharge.
        - Excessive sweating, bad breath, and a metallic taste.
        - Often seen in syphilitic infections or gonorrheal infections.
    - Clinical Features:
        - Yellowish, often offensive discharge.
        - Soreness, swelling, or tenderness of the genital area.
        - Associated with systemic symptoms like fever, swelling of lymph nodes, and profuse sweating.
    - **Management**: Mercurius Solubilis is used for **syphilitic or gonorrheal infections** or when there is **foul-smelling, profuse** discharge.

8. **Kreosote**
    - Indications:
        - Leucorrhea with **burning, offensive** discharge.
        - The discharge may be **yellowish, thin**, or **watery**.
        - Often accompanied by **painful urination, itching**, or **burning** sensations.
    - Clinical Features:
        - Burning, offensive discharge, often yellowish.
        - The discharge can cause **irritation** or **inflammation** of the vaginal mucosa.
        - **Pain** and **irritation** in the genital area.
        - The patient may have a tendency to **feel worse from warmth** or **stress**.

- **Management**: Kreosote is often indicated in cases of **offensive**, **burning** discharge, especially in cases of **vaginal infections**.

9. **Sulphur**
    - Indications:
        - Leucorrhea with itching, burning, or inflammation.
        - Discharge can be watery or yellowish and may have an offensive odor.
        - Often accompanied by eczema, dermatitis, or skin conditions.
        - The patient may have a tendency to be warm, and symptoms may worsen with heat.
    - Clinical Features:
        - Yellowish, watery discharge, possibly with a strong odor.
        - Itching and burning sensations in the genital area.
        - The patient is often flushed, with hot feet and a general sensation of heat.
        - Symptoms tend to worsen in warm rooms or after bathing.
    - **Management**: Sulphur is indicated when **itching**, **burning**, and **offensive discharge** are present, especially when the patient has a **predisposition to skin conditions**.

10. **Silicea**
    - Indications:
        - Leucorrhea with a purulent, yellowish, or pus-like discharge.
        - The patient may have a weak immune system, with a tendency to recurring infections or abscesses.
        - Often used for patients who are delicate, sensitive, and have a tendency to coldness.
    - Clinical Features:
        - Thick, yellow, or greenish discharge, possibly pus-like.
        - Associated with chronic pelvic infections or recurrent vaginal discharge.
        - The patient may feel cold, and symptoms are worse in cold weather.
        - Weakness and **sensitivity to cold** are often present.
    - Management: Silicea is particularly helpful for those with chronic infections or poor resistance to infection.

11. **Graphites**
    - Indications:
        - Leucorrhea with **thick, sticky**, or **glutinous** discharge.
        - The discharge is typically **yellowish** and may have an **offensive odor**.
        - Patients may have **dry skin**, **eczema**, or **cracks** in the skin around the genitals.
    - Clinical Features:

- Thick, yellow, sticky discharge that may be glutinous or stringy.
- Associated with eczema, dryness, and skin cracks.
- The patient often feels cold and may have constipation or hard stools.
- **Management**: Graphites is useful when the discharge is **thick**, **sticky**, and **stringy**, especially in patients with **eczema** or **skin dryness**.

12. Natrum Phos
- Indications:
  - Leucorrhea with a **yellowish, creamy**, or **foul-smelling** discharge.
  - Often seen in cases of gonorrheal infections or chronic vaginal infections.
  - Accompanying symptoms may include **burning** or **itching**.
- Clinical Features:
  - Yellowish, creamy discharge with a strong odor.
  - **Burning** and **itching** in the genital area.
  - The patient may have excessive thirst, digestive disturbances, or a tendency to acidic conditions.
- **Management**: Natrum Phos is indicated for **offensive, creamy discharge** that is associated with **burning** sensations, especially in **chronic infections**.

13. Causticum
- Indications:
  - Leucorrhea with **watery**, **burning**, or **acrid** discharge.
  - Often used for women who experience **vaginal dryness** or **tenderness** with discharge.
  - Patients may have a history of chronic infections or weak pelvic floor muscles.
- Clinical Features:
  - Watery, acrid, or burning discharge that may cause irritation or soreness.
  - The discharge may be offensive and profuse.
  - Accompanying symptoms include soreness in the pelvic region and weakness of the pelvic muscles.
- **Management**: Causticum is indicated when the discharge is **watery**, **acrid**, or **burning**, especially in cases with **vaginal tenderness** or **chronic infections**.

14. Lachesis
- Indications:
  - Leucorrhea with offensive, yellowish, greenish, or purulent discharge.
  - The discharge may be thin or profuse, with a tendency to worsen before menstruation.
  - Often used when there are vascular disturbances or varicosities in the pelvic region.
- Clinical Features:

- o Yellowish or greenish, offensive discharge.
- o Symptoms tend to worsen before menstruation or during physical exertion.
- o The patient may have a tendency to feel congested or experience swelling in the pelvic area.
- o Often worse when the patient is lying down or after sleeping.
- **Management**: Lachesis is helpful in cases where the discharge is **profuse**, **yellowish**, or **greenish**, particularly if there are **vascular changes** or **pre-menstrual exacerbations**.

15. Alumina
- Indications:
  - o Leucorrhea with **thick, dry**, or **mucous** discharge.
  - o The patient may feel **constipated** or have a **dryness** of mucous membranes, including the vagina.
  - o Often seen in women who are **emotionally withdrawn** or **exhausted**.
- Clinical Features:
  - o Thick, dry, or mucous discharge.
  - o Accompanying constipation, dryness of the vagina, and exhaustion.
  - o The patient may feel weary and may have a tendency to withdraw from social situations.
- **Management**: Alumina is useful when the discharge is **thick**, **dry**, or **mucous**, especially when the patient experiences **exhaustion** or **constipation**.

16. Mercurius Vivus
- Indications:
  - o Leucorrhea with **thin**, **watery**, or **mucous discharge** that has a **foul odor**.
  - o Often indicated for gonorrheal infections or syphilitic conditions.
  - o The patient may have a sensitive mouth, swollen glands, and profuse sweating.
- Clinical Features:
  - o Thin, watery, mucous discharge with an offensive odor.
  - o Associated with swollen glands, sore throat, and profuse perspiration.
  - o The discharge may worsen with heat or night-time.
- **Management**: Mercurius Vivus is indicated for **watery, foul-smelling discharge**, particularly in cases related to **gonorrhea** or **syphilitic infections**.

17. Conium Maculatum
- Indications:
  - o Leucorrhea with a **yellowish** or **greenish**, **sticking**, or **stringy** discharge.
  - o Often accompanied by **heavy feeling** in the pelvic region and **tension** in the lower abdomen.
- Clinical Features:

- o Yellowish or greenish, sticky discharge.
- o The patient may experience a feeling of fullness or heavy pressure in the pelvic region.
- o Tension or pain in the lower abdomen is common.
- **Management**: Conium Maculatum is helpful for **sticking**, **stringy**, or **greenish discharge**, particularly in cases where there is a feeling of **pelvic heaviness**.

Malignant Tumours Of Ovary

I. Epithelial Ovarian Tumors

1. **Types:**

Epithelial tumors are the most common type of malignant ovarian cancer, making up about **90%** of all ovarian cancers. They arise from the **epithelial cells** that cover the surface of the ovaries. Key types include:
   - **Serous Carcinoma**: The most common type of ovarian cancer.
   - **Mucinous Carcinoma**: Less common, typically associated with cystic masses filled with mucus.
   - **Endometrioid Carcinoma**: Often associated with endometriosis.
   - **Clear Cell Carcinoma**: A rarer form, often associated with endometriosis.

2. **Aetiology:**
   - **Genetic factors**: Family history of ovarian or breast cancer, including mutations in the **BRCA1/2 genes**.
   - **Hormonal imbalances**: Hormonal therapy or early menarche, late menopause.
   - **Environmental factors**: Exposure to certain chemicals, or long-term use of talcum powder.
   - **Endometriosis**: Increases risk, especially for clear cell carcinoma.

3. **Clinical Features:**
   - Abdominal pain or bloating.
   - **Early satiety** (feeling full quickly).
   - **Urinary symptoms** such as frequency or urgency due to pressure on the bladder.
   - Irregular menstruation.
   - **Weight los**s and **fatigue** in advanced stages.
   - **Ascites** (fluid buildup in the abdomen).

4. **Complications:**
   - **Metastasis**: Spread to other parts of the abdomen, peritoneum, or distant organs.
   - **Peritoneal carcinomatosis**: Malignant spread within the peritoneal cavity.
   - **Obstruction**: Intestinal or urinary tract obstruction from tumor mass effect.
   - **Sepsis**: Due to infection secondary to rupture or treatment.

5. **Diagnosis:**
   - **Transvaginal ultrasound**: Initial imaging tool to assess tumor characteristics.
   - **CT scan/MRI**: Helps in staging and identifying metastasis.

- **CA-125 test**: Elevated in many cases of epithelial ovarian cancer, though not specific.
- **Biopsy**: Confirmatory diagnosis through histopathological examination.

6. **Management:**
   - **Surgery**: Optimal debulking surgery to remove as much of the tumor as possible.
   - **Chemotherapy**: Platinum-based chemotherapy (e.g., **Cisplatin** or **Carboplatin**) is the standard treatment after surgery.
   - **Targeted therapy**: Drugs targeting specific molecules (e.g., **Bevacizumab** for anti-angiogenesis).
   - **Radiation therapy**: Occasionally used, but less common for ovarian cancers.

II. Germ Cell Tumors

1. **Types:**

Germ cell tumors arise from the cells that produce eggs (oocytes) in the ovaries. These tumors are much rarer than epithelial ovarian cancers but occur more commonly in younger women. Types include:
- **Dysgerminoma**: The most common malignant germ cell tumor.
- Endodermal Sinus Tumor (Yolk Sac Tumor).
- Embryonal Carcinoma.
- **Teratoma** (immature).
- Choriocarcinoma.

2. **Aetiology:**
   - **Genetic factors**: In some cases, family history of other cancers or genetic mutations may play a role.
   - **Age**: Germ cell tumors are more common in **adolescent** and **young adult** women.
   - **Elevated hCG levels**: In some cases, these tumors secrete hormones like **human chorionic gonadotropin (hCG)**.

3. **Clinical Features:**
   - Abdominal or pelvic mass.
   - Abdominal pain or bloating.
   - **Menstrual irregularities** or postmenopausal bleeding.
   - **Elevated hCG or AFP** levels (in certain types).
   - **Nausea and vomiting** in cases of large tumors causing torsion.
   - **Early metastasis**: Some types can spread rapidly.

4. **Complications:**
   - **Ovarian torsion**: Twisting of the ovary due to the large mass.
   - **Metastasis**: Particularly to the lungs and liver.

- **Hemorrhage**: Tumor rupture can cause bleeding into the abdomen.
- **Sepsis**: Infected tumors leading to systemic infection.

5. **Diagnosis:**
   - **Ultrasound**: First imaging study to assess the characteristics of the mass.
   - **CT/MRI scans**: To evaluate the extent of the disease.
   - Tumor markers: Elevated levels of hCG, alpha-fetoprotein (AFP), or lactate dehydrogenase (LDH) help in diagnosis and monitoring.
   - **Biopsy**: Confirmation of tumor type through histopathological examination.

6. **Management:**
   - **Surgery**: Laparotomy or laparoscopy for tumor resection.
   - **Chemotherapy**: Often a combination of **etoposide** and **cisplatin**, particularly for dysgerminomas or other non-teratoma types.
   - **Radiation therapy**: Can be used for some germ cell tumor types.
   - **Fertility-sparing surgery**: If the tumor is confined to one ovary, fertility-preserving surgery may be an option for younger patients.

III. Stromal Cell Tumors

1. **Types:**

Stromal tumors arise from the connective tissue of the ovaries, which supports the development of the eggs. Types include:
   - **Granulosa Cell Tumor**: The most common stromal tumor.
   - Thecoma.
   - Fibroma.
   - Sertoli-Leydig Cell Tumor.

2. **Aetiology:**
   - **Hormonal imbalance**: Some tumors, particularly granulosa cell tumors, secrete hormones such as estrogen.
   - **Age**: Granulosa cell tumors are more common in postmenopausal women.
   - **Genetic mutations**: Certain genetic syndromes like **Peutz-Jeghers syndrome** or **Germline mutations** may predispose individuals.

3. **Clinical Features:**
   - Pelvic mass or abdominal bloating.
   - **Hormonal symptoms**: Such as **vaginal bleeding** (from estrogen secretion), **virilization** (due to testosterone secretion), or **precocious puberty** in younger women.
   - Abdominal pain or discomfort from tumor growth.
   - **Menstrual irregularities** in patients with estrogen-secreting tumors.

4. **Complications:**
    - **Metastasis**: Though rare, stromal tumors can spread to the lungs or liver.
    - **Hormonal imbalance**: Leads to menstrual irregularities, endometrial hyperplasia, or atypical uterine bleeding.
    - **Ovarian torsion**: In cases of large tumors or rapid growth.
    - **Sepsis**: Secondary infection due to tumor rupture.

5. **Diagnosis:**
    - **Ultrasound**: First line for detecting ovarian masses.
    - **CT/MRI**: To evaluate the extent of the tumor.
    - Tumor markers: Such as inhibin, estrogen, testosterone, or anti-Müllerian hormone (AMH) for certain types.
    - **Biopsy**: For definitive diagnosis.

6. **Management:**
    - **Surgery**: Complete surgical resection is the mainstay of treatment.
    - **Chemotherapy**: For advanced cases with metastasis, although these tumors tend to respond less to chemotherapy.
    - **Hormonal therapy**: For tumors with hormonal production, medical management may be considered.
    - **Fertility preservation**: In younger women, fertility-sparing surgery may be possible for localized disease.

Homoeopathic Management-

1. **Conium Maculatum (Poison Hemlock)**
    - **Indications**: Conium is indicated when ovarian tumors are **hard**, **painful**, and associated with **induration** (hardening of the tissues). This remedy is useful for **slow-growing tumors** that are **painless** at first but gradually become tender and hard. It may be indicated when there is a **history of hormonal imbalance** or when the patient experiences **mental sluggishness**, **depression**, or **indifference**.
    - Symptoms:
        - Hard, **indurated tumors** or lumps in the ovaries.
        - **Dull, heavy pain** or a sensation of **weight** in the pelvis.
        - Painless growths that become painful over time.
        - Nausea, weakness, and dizziness.
        - Emotional symptoms: Depression, anxiety, irritability, or indifference.
    - **Dosage**: Typically prescribed in **30C** or **200C** potencies, depending on the stage of disease.

2. **Phytolacca Decandra (Pokeweed)**
    - **Indications**: Phytolacca is useful for **fibrocystic ovarian growths** or **malignant tumors** that are associated with **hardness, fibrosis**, and **induration**. It is beneficial in cases where the tumor has a **painful, burning**, or **stinging** sensation. The remedy is also helpful when **breast or ovarian cancer** involves **lymphatic involvement**.
    - Symptoms:
        o **Painful tumors** that feel **hard** and **hot** to touch.
        o **Sharp, burning pain** in the ovarian area or breasts.
        o **Swelling** and **induration** of the lymph nodes.
        o **Severe aching** in the affected area, worsened by movement.
        o **Dosage**: **30C** or **200C**, depending on the severity.

3. **Arsenicum Album (Arsenic Trioxide)**
    - **Indications**: Arsenicum is useful when there is **severe restlessness, weakness, exhaustion**, and **great anxiety** associated with ovarian cancer. The patient may experience a **burning sensation** in the pelvic region, along with **extreme fatigue** and a tendency to feel **cold**. This remedy is also indicated when there is **great fear of death, delirium**, and **restlessness** due to cancer-related complications.
    - **Symptoms:**
        o Extreme fatigue, weakness, and emaciation.
        o Burning pain or stinging in the abdomen.
        o Restlessness, anxiety, and a fear of dying.
        o Coldness in the body, especially the extremities.
        o Digestive issues: Nausea, vomiting, and diarrhea.
    - **Dosage**: Typically prescribed in **30C, 200C**, or **1M** potencies, depending on the severity and constitutional type of the patient.

4. **Carcinosin (Cancer Nosode)**
    - **Indications**: Carcinosin is a **constitutional remedy** for individuals who have a **family history of cancer** or who exhibit **a predisposition** to developing malignancies. It is often used when there is a **deep-seated fear** of cancer or a history of **chronic disease**, especially in those with a **history of hormonal imbalances** or **autoimmune conditions**. It can help in **stabilizing immune function** and **addressing the underlying susceptibility to cancer**.
    - Symptoms:
        o Family history of cancer or precancerous conditions.
        o Mental anxiety about developing cancer.
        o Chronic conditions or a history of autoimmune disease.
        o Deep emotional issues: Resentment, fear of death, or a history of childhood trauma.

- o Hormonal imbalances and reproductive system issues.
- **Dosage**: Carcinosin is often used in **200C** or **1M** potencies, especially in the early stages of treatment for cancer.

5. **Chelidonium Majus (Greater Celandine)**
   - **Indications**: Chelidonium is particularly useful when there is **liver involvement** with ovarian cancer, such as **ascites** or **metastasis to the liver**. It may also help if the patient experiences **bloating**, **digestive issues**, or **jaundice**.
   - Symptoms:
     o **Liver congestion** or **ascites** (fluid accumulation).
     o Yellowing of the skin or sclera (eyes) due to liver issues.
     o Digestive disturbances like nausea, vomiting, or constipation.
     o Pain in the upper abdomen, especially the right side.
   - **Dosage**: Chelidonium is typically given in **30C** or **200C** potencies.

6. **Ruta Graveolens (Rue)**
   - **Indications**: Ruta is helpful for ovarian cancers that are associated with **tissue damage** or **degeneration**. It is particularly beneficial when there is a **feeling of bruising** or **aching** pain around the pelvic area, often linked to **post-surgical healing** or **radiation side effects**.
   - Symptoms:
     o **Achy, bruised** sensation in the pelvic area or lower abdomen.
     o **Stiffness** in the pelvic region, especially after surgery or radiation.
     o Tissue degeneration, cellular breakdown, and weakness.
     o Healing of wounds or incisions after surgery.
   - **Dosage**: Ruta is often prescribed in **30C** or **200C** potencies for pain and healing support.

7. **Natrum Muriaticum (Common Salt)**
   - **Indications**: Natrum muriaticum is useful for individuals who exhibit **emotional suppression** and **grief** related to the diagnosis of cancer. It is helpful when the patient experiences **depression**, **despair**, and **isolates themselves emotionally**. It can also be used when **fluid retention** (ascites) is a concern in ovarian cancer.
   - Symptoms:
     o **Emotional withdrawal**: Difficulty expressing emotions, deep sadness, or grief.
     o **Fluid retention** (ascites or swelling).
     o **Headaches** or **migraines** associated with emotional distress.
     o **Exhaustion** or **weakness**, particularly after emotional strain.
   - **Dosage**: **30C**, **200C**, or **1M** potencies based on symptom severity.

8. **Calcarea Carbonica (Calcium Carbonate)**
    - **Indications**: Calcarea is particularly helpful for individuals who have a **history of cancer**, especially those who are **overweight**, **cold**, and have **metabolic issues**. It is useful when the patient experiences **debilitating fatigue**, **excessive sweating**, and **susceptibility to infections**.
    - Symptoms:
        - Obesity, cold intolerance, and tendency to gain weight.
        - **Excessive perspiration** during sleep or exertion.
        - Fatigue, weakness, and a slow recovery from illness.
        - History of chronic diseases or hormonal imbalances.
    - **Dosage**: **30C**, **200C**, or **1M**, depending on the patient's condition.

9. **Belladonna (Deadly Nightshade)**
    - **Indications**: Belladonna is often used in cases of **sudden, intense pain** associated with ovarian tumors or malignancy. It is particularly helpful for **acute inflammation** and **tumors that cause swelling or pulsation**. The pain may be sharp, stabbing, and aggravated by **touch**, **motion**, or **light**.
    - Symptoms:
        - **Severe, throbbing pain** in the ovarian region.
        - **Hot, inflamed** areas of the abdomen with a tendency to **sweat**.
        - **Pulsating, cramp-like pain** in the pelvis, aggravated by motion or pressure.
        - **Restlessness**, **agitation**, and **delirium** in advanced stages of cancer.
    - **Dosage**: Typically given in **30C**, **200C**, or **1M** potencies, based on the intensity of the symptoms.

10. **Hepar Sulphuris Calcareum (Calcium Sulphide)**
    - **Indications**: Hepar sulphuris is indicated for cases where there is **pus formation** or **suppuration** around the tumor. It is especially helpful in situations where a **tumor has ruptured** or is prone to infection. It is also used for **sharp, splinter-like pain** in the abdomen and **sensitivity** to touch.
    - Symptoms:
        - Tumors with a tendency to abscess or rupture.
        - **Painful lumps** in the ovarian area that are **highly sensitive** to touch.
        - Pus-filled masses or draining abscesses.
        - **Aggravation** of symptoms in cold air or **drafts.**
    - **Dosage**: Typically **30C** or **200C**, depending on the stage of the tumor.

11. **Thuja Occidentalis (White Cedar)**
    - **Indications**: Thuja is particularly useful when there is a history of **wart-like growths** or **sarcoma** in the ovaries. It may also be indicated for **growths** that are

hard, **bony**, and **immovable**. Thuja is frequently used when there is **mental suppression**, **anxiety**, or **guilt**.

- Symptoms:
  o Hard, immovable tumors that feel like warts.
  o Mental exhaustion, guilt, and feelings of unworthiness related to the cancer diagnosis.
  o Growths that are bony, painful, and excessively dry.
  o Symptoms worsened by dampness or cold.
- **Dosage**: Commonly prescribed in **30C**, **200C**, or **1M** potencies.

12. Baryta Carbonica (Barium Carbonate)

- **Indications**: Baryta carbonica is used in cases where there is **weakness** and **immaturity** of the immune system, especially in older women or those who are **physically debilitated**. It is helpful when the patient experiences **slow tumor growth** and shows signs of **premature aging** or **failure to thrive**.
- Symptoms:
  o **Premature aging, mental confusion, or poor concentration.**
  o **Chronic fatigue, weakness, and emaciation.**
  o **Small, immobile tumors in the ovaries with slow progression.**
  o **Swelling and inflammation in the pelvic area.**
- **Dosage**: **30C** or **200C** potencies can be used for constitutional treatment.

13. Natrum Phosphoricum (Sodium Phosphate)

- **Indications**: Natrum phosphoricum is helpful in cases where **tumors are associated with acid-base imbalance** or where the patient has **gastrointestinal issues** such as **bloating** and **indigestion**. It is also useful when there is **fluid retention** (ascites) or **jaundice** due to liver involvement.
- Symptoms:
  o **Bloating, indigestion, or gastrointestinal discomfort.**
  o **Ascites (fluid retention in the abdomen).**
  o **Yellowing of the skin, jaundice, or liver congestion.**
  o **Acidic conditions that aggravate the cancer symptoms.**
- **Dosage**: Typically given in **30C** or **200C** potencies.

14. Calcarea Phosphorica (Calcium Phosphate)

- **Indications**: Calcarea phosphorica is a **constitutional remedy** often indicated for individuals with **bone involvement** in ovarian cancer (e.g., metastatic spread to bones). It is particularly helpful in people who experience **bone pain**, **stiffness**, or **growth disturbances**. It is also used for **mental fatigue** and **poor concentration**.
- Symptoms:
  o **Bone pain, particularly in the lower back or pelvis.**

- Stiffness or difficulty moving, especially after long periods of rest.
- Tiredness, poor memory, and mental sluggishness.
- Delayed healing or growth disturbances in the body.
- **Dosage**: Prescribed in **30C** or **200C**, depending on the condition.

15. Zincum Metallicum (Zinc)
- **Indications**: Zincum metallicum is indicated for **hyperactive nervous systems** or cases of **restlessness** in the later stages of ovarian cancer. It is useful for **tremors**, **weakness**, and **muscle spasms** in advanced disease.
- Symptoms:
  - **Restlessness and tremors in the legs and other parts of the body.**
  - **Weakness in the pelvic area or the lower body.**
  - **Pain and muscle spasms associated with metastatic involvement.**
  - **Fatigue and mental confusion.**
- **Dosage**: **30C** or **200C**, based on the severity of symptoms.

16. Sabina (Juniperus sabina)
- **Indications**: Sabina is useful for **hemorrhaging tumors** in the ovaries, especially when there is **heavy bleeding** or **spotting** due to **cancer**. It can also be used when there is a sensation of **pressure** in the pelvic area and when the patient has **dark, foul-smelling menstrual blood**.
- Symptoms:
  - **Heavy, dark menstrual bleeding or bleeding between periods.**
  - **Painful pressure or aching in the ovarian region.**
  - **Foul-smelling discharge or bleeding.**
  - **Sensation of fullness or heaviness in the abdomen.**
- **Dosage**: Prescribed in **30C** or **200C**, depending on symptoms.

17. Silicea (Silica)
- **Indications**: Silicea is indicated when there is **pus formation**, **chronic infection**, or **draining abscesses** associated with ovarian tumors. It is also useful for patients who experience **weakness** and **slow healing**.
- Symptoms:
  - **Abscesses or pus-filled growths in the ovarian area.**
  - **Chronic infections or a tendency to get infections.**
  - **Weakness, exhaustion, or fatigue after surgery or chemotherapy.**
  - **Delayed healing of tissues and wounds.**
- **Dosage**: **30C** or **200C** potencies.

18. Medorrhinum (Gonorrhea Nosode)
- **Indications**: Medorrhinum is helpful when there is a **family history of cancer**, especially **hormonal cancers**, and in individuals who have **a history of infections**

(such as **gonorrhea**) or **recurrent infections**. It may also be used when there is **extreme fear** of cancer or a deep-seated sense of **guilt**.
- Symptoms:
    - **Family history of cancer or hormonal imbalances.**
    - **Emotional distress with fear or guilt related to cancer.**
    - **History of chronic infections or venereal diseases.**
    - **Mental restlessness and a desire for cold, open air.**
- **Dosage**: Typically prescribed in **200C** or **1M**, depending on the patient's response

Menstrual Cycle

Definition of the Menstrual Cycle

The menstrual cycle is a natural, recurring physiological process that occurs in females of reproductive age. It is regulated by hormonal changes and involves the preparation of the uterus for pregnancy. If pregnancy does not occur, the uterine lining is shed during menstruation. The average cycle lasts 28 days but can range from 21 to 35 days.

Phases of the Menstrual Cycle

The menstrual cycle is divided into **four phases**, each marked by specific hormonal and physiological changes:

1. **Menstrual Phase (Day 1–5)**
   - **Definition:** This phase marks the beginning of the cycle, characterized by the shedding of the uterine lining (endometrium) in the form of menstrual blood.
   - Hormonal Changes:
     - Low levels of **estrogen** and **progesterone** trigger menstruation.
     - Follicle-stimulating hormone (**FSH**) levels begin to rise slightly.
   - Physiological Changes:
     - The uterine lining disintegrates and is expelled through the vagina.
     - Some women experience cramping due to uterine contractions (mediated by prostaglandins).
   - **Symptoms:** Abdominal cramps, fatigue, mood changes, and lightheadedness.

2. **Follicular Phase (Day 1–13)**
   - **Definition:** This phase overlaps with the menstrual phase and continues until ovulation. It involves the maturation of ovarian follicles.
   - Hormonal Changes:
     - Rising levels of **FSH** stimulate the growth of multiple follicles in the ovaries.
     - One dominant follicle becomes the **Graafian follicle**, which produces increasing levels of **estrogen**.
     - Estrogen levels rise sharply toward the end of this phase.
   - Physiological Changes:
     - The endometrium starts to regenerate and thicken under the influence of estrogen.
     - Cervical mucus becomes thinner and more conducive to sperm survival.
   - **Symptoms:** Energy levels may improve, and mood may stabilize due to rising estrogen levels.

3. **Ovulation Phase (Day 14)**
   - **Definition:** Ovulation is the release of a mature egg (oocyte) from the dominant follicle in the ovary.
   - Hormonal Changes:
     o A surge in **luteinizing hormone (LH)**, triggered by high estrogen levels, causes ovulation.
     o FSH also peaks but at lower levels than LH.
     o Estrogen levels peak just before ovulation, then decline.
   - Physiological Changes:
     o The mature follicle ruptures, releasing the egg into the fallopian tube.
     o Cervical mucus becomes clear, stretchy, and slippery, facilitating sperm transport.
     o Basal body temperature increases slightly after ovulation due to rising **progesterone** levels.
   - **Symptoms:** Mild abdominal discomfort (known as mittelschmerz) in some women and increased libido.

4. **Luteal Phase (Day 15–28)**
   - **Definition:** This phase begins after ovulation and lasts until the start of the next menstrual period. The body prepares for possible pregnancy.
   - Hormonal Changes:
     o The ruptured follicle forms the **corpus luteum**, which secretes **progesterone** and small amounts of estrogen.
     o Progesterone levels peak mid-phase to maintain the thickened endometrium.
     o If pregnancy does not occur, the corpus luteum degenerates, and hormone levels drop.
   - Physiological Changes:
     o The endometrium becomes highly vascularized and glandular, ready to support a fertilized egg.
     o If pregnancy does not occur, the endometrial lining begins to break down.
     o Progesterone withdrawal causes the uterine lining to shed (menstruation).
   - Symptoms:
     o Premenstrual symptoms (PMS) like bloating, mood swings, breast tenderness, and irritability occur due to hormonal fluctuations.
     o If pregnancy occurs, **human chorionic gonadotropin (hCG)** is produced to maintain the corpus luteum and hormone levels.

1. **Estrogen:** Stimulates endometrial growth and regulates the early phases of the cycle.

2. **Progesterone:** Maintains the endometrium for implantation and dominates the luteal phase.
3. **FSH:** Stimulates follicle growth and maturation in the ovaries.
4. **LH:** Triggers ovulation and supports the formation of the corpus luteum.

Summary Table

Phase	Hormonal Peak	Key Changes
Menstrual	Low estrogen & progesterone	Uterine lining is shed.
Follicular	Rising FSH, peak estrogen	Follicle growth, endometrial thickening, and cervical mucus changes.
Ovulation	LH surge	Egg release, thin cervical mucus, and slight temperature rise.
Luteal	Peak progesterone	Endometrium is maintained; PMS occurs if pregnancy does not happen.

Irregular Menstrual Cycles

Irregular menstrual cycles refer to variations in the frequency, duration, or intensity of menstrual periods. Normally, a menstrual cycle ranges between **21 and 35 days**, with bleeding lasting 2–7 days. Irregular periods may involve missing periods, cycles longer than 35 days (**oligomenorrhea**), cycles shorter than 21 days (**polymenorrhea**), or heavy/prolonged bleeding (**menorrhagia**).

Common Causes of Irregular Menstrual Cycles

Irregular menstruation can result from a variety of factors, which are broadly classified into physiological, hormonal, and pathological causes:

1. **Hormonal Imbalances**
   - Polycystic Ovary Syndrome (PCOS):
     - A condition where excess **androgens** (male hormones) disrupt ovulation, leading to irregular or missed periods.
   - Thyroid Disorders:
     - **Hypothyroidism** (low thyroid hormones): Can cause heavy or prolonged periods.
     - **Hyperthyroidism** (high thyroid hormones): May cause lighter or infrequent periods.
   - Hyperprolactinemia:
     - Elevated **prolactin** levels suppress ovulation and disrupt the menstrual cycle.

- Perimenopause:
  o Irregular cycles due to fluctuating levels of **estrogen** and **progesterone** as women approach menopause.
- Hypothalamic Dysfunction:
  o Stress, excessive exercise, or significant weight loss affect the hypothalamus, disrupting hormone secretion.

2. **Uterine and Ovarian Conditions**
   - Uterine Fibroids:
     o Noncancerous growths in the uterus can cause heavy bleeding or prolonged cycles.
   - Endometriosis:
     o Growth of uterine-like tissue outside the uterus leads to painful and irregular periods.
   - Pelvic Inflammatory Disease (PID):
     o Infection of the reproductive organs causes inflammation, irregular bleeding, and pain.
   - Premature Ovarian Failure (POF):
     o Early depletion of ovarian follicles leads to irregular or absent periods.

3. **Lifestyle Factors**
   - Stress:
     o Cortisol elevation suppresses normal reproductive hormone function.
   - Extreme Weight Changes:
     o Obesity increases **estrogen** production, while being underweight suppresses ovulation.
   - Excessive Exercise:
     o Athletic amenorrhea occurs due to energy deficits and low hormone levels.
   - Medications:
     o Birth control pills, antipsychotics, or anticoagulants can affect menstrual regularity.

4. **Systemic Medical Conditions**
   - Diabetes Mellitus:
     o Poorly controlled blood sugar affects hormonal balance.
   - Cushing's Syndrome:
     o Elevated cortisol disrupts menstrual cycles.
   - Chronic Kidney or Liver Disease:
     o Impaired metabolism of hormones like estrogen affects the cycle.

5. **Pregnancy-Related Issues**
   - Early Pregnancy:
     o Irregular bleeding may occur during implantation or due to complications.
   - Ectopic Pregnancy:
     o Bleeding and irregularity due to a fertilized egg implanting outside the uterus.
   - Miscarriage:
     o Can cause irregular bleeding.

Allopathic Management of Irregular Menstrual Cycles

Management depends on the underlying cause, severity of symptoms, and reproductive goals. Treatment aims to restore hormonal balance, regularize periods, and address associated conditions.

1. **Hormonal Therapies**
   - Combined Oral Contraceptive Pills (COCPs):
     o Regulate menstrual cycles and reduce heavy bleeding.
     o Common brands contain **estrogen** and **progestin**.
   - Progestin-Only Pills (Mini-Pill):

Useful for women with contraindications to estrogen (e.g., smokers or those with blood clot risks).

   - Progesterone Therapy:
     o Prescribed for women with luteal phase defects or irregular ovulation.
   - Hormonal Intrauterine Devices (IUDs):
     o E.g., **Levonorgestrel-releasing IUD** reduces heavy bleeding and protects the endometrium.

2. **Treatment for Specific Hormonal Disorders**
   - PCOS:
     o **Metformin:** Improves insulin sensitivity and regularizes cycles.
     o **Clomiphene Citrate:** Induces ovulation in women trying to conceive.
     o Anti-androgens (e.g., **spironolactone**) reduce excess male hormones.
   - Thyroid Disorders:
     o **Levothyroxine** for hypothyroidism or antithyroid medications for hyperthyroidism.
   - Hyperprolactinemia:
     o Treated with dopamine agonists like cabergoline or bromocriptine.

3. **Non-Hormonal Medications**
   - Nonsteroidal Anti-Inflammatory Drugs (NSAIDs):
     o Reduce menstrual pain and heavy bleeding.
   - Tranexamic Acid:

- o Prescribed for menorrhagia to reduce blood loss.
- Iron Supplements:
  - o For anemia caused by heavy bleeding.

4. **Lifestyle Modifications**
   - Weight Management:
     - o Obesity or being underweight can disrupt cycles; a balanced diet and regular exercise help.
   - Stress Management:
     - o Yoga, meditation, or counseling to reduce hypothalamic dysfunction.
   - Avoid Excessive Exercise:
     - o Moderate activity levels maintain hormonal balance.

5. **Surgical Interventions (If Required)**
   - Uterine Fibroids:
     - o Managed with **myomectomy** or minimally invasive procedures (e.g., uterine artery embolization).
   - Endometriosis:
     - o **Laparoscopic surgery** to remove endometrial tissue.
   - Polypectomy:
     - o Removal of uterine polyps causing irregular bleeding.

Monitoring and Follow-Up

1. **Tracking Menstrual Cycles:**
   - o Mobile apps or calendars help in identifying patterns and irregularities.
2. **Ultrasound and Hormone Tests:**
   - o Monitor the progress of treatments and evaluate structural or hormonal abnormalities.
3. **Regular Check-Ups:**
   - o Especially for patients with chronic conditions like PCOS or thyroid disease.

Comparative Table of Homeopathic Therapeutics for Irregular Menstruation

Remedy	Key Indications	Associated Symptoms	Mental/Emotional Traits
Pulsatilla Nigricans	**Irregular periods** (delayed, suppressed, or scanty); PCOS; amenorrhea.	Periods are changeable, scanty, or late. Pain is mild. Desire for open air.	Weepy, gentle, emotional; seeks consolation.

Remedy	Key Indications	Associated Symptoms	Mental/Emotional Traits
Sepia Officinalis	**Hormonal imbalance**, amenorrhea, scanty periods, PMS, or menopausal symptoms.	Bearing-down sensation in the pelvis; fatigue and indifference to loved ones.	Indifferent, irritable, exhausted; aversion to family life.
Calcarea Carbonica	**Heavy/profuse bleeding**, delayed or scanty periods; suitable for women with obesity or thyroid dysfunction.	Excessive sweating (especially on the head), cold intolerance, sluggishness.	Fearful, anxious, overwhelmed by responsibilities.
Natrum Muriaticum	**Scanty or irregular periods**; frequent periods; emotional trauma or stress-induced irregularities.	Headaches before/during menstruation; dryness of vagina; craving for salty foods.	Reserved, emotional, sensitive; dislikes consolation.
Lachesis Muta	Irregular, suppressed, or scanty periods; severe PMS with emotional lability.	Symptoms worsen before periods and improve after flow starts. Painful ovaries.	Jealous, talkative, intense; worse with tight clothing.
Magnesia Phosphorica	**Dysmenorrhea** (severe cramping pain); spasmodic uterine pain relieved by warmth and pressure.	Cramping pain that radiates to other parts of the body; better with warm applications.	Nervous, hypersensitive; prefers quiet and warmth.
Cimicifuga Racemosa	**Painful or irregular periods**; associated with emotional disturbances or ovarian conditions.	Pain radiates to the back and thighs; spasmodic contractions.	Depression, fear of impending illness, restlessness.
Sabina	**Heavy or prolonged bleeding** with bright red blood and clots; menorrhagia and miscarriage tendency.	Severe back and abdominal pain during bleeding.	Impatient, nervous, sensitive to music.

Remedy	Key Indications	Associated Symptoms	Mental/Emotional Traits
Thuja Occidentalis	**Irregular or suppressed periods**; PCOS; hormonal imbalances with cystic growths.	Ovarian cysts; warts; oily skin; hair growth in unusual places (hirsutism).	Fixed ideas, secretive, low self-esteem.
Trillium Pendulum	**Heavy bleeding** aggravated by movement and relieved by pressure; uterine fibroids.	Weakness from excessive bleeding; dizziness.	Usually calm but weak and fatigued during periods.
Ignatia Amara	**Stress-related menstrual irregularities**; suppressed or scanty periods due to emotional trauma or grief.	Sighing, lump in the throat; sensitivity to odors; cramping uterine pain.	Grief-stricken, nervous, moody, or prone to emotional extremes.
Apis Mellifica	**Frequent or suppressed periods**, ovarian cysts, or painful menstruation with stinging sensations.	Puffiness or swelling in the genital area; burning or stinging pain.	Irritable, restless, dislikes heat.
Caulophyllum	**Irregular or spasmodic menstruation**; dysmenorrhea with labor-like pain; useful in uterine atony.	Painful contractions and delayed periods.	Irritable, nervous, and restless during pain.
Phosphorus	**Heavy and prolonged periods** with bright red blood; anemia due to excessive bleeding.	Weakness, craving for cold drinks, and dizziness after bleeding.	Sensitive, emotional, friendly, and extroverted.
Graphites	**Scanty, delayed periods**; irregular menses with constipation and obesity; suitable for sluggish individuals.	Dry skin, cold hands and feet; scanty discharge; poor stamina.	Depressed, indecisive, and emotionally reserved.
Belladonna	**Sudden onset of painful menstruation** with heat,	Sudden sharp pain; sensitivity to noise and light.	Restless, easily irritable, and

Remedy	Key Indications	Associated Symptoms	Mental/Emotional Traits
	throbbing, and a flushed face.		oversensitive to stimuli.
Silicea	**Scanty periods**, irregular cycles, or delayed menstruation; useful in undernourished individuals.	Profuse sweating; cold extremities; poor stamina; late puberty.	Shy, timid, and easily fatigued.

Menopause & Syndrome

Definition[menopause]-
Menopause is the stage of life when a woman hasn't had a period for 12 months in a row.

Menopausal syndrome-
Multisystemic symptoms together during menopause due to oestrogen deficiency due to ovarian failure in menopaus

Stages of menopause-

Perimenopause/ climacteric age
The transition to menopause, which can last from a few months to several years. During this time, your ovaries produce less estrogen, and you may experience irregular periods, hot flashes, and night sweats.

Menopause
When there is no longer have a menstrual period for 12 months in a row.Ovaries stop releasing eggs, and your body produces less estrogen.

Postmenopause
The years after menopause, when symptoms usually taper off. However, other health conditions may begin, such as osteoporosis.

Aetiology-

- **Ovarian function**

As a woman ages, her ovaries produce less estrogen and progesterone, and stop releasing eggs.

- **Menstrual cycle changes**

In your 40s, your menstrual periods may become longer or shorter, heavier or lighter, and happen more often or less often.

- **Surgical procedures**

Surgical interventions that involve the ovaries, such as removing both ovaries, can cause menopause.

- **Chemotherapy or hormone therapy**

Drugs used for chemotherapy or hormone therapy for breast cancer can cause menopause.

- **Autoimmune diseases**

Certain conditions, such as rheumatoid arthritis, Crohn's disease, or thyroid disease, can lead to premature menopause.

- **Endometriosis**

Severe endometriosis can cause premature menopause.

- **Family history**

If your mother has a history of premature menopause.

Clinical Features-

1. Night Sweats

Night sweats, assume that it is because of decreased estrogen levels. These falling hormone levels may have an effect on the

hypothalamus, a region in the brain responsible for body temperature regulation.

2. Hot flashes

Many women in menopause experience hot flashes. This symptom can make you sweat heavily, hot and look flushed, especially in the chest, neck, and face. In some cases, women in menopause and perimenopause can experience chills.

3. Mood swings

Due to changes in hormone levels, women in menopause and perimenopause can experience unpredictable mood shifts unrelated to life events .They can suddenly feel angry, weepy, or sad.

4. Irregular Menstrual Cycle

A common sign of perimenopause, the transitional phase before a woman enters menopause, is having irregular periods. Occasionally, a woman may have multiple missed periods until she stops having them entirely.Sometimes there may be chances of METROPATHA HAEMORRHAGICA [heavy prolonged menstruation following prolonged duration amenorrhea]

5. Decreased Libido

Menopause and perimenopause can affect the desire for sex or the Libido. This happens because of lower estrogen and testosterone levels and the shifts in mood. In addition, some women experience low libido levels due to menopause medication.

6. Breast Soreness

Some women experience sore breasts during menopause.

7. **Vaginal Dryness/Senile vaginitis**

One of the more unusual menopause symptoms is lack of natural lubrication. As a woman's hormones drop, blood flow may decrease too. this symptom can make penetrative intercourse difficult and painful.**[DYSPARENIA]**

8. **Tingling Hands and Feet**

Another one of the more unusual menopause symptoms is tingling extremities, most commonly in the hands and the feet. However, some women also feel this sensation in the arms and the legs. Since the hormones are constantly fluctuating, this affects the central nervous system.

9. **Headaches**

One of the most annoying signs of perimenopause is experiencing frequent migraines or headaches (due to a lower estrogen).

10. **Changes in Sense of Taste**

some women experience stronger flavors, along with a dry mouth.

11. **Burning Sensation in the Mouth**

Another unusual menopause symptom is experiencing a burning, tingling, or numbing sensation in or around your mouth.

12. **Bloating**

Bloating happens due to a few reasons including gassiness, water retention, and slower digestion due to stress.

13. **Fatigue**

One of the biggest reasons for fatigue is low sleep quality due to night sweats and hot flashes that keep you from resting.

14. **Joint Pain**

Since estrogen assists in joint lubrication and decreasing inflammation, you may experience aches in the joints.

15. **Different Digestive Changes**

A lot of unusual menopause symptoms are linked to the gut. For instance, women in menopause and perimenopause can experience a "weird" reaction to certain foods and changes in digestion.

16. **Sensations of Electric Shock**

One of the more worrisome signs of perimenopause involves experiencing sensations that feel like electric shocks. Researchers believe this happens due to changes in hormones that affect the nervous system.

17. Muscle Aches and Tension

Women may experience these unusual menopause symptoms due to the same reasons they can experience joint pain.

18. Sleep Issues

Night sweats and hot flashes can keep you awake, resulting in poor sleep.

19. Itchiness

Estrogen is linked to collagen production, and it also hydrates your skin. So, its decline can affect dryness and itchiness, around your vulva or elsewhere on your body.

20. Memory Problems

Compromised sleep and low estrogen levels can affect her memory.

21. Concentration Challenges

Signs of perimenopause also include having a sudden lack of focus. You may experience mental fogginess and trouble concentrating.

22. Brittle Nails

A woman's body in menopause produces less keratin, the substance needed for strong nails.

23. Thinning Hair

You may experience hair thinning or even hair loss due to changes in ovarian hormones.

24. Sudden Urge to Urinate

Women in perimenopause and menopause may experience stress incontinence or frequent/sudden urges to pee. During menopause, a woman's pelvic and bladder muscles may become weaker.

25. Weight Gain

Some women may gain weight due to lower estrogen l
evels and decreased physical activity levels. In addition, if you experience mood changes, your eating patterns can shift too. maintaining a balanced diet and exercise will prevent gain weight.

26. Allergies

One of the rarer menopause symptoms is experiencing new or worsening symptoms of allergies. The reason being is that women in menopause can have histamine spikes (the chemical responsible for allergic reactions).

27. Occasional Dizziness

Fluctuating hormones can influence insulin production, making it more challenging for a woman's body to maintain proper blood sugar levels.

28. Irregular Heartbeat

Women in menopause may also experience arrhythmia.this could also be a symptom of diabetes, high blood pressure, and blocked arteries.

29. Depression

Hormonal changes can trigger depression.

30. Irritability

Lack of sleep and stress can lead to mood shifts.

31. Boosted Body Odor

Due to night sweats and hot flashes, your body odor may change.

32. Panic Disorder

In rare cases, women in menopause can experience frequent panic attacks. However, this symptom can also indicate panic or anxiety disorder.

33. Anxiety

Similar to other mood-related symptoms, changes in hormones can boost anxiety.

34. Osteoporosis

A plunge in estrogen can lead to bone density loss. Your bones can become fragile and easy to fracture.

Complications-

- **Cardiovascular disease**

Women are more likely to develop heart disease and stroke after menopause. This is because estrogen helps keep blood vessels open and maintain a healthy balance of cholesterol.

- **Osteoporosis**

After menopause, women lose bone mass more quickly due to decreased estrogen levels. This can lead to osteoporosis, a condition that causes bones to become brittle and break more easily.

- **Urinary incontinence**

Weakened pelvic floor muscles can cause women to lose control of their bladder. This can happen when coughing, laughing, sneezing, or lifting something heavy.

- **Sexual dysfunction**

Hormonal changes and psychological factors can cause sexual dysfunction, including vaginal dryness, pain during sex, and changes in libido.

- **Cognitive changes**

Some women may experience memory loss, trouble focusing, and other cognitive abnormalities.

- **Weight gain**

Hormonal changes, a decline in physical activity, and changes in metabolism can cause women to gain weight, especially in the stomach region.

- **Oral issues**

Dry mouth and an increased risk for cavities are more common after menopause.

Other health concerns associated with menopause include:
- Breast, ovarian, and endometrial cancer
- Psychiatric symptoms
- Genitourinary syndrome of menopause (formerly called vaginal atrophy)

Diagnosis-

— Follicle-stimulating hormone (FSH) and estrogen (estradiol). FSH goes up and estrogen goes down during menopause.

— Thyroid-stimulating hormone (TSH). Overactive thyroid, called hyperthyroidism, can cause symptoms like those of menopause.

— AMH

Treatment-

— **Hormone therapy.** Estrogen therapy works best for easing menopausal hot flashes. It also eases other menopause symptoms and slows bone loss. estrogen in the lowest dose and for the time needed to relieve symptoms. It's best used by people who are younger than 60 and within 10 years of the onset of menopause.

In patient with uterus, you'll need progestin with estrogen. Estrogen also helps prevent bone loss.

Long-term use of hormone therapy may have some heart disease and breast cancer risks. But starting hormones around the time of menopause has shown benefits for some people.

Vaginal estrogen.

To relieve vaginal dryness, apply estrogen to the vagina using a vaginal cream, tablet or ring. This treatment gives you a small amount of estrogen, which the vaginal tissues take in. It can help ease vaginal dryness, pain with intercourse and some urinary symptoms.

— **Prasterone (Intrarosa).** You put this human-made hormone dehydroepiandrosterone (DHEA) into the vagina. It helps ease vaginal dryness and pain with intercourse.

— **Low-dose medicines to treat depression, called antidepressants.** Some antidepressants may ease menopausal hot flashes. These are called selective

serotonin reuptake inhibitors (SSRIs) and serotonin-norepinephrine reuptake inhibitors (SNRI). A low-dose antidepressant may help manage hot flashes in people who can't take estrogen for health reasons or for those who need an antidepressant for a mood disorder.
- **Gabapentin (Gralise, Neurontin).** Gabapentin is approved to treat seizures, but it also has been shown to help reduce hot flashes. This medicine is useful for people who can't use estrogen therapy and for those who also have nighttime hot flashes.
- **Clonidine (Catapres-TTS-1, Nexiclon XR).** This pill or patch most often treats high blood pressure. It might give some relief from hot flashes. It's not often prescribed for hot flashes because of the possible side effects, such as low blood pressure, headache, sleepiness and constipation.
- **Fezolinetant (Veozah).** This medicine is free of hormones. It treats menopause hot flashes by blocking a pathway in the brain that helps manage body temperature. It's FDA approved for managing menopause symptoms. It can cause abdominal pain, liver problems and make sleep problems worse.
- **Oxybutynin (Oxytrol).** This medicine treats overactive bladder and urinary urge incontinence. It's also been shown to relieve menopause symptoms. But in older adults, it may be linked to cognitive decline.
- Medicines to prevent or treat the bone-thinning condition called osteoporosis. Caalcium & vitamin D supplements to help strengthen bones.
- **Ospemifene (Osphena).** Taken by mouth, this selective estrogen receptor modulator (SERM) medicine treats painful intercourse linked to the thinning of vaginal tissue. This medicine isn't for people who have had breast cancer or who are at high risk of breast cancer.

Lifestyle and home remedies

Many of the symptoms menopause causes go away on their own in time. In the meantime, the following might help:
- Cool hot flashes.
- Dress in layers,
- wear sleeveless tops and wear fabrics that breathe, such as cotton.
- Lower room temperatures and use hand or room fans.
- Put cold packs under your pillow and turn the pillow often so your head is on the cool side.
- It might also help to avoid triggers such as caffeine, alcohol and spicy foods.
- **Ease vaginal pain.** Try a water-based vaginal lubricant (Astroglide, Sliquid, others) or a silicone-based lubricant or moisturizer (Replens, K-Y Liquibeads, others). You can get these without a prescription.

Stay sexually active by yourself or with a partner. This also can ease vaginal discomfort by increasing blood flow to the vagina.

- **Get enough sleep.** Skip caffeine and alcohol, which can make it harder to sleep. Exercise during the day, but not right before bedtime. If hot flashes disturb your sleep, find a way to help manage them so you can get better rest.
- **Find ways to relax.** There's little proof that deep breathing, guided imagery, massage and muscle relaxation can ease menopausal symptoms. But finding ways to relax is good for overall health and may help you cope with menopausal symptoms.
- **Strengthen your pelvic floor.** Pelvic floor muscle exercises, called Kegel exercises, can improve some forms of urinary incontinence.
- **Eat a balanced diet.** Include a variety of fruits, vegetables and whole grains. Limit saturated fats, oils and sugars. Take calcium or vitamin D supplements.
- **Manage weight.** Studies show that being obese is linked to having more and worse hot flashes. Losing weight and keeping it off may help ease them.
- **Don't smoke.** Smoking increases risk of heart disease, stroke, osteoporosis, cancer and a range of other health problems. It also may increase hot flashes and bring on earlier menopause.
- **Exercise regularly.** Get regular physical activity or exercise on most days to help protect against heart disease, diabetes, osteoporosis and other conditions associated with aging.

Alternative medicine

There are many alternative medicines that claim to help ease the symptoms of menopause. But few of them have been proved in studies. Some complementary and alternative treatments that have been or are being studied include:

- **Plant estrogens, also called phytoestrogens.** There are natural estrogens in certain foods. There are two main types of phytoestrogens, called isoflavones and lignans. Soybeans, lentils, chickpeas and other legumes have isoflavones. Flaxseed, whole grains and some fruits and vegetables have lignans.

  It hasn't been proved that the estrogens in these foods can ease hot flashes and other menopausal symptoms. Isoflavones have some weak estrogen-like effects. So if you've had breast cancer, talk with your healthcare provider before taking isoflavone pills.
- **Bioidentical hormones.** These hormones come from plant sources. The term "bioidentical" implies the hormones in the product are chemically the same as those the body makes.

  The Food and Drug Administration (FDA) has approved some bioidentical hormones. But many are mixed in a pharmacy from a healthcare professional's prescription, called compounded. But the FDA doesn't regulate them, so quality and risks could vary.

Bioidentical hormones have not been shown to work better or be safer than other hormone therapy.
- **Cognitive behavior therapy.** This type of therapy can help you change thoughts, feelings and behaviors that aren't healthy. It's been shown to reduce how much menopause symptoms bother you.
- **Black cohosh.** Black cohosh has been popular among many people with menopause symptoms. But there's little proof that black cohosh works. And it can harm the liver and not be safe for people with a history of breast cancer.
- **Yoga.** Yoga might ease menopause symptoms at least as well as other forms of exercise. And balance exercises such as yoga or tai chi can improve strength and help you move better. That may help prevent falls that could lead to broken bones.
- **Acupuncture.** Acupuncture may help to reduce hot flashes in the short term. But research hasn't shown that it helps a lot. More research is needed.
- **Hypnosis.** This mind-body therapy involves a deeply relaxed state and mental images. Hypnotherapy may lower the number of hot flashes and how bad they are for some menopausal people.

Homoeopathic Management-

Homeopathic Remedy	Indications
1. Lachesis	Lachesis is indicated when there are **hot flashes**, **night sweats**, and **mood swings**. It is often prescribed when the patient feels **irritable**, **restless**, or suffers from **headaches** that are worse after sleep. Symptoms worsen with **heat**, tight clothing, or around **menstruation** time. It is also helpful when **menstrual irregularities** are present before menopause.
2. Sepia	Sepia is often used when there are **fatigue**, **irritability**, and a feeling of being **overwhelmed**. It is indicated for **hot flashes**, especially when they are accompanied by **vaginal dryness** and **loss of libido**. Women who need Sepia may also experience **mood swings**, a sense of **indifference**, and **depression**. It is beneficial for **hormonal imbalances** during perimenopause.
3. Pulsatilla	Pulsatilla is helpful when there are **mood swings, weepiness**, and **tearfulness** during menopause. It is particularly useful for women who feel **clingy** and **desire company** during emotional upheaval. Symptoms are often relieved by **cool air** and worsened in a **stuffed room**. Pulsatilla is suitable for those experiencing **irregular menstrual cycles** or **delayed periods**.

Homeopathic Remedy	Indications
4. Cimicifuga (Actaea racemosa)	This remedy is often used for **hot flashes, headaches**, and **nervous tension** associated with menopause. It can help in cases of **muscular pain** or **joint stiffness** that often occur during menopause. Women experiencing **irritability, mood swings**, or **nervous exhaustion** benefit from Cimicifuga. It's helpful for those who feel **overwhelmed** by the physical changes in their body.
5. Sulphur	Sulphur is indicated when there are **hot flashes**, especially at **night**, accompanied by a **sensation of heat** in the head and body. It is useful for women experiencing **itching, dry skin**, and **sweating**, especially when these symptoms worsen at **night**. Additionally, it can help with **irritability** and **anxiety**. Sulphur is often needed by women with **chronic skin conditions** during menopause.
6. Natrum Muriaticum	This remedy is ideal for women who are experiencing **emotional withdrawal, moodiness**, and **sensitivity** during menopause. It helps with **headaches**, especially those that are **stress-induced**, and is beneficial for women who feel **isolated** or **depressed**. Natrum Muriaticum is also helpful when there is **hot flushes, vaginal dryness**, or **dry skin**.
7. Ignatia Amara	Ignatia is indicated for those experiencing **emotional stress, grief**, and **mood swings** during menopause. Women in need of this remedy may feel **mentally confused, anxious**, and have **nervous symptoms** like **tremors**. It is useful for those who are going through emotional **upheavals** and **tears** or feel as though they are **unable to cope**.
8. Thyroidinum	This remedy is used for symptoms of **hypothyroidism** associated with menopause, such as **fatigue, weight gain**, and **constipation**. It can help when the **metabolism slows down**, leading to **coldness, dry skin**, and **hair loss**. Thyroidinum is also helpful in correcting **hormonal imbalances** and boosting **energy levels**.
9. Calcarea Carbonica	Indicated for women who feel **overburdened, anxious**, and **exhausted** by the menopausal transition. Calcarea Carbonica is useful when there is **weight gain, fluid retention**, and **heavy perspiration**, particularly **at night**. Women with **low energy, weak bones**, and **poor tolerance to cold** often need this remedy. It can help in **balancing hormones** and addressing **bone health**.

Homeopathic Remedy	Indications
10. Graphites	Graphites is useful for women who experience **dry skin**, **itching**, and **cracking** of the skin during menopause. It can also address **constipation**, **moodiness**, and a feeling of being **physically and emotionally drained**. The remedy is beneficial when there is a **tendency to be overweight**, especially around the abdomen, and **hormonal imbalance**. It is also indicated when there is **vaginal dryness** and **painful intercourse**.

Menorrhagia

Definition: Menorrhagia refers to excessive or abnormally heavy menstrual bleeding that lasts longer than the usual duration of menstruation (typically more than 7 days) or involves the loss of more than 80 milliliters of blood per cycle. This condition can be both physically and emotionally distressing and may interfere with a woman's daily activities.

Types of Menorrhagia:

1. Primary Menorrhagia:
- Occurs in the absence of any underlying gynecological condition. It is often due to hormonal imbalances, particularly anovulation (lack of ovulation).
- More common in adolescents or women approaching menopause.

2. Secondary Menorrhagia:
- Caused by an underlying condition such as fibroids, endometrial polyps, adenomyosis, or medical conditions like thyroid disorders or bleeding disorders.
- More common in women over 30.

3. Ovulatory Menorrhagia:
- Heavy bleeding occurs during ovulation, often due to a hormonal imbalance where the estrogen levels rise excessively without adequate progesterone levels to balance the endometrial growth.

4. Anovulatory Menorrhagia:
- Heavy menstrual bleeding without ovulation, often seen in women with conditions like polycystic ovary syndrome (PCOS) or thyroid dysfunction. The absence of ovulation leads to irregular or heavy bleeding.

Clinical Features of Menorrhagia:
- **Heavy Bleeding**: The most prominent feature is excessive blood flow, which may involve soaking through a pad or tampon every 1-2 hours for several hours.
- **Prolonged Menstrual Periods**: A menstrual cycle that lasts longer than 7 days.
- **Clotting**: Passing large blood clots (greater than 2.5 cm in diameter) is common in cases of menorrhagia.
- **Fatigue and Weakness**: As a result of prolonged blood loss, many women may experience fatigue, dizziness, or weakness, which can lead to anemia.
- **Pelvic Pain**: Some women experience lower abdominal cramping or pelvic discomfort, which may be associated with fibroids, adenomyosis, or other conditions.

- **Irregular Cycles**: Menstrual cycles may become irregular with variable flow patterns, especially in cases involving hormonal imbalances.

Complications of Menorrhagia:

1. **Anemia:**
   - The most common complication, caused by the significant loss of red blood cells leading to iron deficiency. Symptoms include fatigue, paleness, dizziness, and shortness of breath.

2. **Infection:**
   - If the bleeding is related to a structural problem like fibroids, polyps, or endometrial hyperplasia, it can increase the risk of infections.

3. **Infertility:**
   - Conditions such as fibroids or endometrial hyperplasia, which cause menorrhagia, can lead to infertility or difficulty in conceiving.

4. **Psychological Stress:**
   - Chronic heavy bleeding may cause significant emotional distress, leading to anxiety, depression, and a decreased quality of life.

5. **Endometrial Cancer:**
   - In postmenopausal women or those with prolonged untreated menorrhagia, the condition may be linked to endometrial cancer or hyperplasia, which can become precancerous.

Diagnosis of Menorrhagia:

1. **History and Physical Examination:**
   - A detailed history of the menstrual cycle (duration, frequency, amount of bleeding) and physical examination to assess for signs of anemia, pelvic masses, or uterine abnormalities.

2. **Blood Tests:**
   - **Complete Blood Count (CBC)** to assess for anemia (low hemoglobin or hematocrit).
   - **Thyroid Function Tests** to check for thyroid abnormalities that could be contributing to the condition.
   - **Coagulation Profile** to rule out bleeding disorders (e.g., von Willebrand disease).

3. **Ultrasound:**
   - **Transvaginal Ultrasound** is commonly used to detect uterine abnormalities such as fibroids, polyps, or adenomyosis. It also helps evaluate the thickness of the endometrial lining.

4. **Endometrial Biopsy:**
    - Performed to obtain a tissue sample from the lining of the uterus, particularly in women over 40, or when postmenopausal bleeding is suspected, to rule out endometrial cancer or hyperplasia.

5. **Hysteroscopy:**
    - A minimally invasive procedure that allows the doctor to directly view the inside of the uterus and diagnose conditions such as fibroids, polyps, or adhesions.

6. **MRI:**
    - In certain cases, especially if the ultrasound is inconclusive or to assess larger fibroids or complex uterine abnormalities, an MRI may be recommended.

Modern Management of Menorrhagia:

1. **Medical Management:**
    - Hormonal Therapy:
        - **Oral Contraceptives**: Birth control pills containing both estrogen and progestin can help regulate the menstrual cycle and reduce bleeding.
        - **Progestin-only Therapy**: IUDs like Mirena or oral progestins can help reduce bleeding by thinning the endometrial lining.
        - **GnRH Agonists**: Medications like leuprolide that block the production of estrogen and progesterone, leading to a temporary "menopausal" state and reduced bleeding.
    - Nonsteroidal Anti-Inflammatory Drugs (NSAIDs):
        - Medications like ibuprofen or naproxen can reduce bleeding and alleviate pain associated with menorrhagia.
    - **Desmopressin**: For women with bleeding disorders (e.g., von Willebrand disease), this medication helps in increasing clotting factor levels to control bleeding.
    - **Tranexamic Acid**: An antifibrinolytic medication that helps reduce excessive bleeding by inhibiting the breakdown of blood clots.

2. **Surgical Management:**
    - **Dilation and Curettage (D&C)**: A procedure to scrape the uterine lining, often used when there are abnormal growths like polyps or if a biopsy is needed.
    - **Endometrial Ablation**: A procedure that destroys the endometrial lining to reduce or stop bleeding. This is a less invasive option for women who have completed childbearing.
    - **Hysterectomy**: Removal of the uterus, which may be recommended in severe cases, especially when other treatments fail or when the condition is linked to uterine cancer.

3. **Blood Transfusion:**
   o For severe cases where significant blood loss has occurred, a blood transfusion may be required to replenish red blood cells and prevent anemia.

Homeopathic Therapy for Menorrhagia

Homeopathic Remedy	Indications/Use	Effectiveness
Cinchona Officinalis	For excessive bleeding with weakness and fatigue, often after prolonged blood loss.	Helps replenish energy and improve blood circulation.
Phosphorus	For heavy, profuse menstrual bleeding, often with faintness, and exhaustion.	Effective for profuse bleeding with a feeling of weakness.
Secale Cornutum	For uterine hemorrhage with coldness, weakness, and dry mucous membranes.	Used for hemorrhages with a cold feeling or weakness.
Ipecacuanha	For continuous, unrelenting bleeding, often accompanied by nausea and vomiting.	Beneficial when bleeding is unremitting and accompanied by nausea.
Arnica Montana	For post-traumatic bleeding or bleeding after surgery or childbirth.	Ideal for bleeding following injury or surgical procedures.
Tarantula Hispanica	For heavy, irregular bleeding with restlessness and emotional agitation.	Useful for emotional distress accompanying irregular bleeding.
Carbo Vegetabilis	For bleeding with weakness, dizziness, and a sensation of collapse or fainting.	Helps in cases of exhaustion and weakness related to blood loss.
Lachesis	For bleeding with a feeling of fullness in the pelvic area, often with hot flashes.	Effective for bleeding linked with menopausal symptoms or fullness in the pelvis.
Belladonna	For sudden, intense bleeding with throbbing pain, hot flashes, or fever.	Effective for acute, intense bleeding with accompanying fever or throbbing.
Alumina	For uterine hemorrhage in women who are weak, exhausted, and dry.	Helpful for long-standing menorrhagia with physical weakness.

Comparative Management in Modern Medicine vs. Homeopathy:

Aspect	Modern Medicine	Homeopathic Treatment
Mechanism	Treats the underlying cause (e.g., hormonal imbalances, fibroids).	Focuses on restoring the body's natural balance and self-healing.
Treatment Approach	Based on specific diagnoses (e.g., hormone therapy, surgery).	Holistic approach based on individual symptoms (physical and emotional).
Duration of Treatment	Often short-term for acute cases, but long-term for chronic menorrhagia.	Long-term management and prevention, with periodic adjustments.
Side Effects	Risk of side effects from medications or surgical procedures.	Minimal side effects when remedies are tailored to the individual.
Effectiveness	High effectiveness, especially for treating underlying causes.	Varies depending on individual cases, but often used as complementary therapy.

Metrorrhagia

Definition: Metrorrhagia refers to abnormal bleeding from the uterus that occurs between menstrual periods, often in the form of irregular or prolonged spotting. It is different from menorrhagia (excessive menstrual bleeding) and can occur at any time during the menstrual cycle. Metrorrhagia can be a sign of an underlying gynecological disorder and requires medical evaluation.

Types of Metrorrhagia:

1. **Acute Metrorrhagia:**
   - Characterized by sudden, heavy, irregular bleeding, often requiring immediate medical attention.
   - It may be associated with trauma, infections, or hormonal disturbances.

2. **Chronic Metrorrhagia:**
   - Prolonged or recurrent irregular bleeding that persists for several months.
   - Typically linked to underlying conditions like fibroids, polyps, or endometrial hyperplasia.

3. **Ovulatory Metrorrhagia:**
   - Occurs around the time of ovulation, often due to hormonal fluctuations or an imbalance in estrogen and progesterone levels.
   - May present as light bleeding or spotting.

4. **Postmenopausal Metrorrhagia:**
   - Abnormal bleeding that occurs after a woman has entered menopause.
   - This requires further investigation, as it can be indicative of serious conditions such as endometrial cancer or atrophic vaginitis.

Aetiology (Causes) of Metrorrhagia:

1. **Hormonal Imbalance:**
   - **Anovulation**: Occurs when the ovaries fail to release an egg, causing irregular menstrual cycles and irregular bleeding.
   - **Polycystic Ovary Syndrome (PCOS)**: A hormonal disorder that leads to irregular periods and metrorrhagia.
   - **Thyroid Disorders**: Hypothyroidism or hyperthyroidism can lead to menstrual irregularities, including metrorrhagia.

2. **Structural Abnormalities:**
   - **Uterine Fibroids**: Non-cancerous growths in the uterus that can cause abnormal bleeding.
   - **Uterine Polyps**: Benign growths in the endometrial lining that can cause irregular bleeding.
   - **Endometrial Hyperplasia**: Thickening of the uterine lining, which can lead to abnormal bleeding.
   - **Endometriosis**: When endometrial tissue grows outside the uterus, it can cause bleeding and pain.

3. **Infections:**
   - **Pelvic Inflammatory Disease (PID)**: Infections in the reproductive organs can lead to abnormal bleeding.
   - **Cervicitis**: Inflammation of the cervix, often due to infection, may cause metrorrhagia.

4. **Medications:**
   - **Oral Contraceptives**: Hormonal birth control pills can sometimes cause irregular bleeding, especially during the first few months of use.
   - **Anticoagulants**: Blood-thinning medications can cause abnormal bleeding.

5. **Cancerous Conditions:**
   - **Endometrial Cancer**: A type of cancer that affects the lining of the uterus and can cause irregular bleeding, especially postmenopausal.
   - **Cervical Cancer**: May cause abnormal bleeding between periods or after intercourse.

6. **Trauma or Injury:**
   - Injury to the uterus or cervix, such as after childbirth, medical procedures, or sexual activity, can lead to irregular bleeding.

Clinical Features of Metrorrhagia:

- **Irregular Bleeding**: Occurs between periods, which may be light, heavy, or sporadic.
- **Spotting**: Light bleeding or discharge between menstrual cycles.
- **Prolonged Menstrual Periods**: In some cases, the bleeding lasts longer than usual.
- **Pain**: Some women may experience lower abdominal pain or discomfort, often associated with underlying conditions like fibroids or endometriosis.
- **Pelvic Pressure**: A feeling of fullness or heaviness in the pelvic region, often associated with structural causes like fibroids or polyps.
- **Fatigue and Anemia**: Prolonged or excessive bleeding may result in fatigue and signs of anemia (e.g., paleness, dizziness).

Complications of Metrorrhagia:

1. **Anemia**: Chronic or excessive bleeding can lead to a decrease in red blood cells, causing fatigue, weakness, and shortness of breath.
2. **Infertility**: Conditions like endometriosis, fibroids, or polyps may contribute to infertility or difficulty conceiving.
3. **Endometrial Cancer**: Postmenopausal metrorrhagia can be an early sign of endometrial cancer.
4. **Emotional Stress**: Chronic metrorrhagia can cause emotional and psychological stress, leading to anxiety or depression.
5. **Pelvic Infections**: Abnormal bleeding caused by infections can lead to complications like pelvic inflammatory disease (PID).

Diagnosis of Metrorrhagia:

6. **History and Physical Examination**: A thorough history of menstrual cycles, sexual activity, and any associated symptoms is essential. Pelvic examination to assess for masses, tenderness, or abnormalities in the cervix or uterus.
7. **Ultrasound**: Transvaginal ultrasound to visualize the uterine lining, fibroids, polyps, or other structural abnormalities.
8. **Pap Smear**: To rule out cervical infections or cancer, especially if metrorrhagia is associated with post-coital bleeding.
9. **Endometrial Biopsy**: Performed to examine the endometrial lining, especially in cases of postmenopausal bleeding, to rule out endometrial cancer or hyperplasia.
10. **Hysteroscopy**: Direct visualization of the uterine cavity to assess for polyps, fibroids, or other abnormalities.
11. **Blood Tests**: Hormonal levels (e.g., thyroid function tests, progesterone levels) and a complete blood count (CBC) to assess for anemia.

Modern Management of Metrorrhagia:

1. **Medical Management**:
   - **Hormonal Therapy**: Oral contraceptives or progestin therapy to regulate the menstrual cycle and reduce bleeding.
   - Non-Steroidal Anti-Inflammatory Drugs (NSAIDs): Used to reduce pain and inflammation.
   - **Progestin Therapy**: Can be used in cases of anovulation or uterine abnormalities to control bleeding.
   - **Intrauterine Device (IUD)**: Hormonal IUDs, such as Mirena, help to reduce bleeding and are effective for women with structural abnormalities like fibroids or endometrial hyperplasia.
   - **Desmopressin**: For patients with bleeding disorders (e.g., von Willebrand disease or platelet dysfunction).

2. **Surgical Management:**
   - **Dilation and Curettage (D&C)**: A procedure where the uterine lining is scraped to diagnose and treat abnormal bleeding.
   - **Hysteroscopy**: Allows for removal of polyps or fibroids within the uterus.
   - **Endometrial Ablation**: A procedure that destroys the uterine lining to reduce or stop abnormal bleeding.
   - **Hysterectomy**: Removal of the uterus, often considered in severe cases of uterine abnormalities or cancer.
3. **Blood Transfusion: In cases of significant blood loss leading to anemia, a blood transfusion may be required.**

Homeopathic Therapy for Metrorrhagia

Homeopathic Remedy	Indications/Use	Effectiveness
Cinchona Officinalis	For bleeding caused by exhaustion, weakness, or anemia. Often used when there is a history of prolonged or heavy bleeding.	Useful for cases of blood loss and fatigue.
Phosphorus	For bright red, profuse bleeding, often with a sensation of weakness or fainting.	Effective for sudden, profuse bleeding with weakness.
Secale Cornutum	For hemorrhages with coldness, weakness, and a feeling of dryness, often in women with uterine conditions.	Helps with excessive bleeding that occurs with a cold feeling in the body.
Ipecacuanha	For continuous bleeding that doesn't stop, often with nausea and a feeling of distress.	Beneficial when bleeding is constant and accompanied by nausea or vomiting.
Arnica Montana	For trauma-induced bleeding, particularly after childbirth or injury.	Effective for post-traumatic bleeding or after surgery.
Tarantula Hispanica	For profuse, irregular bleeding with a sense of restlessness and anxiety.	Used for emotional and physical symptoms that accompany irregular bleeding.
Carbo Vegetabilis	For bleeding with weakness, dizziness, and a sensation of faintness or collapse.	Helps in cases of bleeding associated with weakness or anemia.

Homeopathic Remedy	Indications/Use	Effectiveness
Lachesis	For bleeding that occurs after or during menopause, often with a sense of fullness or pressure in the pelvic region.	Effective for postmenopausal bleeding with emotional disturbances.
Belladonna	For sudden, acute bleeding, especially when it is heavy, with throbbing pain and hot flashes.	Used for sudden onset of heavy bleeding with intense pain or heat.
Alumina	For uterine hemorrhage in women who are weak and have dry, rough skin. Can be useful for chronic conditions with intermittent bleeding.	Helpful for long-standing cases of irregular bleeding with weakness.

New Mechanically Aided Techniques In Male Infertility: Diagnosis & Treatment

Introduction

Male infertility accounts for nearly **50% of infertility cases** worldwide. Recent advances in **mechanically aided techniques** for **diagnosis and treatment** have significantly improved outcomes. These techniques include **advanced semen analysis, sperm retrieval methods, microsurgical procedures, and assisted reproductive technologies (ARTs).**

I. Diagnostic Methods in Male Infertility

1. **Computer-Assisted Semen Analysis (CASA)**
   - **What it is:** A highly precise, automated system that assesses sperm count, motility, morphology, and DNA integrity.
   - **Advantage:** Removes human error, provides detailed sperm quality reports.
   - **Technology Used:** High-resolution imaging, motion tracking software.

2. **Microfluidic Sperm Selection (Lab-on-a-Chip)**
   - **What it is:** A technique using microfluidic devices to separate high-quality sperm from low-quality sperm.
   - **Advantage:** Enhances sperm selection without DNA fragmentation.
   - **Technology Used:** Lab-on-a-chip technology, mimicking the female reproductive tract.

3. **Sperm DNA Fragmentation Test**
   - What it is: Measures DNA integrity using techniques like TUNEL, COMET assay, and SCD (Sperm Chromatin Dispersion test).
   - **Advantage:** Predicts fertilization potential, detects hidden sperm damage.
   - **Technology Used:** Fluorescence microscopy, flow cytometry.

4. **Artificial Intelligence (AI)-Based Sperm Analysis**
   - **What it is:** AI algorithms analyze sperm parameters and predict fertility potential.
   - **Advantage:** Improves accuracy of sperm morphology and motility assessment.
   - **Technology Used:** Deep learning, computer vision.

5. **Testicular Biopsy and Micro-TESE (Microsurgical Testicular Sperm Extraction)**
   - **What it is:** A microscopic procedure to extract sperm from the testes in men with **non-obstructive azoospermia**.
   - **Advantage:** Increases sperm retrieval rates compared to conventional biopsy.
   - **Technology Used:** Operating microscope with 20–25x magnification.

II. Mechanically Aided Therapeutic Methods in Male Infertility

1. **Sperm Retrieval Techniques for Azoospermia**

   A. **Testicular Sperm Aspiration (TESA)**
      - What it is: A needle is inserted into the testis to extract sperm.
      - Indication: Obstructive azoospermia.
      - Technology Used: Fine-needle aspiration under local anesthesia.

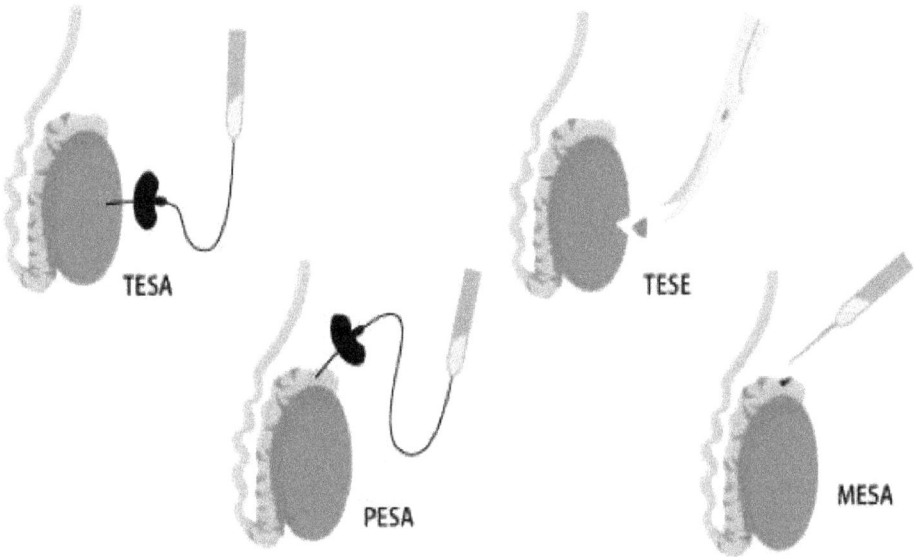

   B. **Percutaneous Epididymal Sperm Aspiration (PESA)**
      - **What it is:** A needle-based aspiration from the epididymis.
      - **Indication:** Obstructive azoospermia (due to vasectomy or congenital absence of vas deferens).
      - **Technology Used:** Ultrasound-guided aspiration.

   C. **Microdissection TESE (Micro-TESE)**
      - **What it is:** A microsurgical procedure to retrieve sperm from seminiferous tubules.
      - **Indication:** Non-obstructive azoospermia.

- **Technology Used:** High-resolution operating microscope.

2. **Advanced Assisted Reproductive Technologies (ARTs)**

    A. **Intracytoplasmic Sperm Injection (ICSI)**

    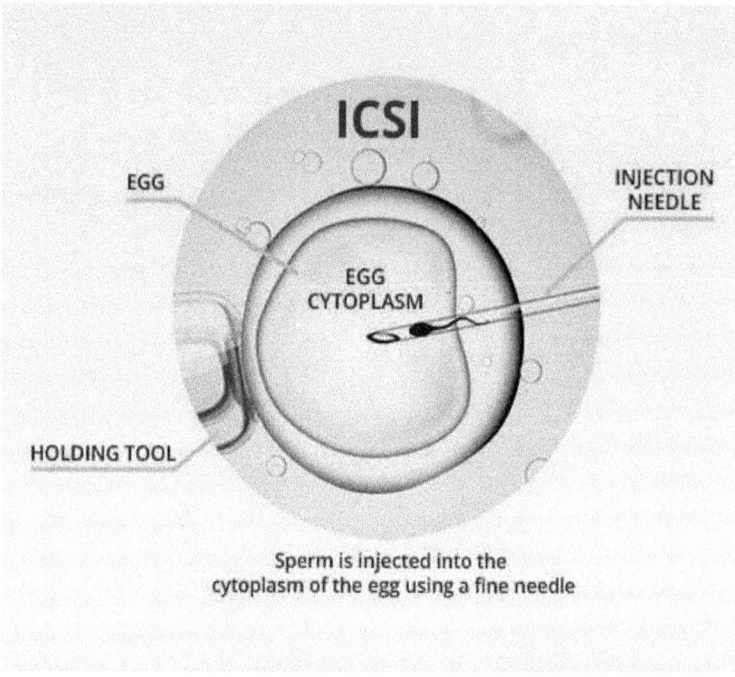

    - **What it is:** A single sperm is directly injected into an egg.
    - **Indication:** Severe male factor infertility (low sperm count, poor motility).
    - **Technology Used:** Micromanipulation system.

    B. **Magnetic-Activated Cell Sorting (MACS) for Sperm Selection**
    - **What it is:** Uses magnetic nanoparticles to remove apoptotic (damaged) sperm.
    - **Advantage:** Increases fertilization success rates.
    - **Technology Used:** Magnetic separation techniques.

    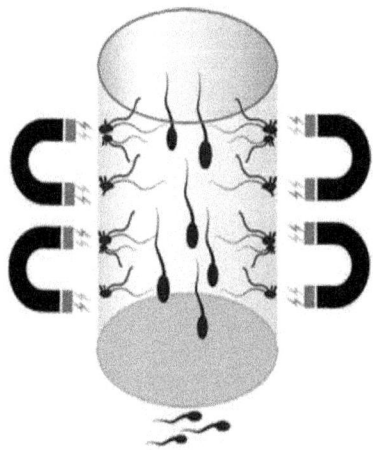

C. Piezo-ICSI (Piezoelectric Intracytoplasmic Sperm Injection)
- **What it is:** Uses micro-pulse technology to inject sperm with minimal damage.
- **Advantage:** Reduces trauma to the egg membrane.
- **Technology Used:** Piezoelectric micromanipulation.

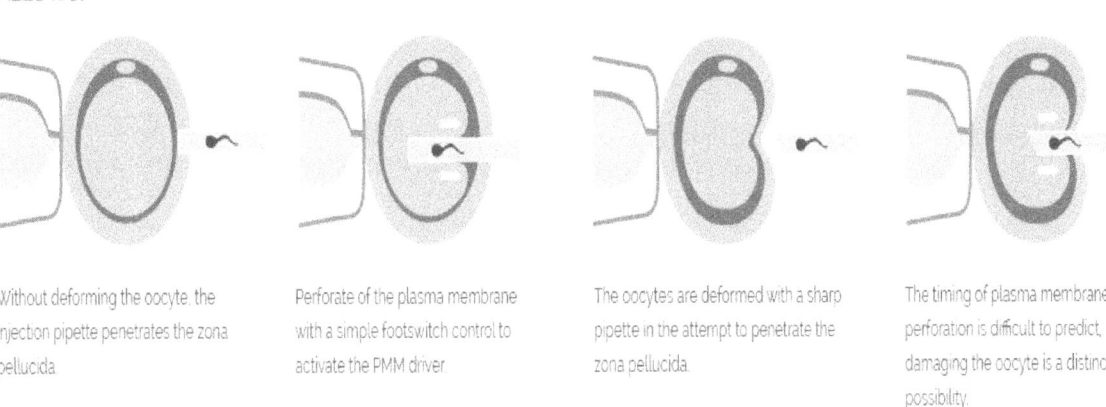

3. Mechanical Therapies for Varicocele Treatment

A. Microsurgical Varicocelectomy
- **What it is:** A high-precision surgical approach to remove varicose veins in the scrotum.
- **Advantage:** Reduces oxidative stress and improves sperm parameters.
- **Technology Used:** Operating microscope, Doppler ultrasound.

B. Embolization of Varicocele
- **What it is:** A non-surgical technique where coils or sclerosing agents block abnormal veins.
- **Advantage:** Minimally invasive, quick recovery.
- **Technology Used:** Fluoroscopy-guided catheterization.

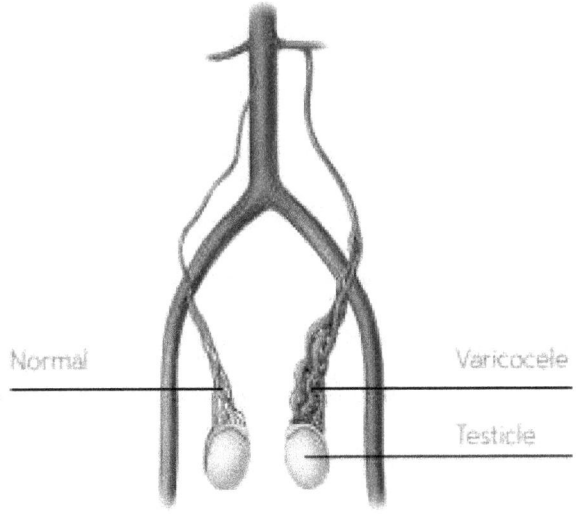

4. **Innovative Sperm Cryopreservation & Preservation Techniques**

   A. **Vitrification (Rapid Sperm Freezing)**
   - **What it is:** Ultra-rapid freezing method preventing ice crystal formation.
   - **Advantage:** Higher post-thaw sperm survival rates.
   - **Technology Used:** Liquid nitrogen (-196°C), cryoprotectants.

   B. **Sperm Sorting Using Microfluidics**
   - **What it is:** Separates best sperm for cryopreservation.
   - **Advantage:** Increases quality of stored sperm.
   - **Technology Used:** Lab-on-a-chip, nanofluidics.

5. **Nanotechnology-Based Approaches**

   A. **Nanoparticle Therapy for Sperm Enhancement**
   - What it is: Uses nanoparticles to deliver antioxidants directly to sperm.
   - **Advantage:** Reduces oxidative stress, improves motility.
   - **Technology Used:** Gold and silver nanoparticles.

   B. **Nano-Encapsulated Drug Delivery for Testicular Disorders**
   - **What it is: Nano-drug carriers** improve drug absorption in testicular tissues.
   - **Indication:** Hormonal disorders affecting sperm production.
   - **Technology Used:** Liposomes, dendrimers.

Comparison of Modern Medicine vs. Homeopathic Management in Male Infertility

Condition	Modern Medicine Management	Homeopathic Management
Low Sperm Count (Oligospermia)	- Clomiphene Citrate 25 mg OD (for hormonal boost) - Letrozole 2.5 mg OD (increases testosterone) - Gonadotropin injections (hCG 2000 IU 3x/week)	- **Agnus Castus 30C** – Boosts testosterone & improves libido - **X-Ray 30C** – Stimulates sperm production
Poor Sperm Motility (Asthenospermia)	- Coenzyme Q10 (200-300 mg/day) - L-Carnitine (2 g/day) - Antioxidants (Vitamin C, E, Zinc, Selenium)	- **Conium Maculatum 30C** – Enhances sluggish sperm motility - **Damiana 30C** – Improves sperm energy & movement

Condition	Modern Medicine Management	Homeopathic Management
Abnormal Sperm Morphology (Teratospermia)	- DNA Fragmentation Repair Therapy - Pentoxifylline (400 mg BID) – Improves blood flow	- **Thuja Occidentalis 30C** – Corrects sperm abnormalities - **Selenium 6X** – Enhances sperm shape
Azoospermia (No Sperm in Semen)	- hCG/hMG Therapy (Stimulates sperm production) - TESE/PESA/Micro-TESE	- **Tribulus Terrestris 30C** – Stimulates testosterone & sperm formation - **Caladium 30C** – Boosts testicular function
Erectile Dysfunction (ED) & Low Libido	- Sildenafil (50 mg PRN) - Tadalafil (5 mg daily) - Testosterone Replacement (if low)	- **Lycopodium 30C** – Treats performance anxiety & weak erection - **Nuphar Luteum 30C** – Improves weak libido
Hormonal Imbalance (Low Testosterone, High FSH/LH)	- Testosterone Gel/Injections - Aromatase Inhibitors (Anastrozole 1 mg OD)	- **Testosterone 6X** – Supports natural hormone balance - **Orchitinum 30C** – Stimulates testes function
Varicocele (Testicular Vein Enlargement)	- Microsurgical Varicocelectomy - Embolization	- **Hamamelis 30C** – Reduces varicocele congestion - **Fluoric Acid 30C** – Strengthens weak veins
Oxidative Stress & Sperm DNA Damage	- NAC (N-Acetylcysteine 600 mg/day) - Resveratrol (500 mg/day)	- **Carcinosin 30C** – Prevents sperm DNA fragmentation - **Selenium 6X** – Strong antioxidant
Retrograde Ejaculation	- Alpha-adrenergic agonists (Ephedrine, Midodrine)	- **Causticum 30C** – Helps proper ejaculation - **Staphysagria 30C** – Treats involuntary semen loss

Condition	Modern Medicine Management	Homeopathic Management
Infections Affecting Fertility (Prostatitis, Epididymitis)	- Antibiotics (Doxycycline, Azithromycin)	- **Medorrhinum 30C** – Treats chronic reproductive infections - **Merc Sol 30C** – Reduces pus & swelling in infections
Autoimmune Male Infertility (Anti-Sperm Antibodies)	- Corticosteroids (Prednisolone) - Immunotherapy	- **Thuja 30C** – Prevents auto-immune sperm destruction - **Silicea 30C** – Improves immune tolerance
Unexplained Infertility	- Assisted Reproductive Technologies (ICSI, IMSI)	- **Natrum Muriaticum 30C** – Balances reproductive hormones - **Sulphur 30C** – Enhances overall reproductive health

Obstrectric Fistula

Definition-
- Abnormal communication between two epithelial surfaces is called fistula
- Obstetric Fistula:-

Genitourinary fistula or genito-rectal fistula related to labor and delivery.
- V VF:-

abnormal connection between bladder &vagina, leakage of urine via vagina.
- RVF :-

abnormal connection between rectum &vagina, leakage of feces via vagina

Types Of Fistula:-
There are several possible types of obstetric fistula. These include the following.
1. Vesicovaginal fistula (VVF), between the bladder and vagina
2. Urethrovaginal fistula (UVF), between the urethra (bladder outlet) and vagina
3. Ureterovaginal fistula, between the ureters (kidney tubes) and the vagina
4. Rectovaginal fistula (RVF), between the rectum and vagina.
5. Vesicouterine fistula, between the bladder and the uterus (womb)

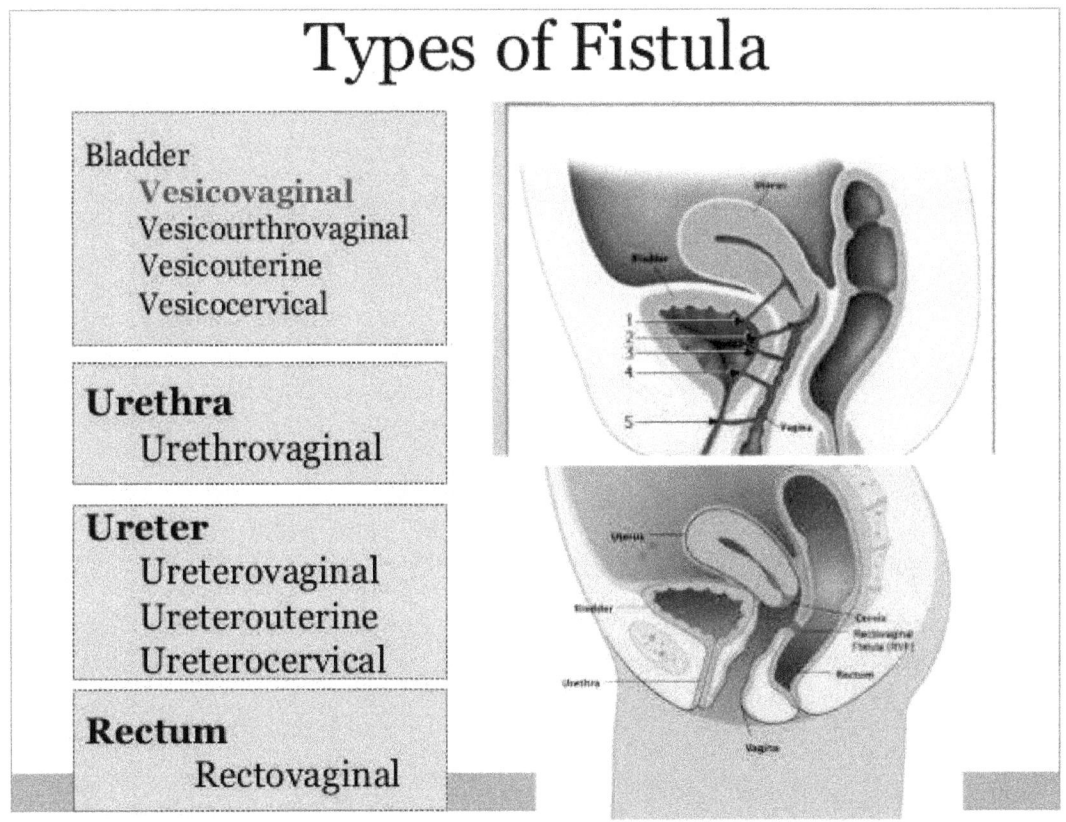

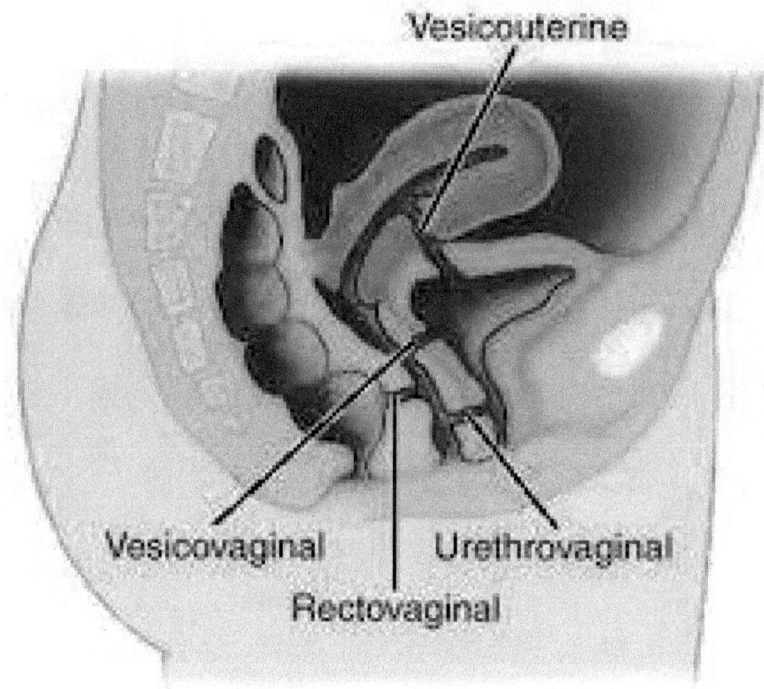

Aetiology:-

— Cancer or radiation treatment from cancer
— Poorly repaired episiotomy after a complicated delivery or injury during a caesarian section or destructive delivery).
— Coital trauma during forcefull intercourse
— Sexual violences / Rape
— Infection (specifically lymphogranuloma venereum)
— Female genital mutilation.
— Obstructed labour.
— LARGER babies, obstructed labour due to CPD.
— Poverty, illiteracy and lack of education about reproductive health, including family planning, nutrition And safe maternity care.

Clinical Features :-

In vascicovaginal fistula-

— -Incontinance of urine.
— -Uncontrolled passage of urine from vagina.
— -Excoriation of skin around the vulva.
— -Recurrent cystitis or UTI
— - Unexplained fever, hematuria, flank discomfort and suprapubic pain.

In rectocele-
- Flatulence and or fecal incontinence
- Foul-smelling vaginal discharge.
- Passing of flatus and stool through vagina.
- Vaginal noise while sitting or walking.

In every type-
- -Decubitus ulcers
- -Psychosocial problems- social recluse; depression, low self-esteem and insomnia.

Complications :-

here are many possible complications of obstetric fistula and/or complications of fistula repair and inch.
- Recurrent fistula that increases with complicated cases.
- Infections: wound, urinary tract infections,
- overactive bladder
- incomplete voiding.
- sexual problems
- obstruction to kidney drainage
- bladder contracture
- Vaginal narrowing, dysparenia
- Nerve complications (drop-foot)
- Psychological trauma
- Social isolation,
- Divorce .

OTHER Psychosocial Complications-
- Depression and anxiety
- Social isolation
- >50% of women with obstetric fistula have been abandoned by their husbands
- Depression and grief related to infertility
- Inability to concentration N work.
- Stigmatization.

Investigations- -
- Urine and stool leaking from vagina
- Contrast tests. A venography or a barium anema can help identity a fistula located in the upper rectum. These tests use a contrast material to show the bladder, vagina, bowel on an X-ray image

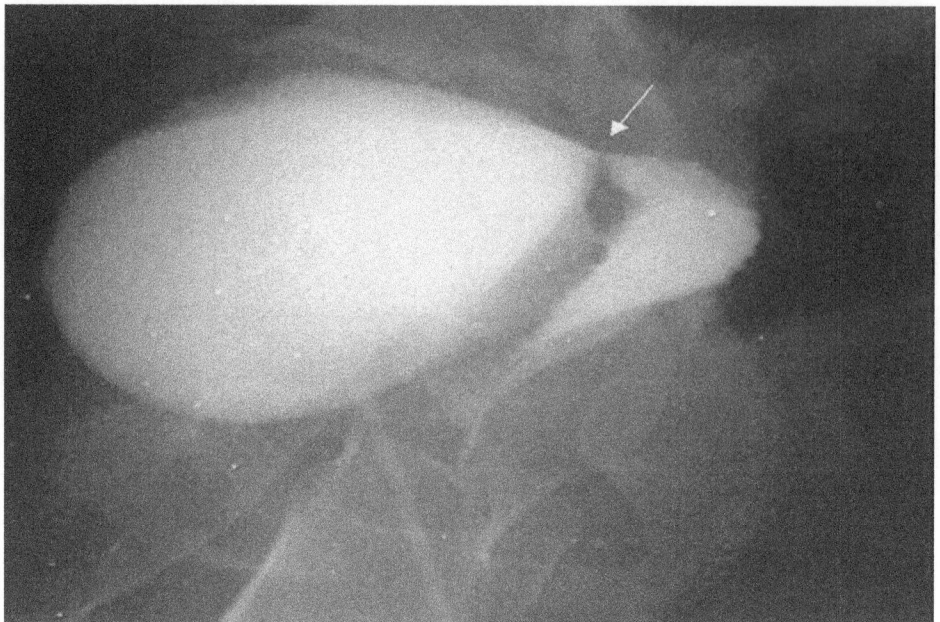

FIG. USG FISTULA

— Cystoscopy
— Rectoscopy
— Sigmoidoscopy

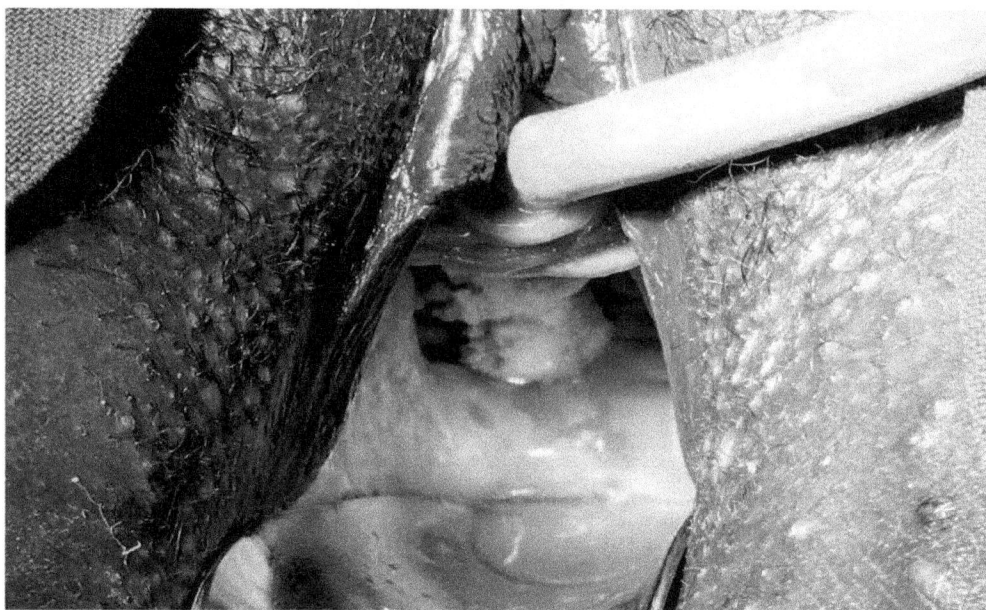

— Blue dye test. This test involvos placing a tampon into your vagina, then blue dye into your rectum in rectovaginal fistula and through urethra via catheter. Blue staining on the tampon indicates a fistula.
— Computerized tomography (CT) scan.
The CT scan can help locato a fistula and determine its cause.

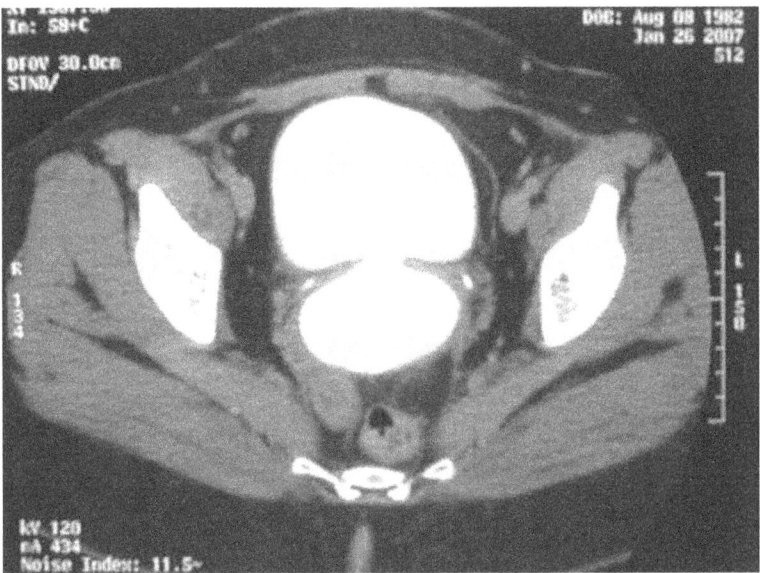

Fig. CT fistula

[filling of contrast in both uterus and bladder ,showing in between tract]

— Magnetic resonance imaging (MRI). This test creates images of soft tissues in your body MRI can show the location of a fistula, whether other pelvic organs are involved.

— Anorectal ultrasound.

— This test can evaluate the structure of your anal sphincter and may show childbirth-related injury

— Anorectal manometry. This test measures the sensitivity and function of rectum and can give information about the rectal sphincter and your ability to control stool . This test does not locate fistulas, but may help in planning the fistula repair

Management :-

— Sewing a fistula plug or patch of biologic tissue into the fistula allow your tissue to grow into the patch and heal the fistula.

— Using a tissue graft of healthy tissue over the fistula opening.

Homoeopathic Management :-

For VVF-

Involuntary passage of urine while laughing,walking and coughing.-nat mur, causticum, puls, arg.nit.

— nat.mur due to cystocele, vvf around climacteric age.

— causticum,due to bladder paralysis, sphincter weakness following birth injuries, surgical operations.

— pulsatilla, with supreesed menses at puberity.

— arg.nit,with great nervousness and examination funk.lack of detrusor muscle power.

Paralysis of bladder after fright- opium

For RVF-
- Berberis V.
— Constant urge to pass stool
— PaIn and burning anus and perineum (area betwoen the anus and vulva in women
— Symptoms aggravate on standing constant at one place for long and with compass movements during exercise
- Causticum-
— complaints due to muscular and sphincter paralysis.
— hard,knotty stool, greesy.
— Hard stool like sheeps dung.
— stool can pass only in standing position.
— Soreness and rawnwss of rectum with constant ineffectual desire.
- Silicea-

-Silicea works well for the treatment of abscesses, spasms, epilepsy and distended a bdomen .

-All types of fistula like anal fistula fistulous uker in breasts, boits arnd tstulours tracts under the skin.

-All diseases related to pus formation

-sensation as if sand in rectum.

-stools partially expels and partially recedes back,remains prolong into rectum,leads to constipation and piles.

-fistula alternate with chest complaints.[berb.,cal.phos]

-Strainng and stinging pain in rectum

-new moon, fullmoon aggravation,during washing

-Symptoms aggravated in cold weather, in the morning. -- However, the complaints improves in summer and it timid or wet weather.

Hydrastis Canadens-

Watery slimy mucus from rectum and vagina.
— Calcarea Phosphorica-
— Forgetfulness
— Weak digestion
— crawling sensati0n

- Symptoms worsen in cold and condition in the dry and warm weather and especially n summer

Nitricum Acid-

- Corroding ulcers with foul, acrid, offensive dicharhes, bleeding ulcers.
- decubitus ulcers and PID following fistulas.
- pungent,strong horse smelling urine.
- Pain while passing stool

Staphysagria-

- Staphysagria is used for the management of genito urinary conditions it works well in sensitive individuals who are easily annoyed and exhibit violent outbursts of passion.
- Honeymoon cystitis,UTI –FISTULAS FOLLOWING RECURRENT SEXUAL INTERCOURSE,FORCIBLE SEX OR RAPE.
- Sunken eyes and a tendency to get styes
- Colicky pain on being angry Bleeding gums and black crumbling teeth
- Constipation
- Hemorrhoids with stiching pains like with sharp object.
- Carbo Veg._
- Carbo vegetables is given to lary and sluggish people who are overweight or fat, hyperventilate patents
- like to have all the windows open.
- Hair fall with itchy scalp
- Sudden memory loss
- Heavy and constricted feeling in the head • Contracting pain in the stomach that extends up to the
- Bleeding from nose and gums
- Slow digestion resulting in rotting of food in stomach
- Inability to wear tight clothing
- Abdominal distention
- Itching and burning in rectum and porineum
- Burning in the anus area
- Bluish, burning piles with pain ater passing stool
- worsen in damp and warm weather in the evening and night, on consuming cold food, costly, butter or wine.
- Symptoms improve in cold, after burping

PAP Smear

Papanicolaou test=PAP TEST
A test that looks for abnormal cells in the cervix the presence of precancerous or cancerous cells

Alternate Names
- Papanicolaou Test
- Papanicolaou smear
- PAP Test
- Cervical Smear
- Cervical Screening

Types
- Smear Test two acceptable techniques for collecting the Pap Smear: liquid-based and conventional.

Indications for Pap Smears
- Women aged 21-65 should get a Pap smear every 3 years, or every 5 years if combined with an HPV test.
- Women who have had a hysterectomy with removal of the cervix do not need to get Pap smears.
- Women who have had the HPV vaccine still need to get Pap smears as the vaccine does not protect against all types of HPV.
- Women who have had abnormal Pap smear results in the past may need to get Pap smears more frequently.

Contraindications for Pap Smears
- Women who are pregnant should not get Pap smears as it can cause bleeding.
- Women who have had a total hysterectomy (removal of the uterus and cervix) do not need to get Pap smears.
- Women who have had a recent Pap smear (within the past 6 months) do not need to get another one.
- Women who have a bleeding disorder or are taking blood thinners should talk to their healthcare provider before getting a Pap smear.

CURRENT CERVICAL CANCER SCREENING RECOMMENDATIONS	
Age 20 or younger	No screening required
21-29	Pap test every 3 years; no HPV screening
30-65	Pap test every 3 years, or a Pap test and HPV test together every 5 years
66 or older	No more screening needed if you've had 3 normal Pap tests or 2 normal HPV tests in a row

Source: CDC

Contraindications & Risk Factors

There are no absolute contraindications for performing a PAP Smear other than the following:
- During menstruation
- Presence of active vaginal/cervical infection; treatment is needed before a PAP Smear is done

Investigations before the procedure

There are no other investigations required before performing a PAP Smear.

Pre procedure advice

The following are advised before performing the test:
Avoiding vaginal intercourse 48 hours before the test
- Avoiding douching 48 hours before the test
- Avoiding medicinal or contraceptive vaginal creams 48 hours before the test
- Avoiding the use of tampons 48 hours before the test

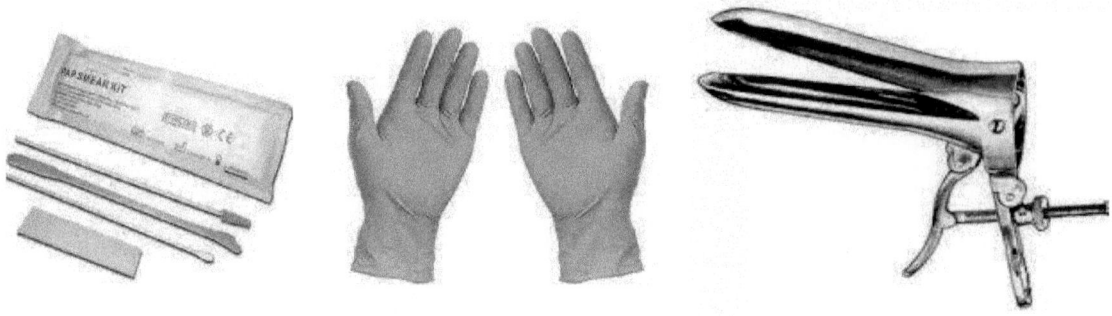

Instrument required-
Gloves
Gynae bed
Cusco speculum
Glass slides
Wooden spatula
Cytology brush
Cytology bud

Procedure Details
A Pap test is an outpatient procedure and does not need admission.
• **Anaesthesia:** No anaesthesia is required for a PAP test
Duration: This test takes 2-3 min to perform.
The individual is asked to lie on their back on the examination table with their feet in foot stirrups and the tailbone at the table's edge. A metal or a plastic speculum is placed in the vagina to examine the cervix. A cervical broom or spatula is placed on the cervix and rotated in one direction to obtain the cells from the cervix. A cervical brush and a spatula may also be used to get the cells from the cervix. The specimen obtained is transferred to a liquid cytology vial or a glass slide labelled and sent to a laboratory for microscopic examination.

Post-procedure advice
The procedure is performed on an outpatient basis, and the individual can leave immediately after and resume their normal activities. Interpretation of test results based on the presence of abnormal cells is done as -
Complications-
No major complications.
Mild pain   Scanty bleeding and discomfort
Result-

Bethesda Classification for cervical squamous cell dysplasia	
Smear Findings	Interpretation
Negative for intra-epithelial lesions or malignancy	Normal Smear
Atypical squamous cells of undetermined significance (ASCUS)	Abnormal squamous cells but do not meet the criteria for a squamous intra-epithelial lesion
Low-grade squamous intra-epithelial lesion (LSIL)	Mildly abnormal cells, changes attributable to HPV
High-grade squamous intra-epithelial lesions (HSIL) with features suspicious for invasion	Moderate to severely abnormal squamous cells
Carcinoma	The possibility of carcinoma is high enough to warrant evaluation

Limitations of conventional PAP smear

- False-negative results as high as 20-30% have been reported, which occurred due to clumping of cells when the cells are not uniformly spread on the glass slide.
- Sometimes, other contents of the cervical specimen such as blood, bacteria and yeasts contaminate the sample and prevent the detection of abnormal cells.
- If exposed to air for too long before being fixed on the slide, cervical cells can become distorted.

New technique – Liquid-Based Cytology (LBC

In order to minimize the number of false-negative results, Liquid Based Cytology is now the preferred method of sample collection where a cervical brush is used to
collect the specimen, which provides almost twice as many epithelial cells. The samples are collected directly in a preservative solution and slides are prepared meticulously avoiding any uneven manual smearing and thus reducing human error while interpretation. LBC has got a higher sensitivity and specificity than Pap smear as the cellular structure is better preserved because the cells are fixed immediately
Result sensitivity is higher than conventional PAP Smear .

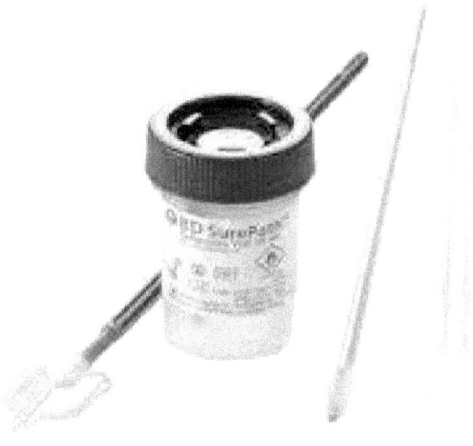

— cytology broom
— liquid base container & Plastic spatulA

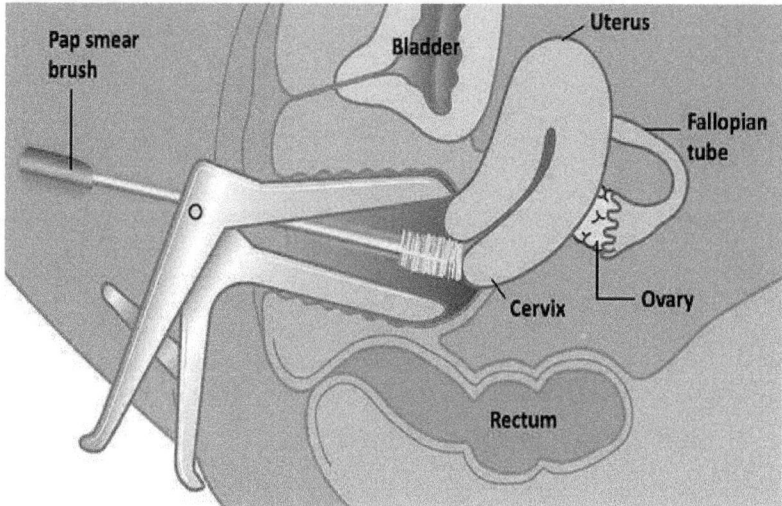

Peocedure Of PAP Smear

Pelvic Inflammatory Disease (PID)

Definition
Pelvic Inflammatory Disease (PID) is an **infection and inflammation of the female reproductive organs**, including the cervix, uterus, fallopian tubes, ovaries, and surrounding pelvic structures.

Types of PID
PID can be classified based on its cause and clinical presentation:

1. **Acute PID**
   - **Rapid onset** of severe symptoms like lower abdominal pain, fever, and vaginal discharge.
   - Commonly caused by Neisseria gonorrhoeae and Chlamydia trachomatis (STIs).
   - Requires **immediate medical treatment** to prevent complications.

2. **Chronic PID**
   - Long-standing infection with mild or intermittent symptoms.
   - Can be due to untreated or recurrent infections.
   - Leads to adhesions, scarring, and chronic pelvic pain.

3. **Subclinical PID**
   - Asymptomatic or mild symptoms that go unnoticed.
   - Diagnosed incidentally during infertility workup or laparoscopy.

Another classification according to part involved
Cervicitis
Endomeritis
Salphingitis
Ovaritis

Common Causes of PID
PID can be caused by infectious (organic) or non-infectious (non-organic) factors.

1. **Organic (Infectious) Causes**

Caused by bacteria, mainly sexually transmitted pathogens:

   A. **Sexually Transmitted Infections (STIs)**
   - **Neisseria gonorrhoeae** (gonorrhea) – Causes rapid, severe infection.
   - **Chlamydia trachomatis** (chlamydia) – More common, often asymptomatic.
   - **Mycoplasma genitalium** – Emerging cause of PID.

B. Non-STI Bacteria (Opportunistic Infections)
- **Escherichia coli** – Can ascend from the gastrointestinal tract.
- **Bacteroides, Peptostreptococcus, Gardnerella vaginalis** – Normal vaginal flora that become pathogenic in certain conditions.
- Actinomyces israelii – Associated with long-term intrauterine device (IUD) use.

C. Post-Procedure Infections
- Post-abortion or post-childbirth infections (especially after C-section).
- **After gynecological procedures** (e.g., hysteroscopy, IUD insertion, endometrial biopsy).

2. Non-Organic (Non-Infectious) Causes
These causes are less common but can mimic PID symptoms:
- **Endometriosis** – Ectopic endometrial tissue causing inflammation.
- **Pelvic Congestion Syndrome** – Due to varicose veins in the pelvis.
- **Foreign Body Reaction** – Due to retained tampon, IUD, or surgical material.

Common Clinical Features of PID
The symptoms vary depending on whether the infection is **acute, chronic, or subclinical**.

1. Acute PID
- Lower abdominal/pelvic pain (most common symptom).
- Fever (>38°C or 100.4°F).
- **Abnormal vaginal discharge** (purulent, foul-smelling).
- Pain during intercourse (dyspareunia).
- Painful urination (dysuria).
- Irregular menstrual bleeding.
- **Nausea and vomiting** (in severe cases).

2. Chronic PID
- Mild, persistent pelvic pain.
- Irregular menstrual cycles.
- Low-grade fever or malaise.
- Pain during intercourse and ovulation.
- Difficulty conceiving (infertility) due to tubal damage.

3. Subclinical PID
- Often **asymptomatic** or presents with mild, vague symptoms like:
  - Mild lower abdominal discomfort.
  - Unusual vaginal discharge.
  - Slight menstrual irregularities.

Complications of PID

If untreated, PID can lead to severe reproductive health issues:
1. **Infertility** – Scarring of fallopian tubes prevents fertilization.
2. **Ectopic Pregnancy** – Damaged tubes increase the risk of implantation outside the uterus.
3. **Chronic Pelvic Pain** – Due to adhesions and ongoing inflammation.
4. **Tubo-Ovarian Abscess (TOA)** – A pus-filled pocket that requires emergency treatment.
5. **Fitz-Hugh-Curtis Syndrome** – Perihepatitis causing **right upper quadrant pain** and adhesions between the liver and diaphragm.

Common Allopathic Management of PID

Treatment depends on **severity and cause**:

1. Mild to Moderate PID (Outpatient Treatment)

First-line antibiotics:
- Ceftriaxone (IM) + Doxycycline (oral) + Metronidazole (oral) for 14 days
- Alternative: Azithromycin instead of Doxycycline

2. Severe PID or Hospitalization (IV Therapy)
- Ceftriaxone IV + Doxycycline IV + Metronidazole IV
- If abscess or no response: Add **Clindamycin or Gentamicin**.

3. Surgical Management (if needed)
- Drainage of Tubo-Ovarian Abscess (TOA).
- Laparoscopic adhesiolysis for chronic pain.
- Hysterectomy (last resort) in severe cases.

Homeopathic Therapeutics for PID

Homeopathy focuses on reducing inflammation, improving immunity, and alleviating pain.

1. Acute PID Treatment
- **Belladonna** – Sudden onset with high fever, throbbing pain, and tenderness.
- **Apis Mellifica** – Pelvic inflammation with burning pain, swelling, and ovarian tenderness.
- **Arsenicum Album** – Restlessness, burning discharge, and exhaustion.

2. Chronic PID & Infertility
- **Sepia** – Deep pelvic pain, irregular menses, and hormonal imbalance.
- **Pulsatilla** – Mild, wandering pain with delayed or suppressed periods.
- **Thuja Occidentalis** – Chronic infections, history of STDs, and warty growths.

3. **PID with Heavy Discharge**
   - **Kreosotum** – Yellow, offensive-smelling vaginal discharge with itching.
   - **Medorrhinum** – Thick, fishy-smelling vaginal discharge with burning.
4. **Pelvic Pain and Adhesions**
   - **Lachesis** – Left-sided pain, intolerance to tight clothing.
   - **Cimicifuga** – Sharp, spasmodic pain in the uterus and ovaries.
   - **Platinum Metallicum** – Neuralgic pain with ovarian involvement.
5. **Post-Surgical or Post-IUD Infection**
   - **Hepar Sulphur** – Abscess formation, pus discharge, painful touch.
   - **Silicea** – Chronic suppuration, recurrent abscesses.

Comparative Table of Homeopathic Remedies PID-

Remedy	Indications
Sepia	Chronic cervicitis, yellow-green discharge, bearing-down sensation
Kreosotum	Offensive, acrid vaginal discharge causing itching and burning
Medorrhinum	Thick, fishy-smelling discharge, history of STDs
Natrum Mur	Excessive white discharge, dryness, worse after intercourse
Hydrastis Canadensis	Thick, ropy, tenacious yellow discharge, chronic inflammation
Borax	Profuse, white, albuminous discharge with burning pain
Cantharis	Intense burning pain during urination, raw inflamed cervix
Merc Sol	Profuse, purulent discharge with ulcers on cervix
Pulsatilla	Thick, creamy discharge, worsens with heat, better in open air
Thuja Occidentalis	Chronic cervicitis with warty growths, linked to HPV

Cervicitis

Definition

Cervicitis is the **inflammation of the cervix** (the lower part of the uterus that opens into the vagina), caused by **infections, irritants, or hormonal imbalances**. It can be **acute** or **chronic** and may lead to complications if untreated.

Types of Cervicitis

Cervicitis is classified into **infectious** and **non-infectious** causes:

1. Infectious Cervicitis

Caused by bacteria, viruses, fungi, or protozoa, often through **sexual transmission**.

- **Chlamydia trachomatis** – Most common bacterial cause.
- **Neisseria gonorrhoeae** – Leads to severe cervicitis.
- **Trichomonas vaginalis** – Protozoal infection causing irritation.
- Candida albicans – Fungal infection leading to candidal cervicitis.
- **Herpes Simplex Virus (HSV-2)** – Causes ulcerative cervicitis.
- **Human Papillomavirus (HPV)** – Can cause chronic cervicitis and cervical dysplasia.

2. **Non-Infectious Cervicitis**

Caused by chemical or mechanical irritation, such as:
- **Allergic reactions** – To spermicides, latex condoms, douches.
- Irritation from foreign bodies – Tampons, diaphragms, IUDs.
- **Hormonal changes** – Estrogen deficiency can lead to **atrophic cervicitis**.

Feature	Candidal Vaginitis	Trichomonal Vaginitis
Causative Agent	Candida albicans (fungus)	Trichomonas vaginalis (protozoa)
Mode of Transmission	Overgrowth of normal flora	Sexual contact
Discharge	Thick, white, "cottage cheese-like"	Frothy, greenish-yellow
Odor	Odorless	Foul-smelling, fishy odor
Vaginal pH	<4.5 (acidic)	>4.5 (alkaline)
Inflammation	Intense vaginal itching, erythema	Strawberry cervix (petechiae)
Associated Symptoms	Burning sensation, dysuria	Dysuria, dyspareunia
Microscopy	Budding yeast, pseudohyphae	Motile, flagellated protozoa
Treatment	Antifungals (fluconazole)	Metronidazole or tinidazole

Differentiating table between viral, bacterial, fungal, and parasitic cervicitis based on various key clinical features:

Feature	Viral Cervicitis	Bacterial Cervicitis	Fungal Cervicitis	Parasitic Cervicitis
Common Causes	- Herpes Simplex Virus (HSV)	- Neisseria gonorrhoeae (Gonorrhea)	- Candida albicans	- Trichomonas vaginalis

Feature	Viral Cervicitis	Bacterial Cervicitis	Fungal Cervicitis	Parasitic Cervicitis
	- Human Papillomavirus (HPV)	- Chlamydia trachomatis	- Other Candida species	- Entamoeba histolytica
Incubation Period	- 2–12 days for HSV	- 2–7 days for gonorrhea	- Few days to weeks	- 5–28 days (for Trichomoniasis)
Symptoms	- Painful ulcers or vesicles on cervix	- Yellow, purulent, foul-smelling discharge	- Thick, white, cheesy vaginal discharge	- Frothy, greenish-yellow vaginal discharge with a foul odor
	- Itching, burning, or discomfort during urination	- Lower abdominal pain, dysuria, and vaginal discharge	- Itching, irritation, burning sensation in the vagina	- Vaginal itching, burning, and discomfort during intercourse
	- Asymptomatic in some cases (HPV)	- Asymptomatic in some cases (Chlamydia)	- Often asymptomatic	- Often asymptomatic (especially in women)
Discharge Characteristics	- Clear, watery or bloody	- Purulent, thick, yellow, or greenish discharge	- Thick, white, clumpy, cottage cheese-like discharge	- Frothy, greenish-yellow, foul-smelling discharge
Pain	- Mild to moderate discomfort	- Pelvic pain, pain during intercourse, dysuria	- Vaginal itching or soreness, discomfort	- Burning, itching, and discomfort during intercourse
Vaginal pH	- Usually normal or slightly acidic	- Usually >4.5 (alkaline)	- pH >4.5, often mildly acidic	- pH >4.5 (alkaline)
Microscopic Examination	- Presence of **multinucleated**	**- Gram-negative diplococci,**	- Yeast cells or pseudohyphae	**- Trichomonads** (motile,

Feature	Viral Cervicitis	Bacterial Cervicitis	Fungal Cervicitis	Parasitic Cervicitis
	giant cells, viral inclusions	polymorphonuclear leukocytes		flagellated protozoa)
Laboratory Diagnosis	- PCR or culture for **HSV** or **HPV**	- Gram stain: Gonococci and Chlamydia culture	- **KOH prep** to identify **Candida**	- Wet mount microscopy for Trichomonas vaginalis
Systemic Symptoms	- Fever, malaise, headache (in severe cases)	- Fever, malaise, joint pain (in severe cases)	- Rarely systemic symptoms	- Rarely systemic symptoms
Treatment	- **Acyclovir** for HSV, **Vaccination** for HPV	- **Antibiotics** (e.g., Ceftriaxone, Azithromycin)	- Antifungal treatments (e.g., Fluconazole)	- Antiprotozoal medications (e.g., Metronidazole)
Complications	- Recurrent infections, **cervical cancer (HPV)**	- Pelvic Inflammatory Disease (PID), infertility	- Chronic vaginal infections, PID	- PID, premature birth, low birth weight
Prevention	- Safe sex, **vaccination** for HPV	- Safe sex, regular screening for **gonorrhea** and **chlamydia**	- Safe sex, proper hygiene	- Safe sex, regular screening for **Trichomoniasis**

Clinical Features of Cervicitis
- **Vaginal discharge** (purulent in bacterial infections, watery in viral infections).
- **Postcoital bleeding** (bleeding after intercourse).
- **Dysuria** (painful urination).
- Pelvic discomfort or lower abdominal pain.
- **Dyspareunia** (pain during intercourse).
- Cervical erythema, edema, and friability (bleeding on touch).

Complications of Cervicitis
1. **Pelvic Inflammatory Disease (PID)** – If untreated, infection ascends to the uterus and fallopian tubes.
2. **Infertility** – Due to damage to cervical mucus and scarring.

3. **Ectopic Pregnancy** – Tubal damage increases the risk.
4. **Chronic Pelvic Pain** – Due to persistent inflammation.
5. **Increased Risk of HIV and STIs** – Inflamed cervix is more susceptible to infections.

Diagnosis of Cervicitis

1. **Physical Examination**
   - Speculum Exam – Shows red, inflamed cervix with discharge.
   - Strawberry Cervix – Seen in Trichomonas infection.

2. **Laboratory Tests**
   - NAAT (Nucleic Acid Amplification Test) – Detects Chlamydia, Gonorrhea, Trichomonas.
   - Wet Mount Microscopy – Identifies Trichomonas (motile protozoa) or Candida (pseudohyphae).
   - pH Test – pH >4.5 suggests Trichomonas or Bacterial Vaginosis.
   - Pap Smear – Detects HPV-related changes.

Allopathic Management of Cervicitis

1. **Antibiotic Therapy (Based on Cause)**
   - **Chlamydia** → Doxycycline 100 mg BID x 7 days OR Azithromycin 1g single dose.
   - **Gonorrhea** → Ceftriaxone 500 mg IM + Doxycycline 100 mg BID x 7 days.
   - **Trichomonas** → Metronidazole 2g single dose OR 500 mg BID x 7 days.
   - **Candidiasis** → Fluconazole 150 mg single dose OR Clotrimazole vaginal tablets.

2. **Antiviral Therapy (For HSV)**
   - Acyclovir 400 mg TID x 7-10 days for herpes cervicitis.

3. **Symptomatic Management**
   - **NSAIDs (Ibuprofen)** – For pain and inflammation.
   - **Sitz baths** – To relieve discomfort.

Homeopathic Therapeutics for Cervicitis

1. **Belladonna**
   - Key Indications:
     - Acute inflammation of the cervix with throbbing pain.
     - Redness, heat, and swelling in the cervix and vaginal area.
     - Fever, headache, restlessness, and sensitivity to light.
     - Pain worsened by movement or touch.
     - Right-sided cervicitis.

- Best for: Acute infections, often associated with gonorrhea, chlamydia, or cervical trauma.

2. **Apis Mellifica**
   - Key Indications:
     - Swollen, inflamed cervix with a sensation of stinging pain.
     - Excessive vaginal discharge that is watery, yellowish, or milky.
     - Pain worse from warmth and relieved by cold applications.
     - Sensitive, sore vagina and cervix, worse with touch.
     - Burning sensations during urination.
   - Best for: Acute cervicitis with inflammation and swelling, often with infection.

3. **Mercurius Solubilis**
   - Key Indications:
     - Pus-like, yellow, foul-smelling discharge from the cervix.
     - Cervix is swollen, inflamed, and very sensitive to touch.
     - Excessive salivation, metallic taste in the mouth, and bad breath.
     - Night sweats with chronic infections.
       - Right-sided cervicitis.
   - Best for: Gonorrheal cervicitis or chronic infections with pus and foul-smelling discharge.

4. **Pulsatilla**
   - Key Indications:
     - Cervical pain, often with yellowish, non-irritating discharge.
     - Emotionally sensitive, weepy, and changeable mood.
     - Menstrual irregularities, scanty or delayed menses.
     - Pain shifting from one side of the cervix to the other.
       - Worse in warm rooms, better in fresh air.
   - Best for: Cervicitis due to hormonal changes, emotional upset, or vaginal infections.

5. **Nitric Acid**
   - Key Indications:
     - Severe, excoriating pain in the cervix, especially when touched or during intercourse.
     - Chronic discharge with foul odor, stinging pain, and ulceration in the cervix.
     - Burning and itching sensations, with a tendency to chronic irritation.
       - Pain radiating to the lower back.
   - Best for: Chronic cervicitis with ulceration and foul-smelling discharge.

Some other drugs-

1. **Acute Cervicitis (Infectious)**
   - **Medorrhinum** – For STDs with thick, offensive discharge.
   - **Cantharis** – Burning, painful urination with inflammation.
   - **Kreosotum** – Acrid, yellow, foul-smelling discharge.

2. **Chronic Cervicitis**
   - **Sepia** – Chronic cervicitis with **yellow-green discharge**, dragging pain.
   - **Hydrastis Canadensis** – Tenacious mucus, chronic inflammation.

3. **Cervicitis with Candida Infection**
   - **Borax** – Thick, white discharge with burning.
   - **Pulsatilla** – Creamy discharge, worsens with heat.

4. **Cervicitis with Trichomoniasis**
   - **Thuja Occidentalis** – Chronic, persistent cervicitis, linked to HPV.
   - **Natrum Mur** – Dryness, painful intercourse, excessive mucus.

5. **Cervicitis with Ulcers (Herpetic)**
   - **Merc Sol** – Ulceration, profuse discharge, offensive smell.
   - **Nitric Acid** – Sharp pains, fissures, offensive discharge.

Endometritis –

Definition

Endometritis is the **inflammation of the endometrium** (the inner lining of the uterus), typically caused by **infection**. It can be **acute** (sudden onset, severe symptoms) or **chronic** (long-standing, mild symptoms). It is commonly associated with **postpartum infections, sexually transmitted infections (STIs), or gynecological procedures**.

Types of Endometritis

1. **Acute Endometritis**
   - Rapid onset of symptoms such as fever, lower abdominal pain, and foul-smelling vaginal discharge.
   - Most commonly occurs **after childbirth (postpartum endometritis)**, miscarriage, or invasive procedures.
   - Usually caused by bacterial infections (polymicrobial).

2. **Chronic Endometritis**
   - Persistent low-grade inflammation of the endometrium.
   - Often linked to untreated STIs (Chlamydia, Gonorrhea) or tuberculosis.
   - Can cause infertility, recurrent miscarriages, and abnormal uterine bleeding.

Causes of Endometritis

1. **Infectious Causes (Organic)**
   - **Postpartum Infection** – Occurs after vaginal delivery or **C-section**.
   - STIs – Chlamydia trachomatis, Neisseria gonorrhoeae, Mycoplasma hominis.
   - Polymicrobial Infections – Escherichia coli, Bacteroides, Streptococcus, Peptostreptococcus.
   - **Tuberculosis (TB Endometritis)** – Chronic, often associated with pelvic TB.
   - **Post-Abortion Infection** – Due to incomplete evacuation of products of conception.
   - **Intrauterine Device (IUD) Infections** – Can cause chronic low-grade inflammation.

2. **Non-Infectious Causes (Non-Organic)**
   - **Chemical Irritants** – Douches, contraceptive creams.
   - **Foreign Bodies** – Retained fetal tissue, IUD, surgical material.
   - **Autoimmune Conditions** – Chronic inflammatory diseases affecting the endometrium.

Clinical Features of Endometritis

1. **Acute Endometritis**
   - Fever (>100.4°F or 38°C).
   - **Lower abdominal pain** (cramping, tenderness).
   - Foul-smelling vaginal discharge (yellow, green, or brown).
   - Heavy or prolonged menstrual bleeding.
   - Painful intercourse (dyspareunia).
   - Malaise, nausea, and vomiting (severe cases).

2. **Chronic Endometritis**
   - Mild pelvic pain.
   - Intermenstrual spotting or irregular bleeding.
   - Infertility or repeated miscarriages.
   - Vague discomfort and mild fever.
   - No significant discharge or foul odor (in many cases).

Complications of Endometritis

1. **Pelvic Inflammatory Disease (PID)** – Infection spreads to fallopian tubes and ovaries.
2. **Infertility** – Chronic inflammation causes scarring and adhesions.
3. **Septicemia (Sepsis)** – If untreated, infection spreads to the bloodstream.
4. **Adhesions and Asherman's Syndrome** – Scar tissue formation inside the uterus.

5. **Ectopic Pregnancy** – Damaged endometrium increases the risk.

Diagnosis of Endometritis

1. **Clinical Examination**
   - Speculum Exam – Shows tender uterus, cervical motion tenderness, purulent discharge.
   - Bimanual Pelvic Exam – Detects uterine tenderness and enlargement.

2. **Laboratory Tests**
   - CBC (Complete Blood Count) – Elevated WBC count suggests infection.
   - **Endometrial Biopsy** – Confirms **chronic endometritis** by detecting plasma cells.
   - Vaginal and Cervical Swabs – Tests for Chlamydia, Gonorrhea, Mycoplasma.
   - **Blood Cultures** – If sepsis is suspected.
   - PCR Tests (for Tuberculosis Endometritis) – Used in endemic areas.

3. **Imaging Studies**
   - Ultrasound (USG) – Detects thickened endometrium, retained tissue, or fluid collection.
   - **Hysteroscopy** – Visualizes chronic inflammatory changes and adhesions.

Allopathic Management of Endometritis

1. **Antibiotic Therapy (Based on Cause)**
   - Mild to Moderate Cases (Oral Therapy)
     - Doxycycline 100 mg BID x 14 days (for Chlamydia).
     - Azithromycin 1g single dose (alternative to doxycycline).
     - Metronidazole 500 mg BID x 14 days (for anaerobic bacteria).
   - Severe Cases (IV Therapy & Hospitalization)
     - **Clindamycin + Gentamicin IV** (for polymicrobial infection).
     - **Ampicillin-Sulbactam IV** (for postpartum endometritis).

2. **Antiviral Therapy (For HSV Endometritis)**
   - Acyclovir 400 mg TID x 7-10 days.

3. **Tuberculosis Endometritis**
   - Anti-TB Therapy (ATT) for 6 months.

4. **Surgical Management**
   - **Dilation and Curettage (D&C)** – For retained fetal tissue.
   - **Hysteroscopic Adhesiolysis** – For chronic endometritis with adhesions.

Homeopathic Management of Endometritis

1. **Pulsatilla**
   - Key Indications:
     - Painful, delayed menses with a heavy or scanty flow.
     - Thick, yellowish, or greenish discharge with cramping pain.
     - Emotional, tearful, and weepy, especially before or after menstruation.
     - Worse in warm rooms, better in fresh air.
   - Best for: Endometritis with hormonal imbalances, especially in young girls or women with delayed or painful periods.

2. **Belladonna**
   - Key Indications:
     - Acute endometrial inflammation with severe throbbing pain in the lower abdomen.
     - High fever, pulsations, and swelling in the pelvic area.
     - Extreme sensitivity to touch or movement.
     - Thirst, dry mouth, and hot, flushed skin.
   - Best for: Acute infections of the endometrium with fever, swelling, and sharp pain. Typically linked to bacterial causes.

3. **Lachesis**
   - Key Indications:
     - Chronic endometritis with heavy menstrual bleeding, and dark, offensive discharge.
     - Left-sided pelvic pain, often associated with severe cramping.
     - Menorrhagia with bloody discharge and pelvic congestion.
     - Sensitive to touch around the abdomen, especially tight clothing.
   - Best for: Chronic endometrial inflammation, heavy periods, and pelvic congestion.

4. **Kali Carbonicum**
   - Key Indications:
     - Deep, aching pain in the lower abdomen, aggravated by walking or standing.
     - Pelvic heaviness, worse before menstruation.
     - Delayed menstruation, dark-colored discharge with extreme weakness.
     - Better by resting and applying warmth.
   - Best for: Chronic endometritis with deep, aching pain and irregular menses.

5. **Mercurius Solubilis**
   - Key Indications:
     - Foul-smelling, yellowish vaginal discharge, with excessive sweating.

- Painful menstruation with a profuse, offensive discharge.
- Cervical erosion, ulceration, and tenderness.
- Night sweats, foul breath, and metallic taste.
- Best for: Chronic endometritis, especially if associated with STIs or persistent infections.

Some other drugs-

1. **Acute Endometritis (Infectious Cases)**
   - **Belladonna** – Sudden high fever, throbbing pelvic pain.
   - **Kreosotum** – Profuse, acrid vaginal discharge causing **severe irritation**.
   - **Arsenicum Album** – Weakness, burning pains, foul-smelling lochia.

2. **Chronic Endometritis (With Infertility)**
   - **Sepia** – Prolonged inflammation, painful intercourse, yellow-green discharge.
   - **Hydrastis Canadensis** – Persistent mucus discharge, chronic inflammation.
   - **Pulsatilla** – Creamy, thick discharge, worsens with heat.

3. **Endometritis with Heavy Discharge**
   - **Merc Sol** – Purulent, offensive-smelling discharge.
   - **Sulphur** – Recurring endometrial inflammation, itching, burning.

4. **Postpartum Endometritis**
   - **Arsenicum Album** – Foul-smelling lochia, exhaustion.
   - **Cantharis** – Intense burning pain, frequent urination.

5. **Endometritis with Ulceration (Herpetic or HPV-related)**
   - **Thuja Occidentalis** – Warty growths, chronic infections.
   - **Nitric Acid** – Sharp, stitching pains, ulcers on cervix.

Salphingitis –

Definition

Salpingitis is the inflammation of one or both fallopian tubes, usually caused by a bacterial infection. It is a major cause of tubal factor infertility and can lead to ectopic pregnancy, chronic pelvic pain, and pelvic inflammatory disease (PID) if untreated.

Types of Salpingitis

1. **Acute Salpingitis**
   - Rapid onset of symptoms, including fever, pelvic pain, and purulent vaginal discharge.
   - Usually caused by bacterial infections such as Chlamydia trachomatis and Neisseria gonorrhoeae.

2. **Chronic Salpingitis**
   - **Long-term, low-grade inflammation** with mild or intermittent symptoms.
   - Leads to tubal scarring, adhesions, and infertility.
   - Often asymptomatic until complications arise.

Causes of Salpingitis

1. **Infectious Causes (Organic)**
   - Sexually Transmitted Infections (STIs)
     - **Chlamydia trachomatis** – Most common cause of salpingitis.
     - **Neisseria gonorrhoeae** – Leads to severe purulent inflammation.
     - Mycoplasma hominis & Ureaplasma urealyticum – Can cause chronic salpingitis.
   - Non-STI Infections
     - **Escherichia coli** – Postpartum or post-abortion infections.
     - **Bacteroides & Peptostreptococcus** – Anaerobic bacteria from vaginal flora.
     - **Mycobacterium tuberculosis** – Tuberculous salpingitis, common in endemic areas.
   - Post-Surgical & Postpartum Infections
     - Following gynecological procedures – D&C, hysteroscopy, IUD placement.

2. **Non-Infectious Causes (Non-Organic)**
   - **Endometriosis** – Endometrial tissue in the tubes causes chronic inflammation.
   - **Chemical Irritants** – Douching, intrauterine contraceptive devices (IUDs).
   - **Pelvic Congestion Syndrome** – Chronic inflammation due to venous stasis.

Clinical Features of Salpingitis

1. **Acute Salpingitis**
   - **Lower abdominal pain** (bilateral, dull or sharp).
   - Fever (>38°C or 100.4°F).
   - **Purulent vaginal discharge** (yellow, green, or foul-smelling).
   - Dyspareunia (pain during intercourse).
   - Dysuria (painful urination).
   - **Nausea & vomiting** (in severe infections).
   - **Cervical motion tenderness** (on bimanual examination).

2. **Chronic Salpingitis**
   - Mild or intermittent pelvic pain.
   - **Irregular menstruation** (spotting, prolonged periods).
   - **Infertility** (due to tubal blockage).
   - Low-grade fever, malaise.

Complications of Salpingitis

1. **Pelvic Inflammatory Disease (PID)** – Infection spreads to uterus and ovaries.
2. **Tubal Infertility** – Chronic inflammation causes fibrosis and tubal obstruction.
3. **Ectopic Pregnancy** – Damaged tubes prevent normal implantation in the uterus.
4. **Tubo-Ovarian Abscess (TOA)** – Collection of pus in fallopian tubes and ovaries.
5. **Peritonitis** – If infection spreads into the peritoneal cavity.

Diagnosis of Salpingitis

1. Clinical Examination

- Bimanual Pelvic Exam – Reveals tender fallopian tubes, cervical motion tenderness.
- Speculum Exam – Purulent cervical discharge.

2. Laboratory Tests

- Complete Blood Count (CBC) – Elevated WBC count (suggests infection).
- Cervical/Vaginal Swabs – NAAT for Chlamydia, Gonorrhea, Mycoplasma.
- **Blood Cultures** – If sepsis is suspected.

3. Imaging Studies

- Transvaginal Ultrasound (TVUS) – Detects fluid-filled fallopian tubes, abscesses.
- Hysterosalpingography (HSG) – Checks for tubal blockage in chronic cases.
- **MRI/CT Scan** – Used if complications like **tubo-ovarian abscess** are suspected.
- Laparoscopy – Gold standard for definitive diagnosis, detects tubal adhesions.

Allopathic Management of Salpingitis

1. **Antibiotic Therapy (Based on Cause)**
   - Mild to Moderate Cases (Oral Therapy)
     - Doxycycline 100 mg BID x 14 days (for Chlamydia).
     - **Azithromycin 1g single dose** (alternative to doxycycline).
     - Metronidazole 500 mg BID x 14 days (for anaerobic bacteria).
   - Severe Cases (IV Therapy & Hospitalization)
     - Ceftriaxone 1g IV + Doxycycline + Metronidazole.
     - **Gentamicin + Clindamycin IV** (for polymicrobial infections).

2. **Tuberculosis Salpingitis**
   - Anti-TB Therapy (ATT) for 6 months.

3. **Surgical Management**
   - **Laparoscopic Drainage** – If tubo-ovarian abscess is present.
   - **Salpingectomy** – Removal of irreversibly damaged tubes.

Homeopathic Therapeutics for Salpingitis

1. **Apis Mellifica**
   - Key Indications:
     - Pain and swelling in the pelvic region, especially in the lower abdomen.
     - Right-sided or bilateral salpingitis with stinging pain.
     - Pain worse from heat and better from cold.
     - Thirstless, swollen abdomen, frequent urination.
   - Best for: Acute or subacute salpingitis with swelling and stinging pain.

2. **Belladonna**
   - Key Indications:
     - Sudden, intense, throbbing pain in the lower abdomen and pelvis.
     - Fever, hot flashes, and sensitive abdomen.
     - Pain worsens with touch or motion.
     - Thirst, dryness of mouth, and restlessness.
   - Best for: Acute salpingitis with fever, severe pain, and heat.

3. **Lachesis**
   - Key Indications:
     - Sharp, left-sided salpingitis with pain extending to the thighs.
     - Chronic pelvic congestion, dark, offensive discharge, and heavy menstruation.
     - Irritable, intolerant to tight clothing.
     - Pain worse after sleep and better with profuse discharge.
   - Best for: Chronic salpingitis, pelvic congestion, and irregular, heavy periods.

4. **Mercurius Solubilis**
   - Key Indications:
     - Profuse, yellowish, foul-smelling vaginal discharge.
     - Pelvic tenderness, especially bilateral.
     - Pain and swelling in the fallopian tubes with night sweats.
     - Swollen, inflamed cervix, and painful menstruation.
   - Best for: Chronic salpingitis with pus-like discharge and systemic symptoms like sweating.

5. **Pulsatilla**
   - Key Indications:
     - Cyclic, cramp-like pain in the lower abdomen, especially during menstruation.
     - Yellowish, non-irritating discharge and pain shifting sides.
     - Worse in warm rooms, better in fresh air.
     - Emotionally sensitive, tears easily, and mood swings.

- Best for: Salpingitis due to emotional stress, hormonal imbalance, or chronic infections

More Homeopathic drugs in Management of Salpingitis

1. **Acute Salpingitis (Infectious Cases)**
   - Belladonna – Sudden high fever, throbbing pelvic pain.
   - **Kreosotum** – Profuse, acrid vaginal discharge causing **severe irritation**.
   - Arsenicum Album – Weakness, burning pains, foul-smelling discharge.

2. **Chronic Salpingitis (With Infertility)**
   - Sepia – Dragging pain, yellow-green discharge, sterility.
   - Hydrastis Canadensis – Persistent mucus discharge, chronic inflammation.
   - Pulsatilla – Creamy, thick discharge, worse with heat.

3. **Salpingitis with Heavy Discharge**
   - Merc Sol – Purulent, offensive-smelling discharge.
   - Sulphur – Recurring endometrial inflammation, itching, burning.

4. **Postpartum or Post-Abortion Salpingitis**
   - Arsenicum Album – Foul-smelling lochia, exhaustion.
   - Cantharis – Intense burning pain, frequent urination.

5. **Salpingitis with Ulceration (Tuberculous or HPV-related)**
   - Thuja Occidentalis – Warty growths, chronic infections.
   - Nitric Acid – Sharp, stitching pains, ulcers on cervix.

Ovaritis –

Definition

Ovaritis (oophoritis) is the inflammation of one or both ovaries, often caused by bacterial, viral, or autoimmune factors. It is commonly associated with Pelvic Inflammatory Disease (PID), mumps virus, or chronic inflammatory conditions. If untreated, it may lead to ovarian abscess, infertility, and hormonal imbalances.

Types of Ovaritis

1. **Acute Ovaritis**
   - Sudden onset of severe lower abdominal pain.
   - Often due to bacterial infections, especially STIs (Chlamydia, Gonorrhea).
   - May be associated with high fever, nausea, and purulent discharge.

2. **Chronic Ovaritis**
   - Long-standing, low-grade inflammation of the ovaries.
   - Leads to infertility, irregular menstrual cycles, and pelvic pain.

- Often occurs after repeated infections or autoimmune disorders.

3. **Autoimmune Oophoritis**
   - Immune system attacks ovarian tissue, leading to ovarian failure.
   - Associated with Addison's disease, thyroid disorders, and premature ovarian insufficiency (POI).

Causes of Ovaritis

1. **Infectious Causes (Organic)**
   - Sexually Transmitted Infections (STIs)
     - **Chlamydia trachomatis** – Most common bacterial cause.
     - **Neisseria gonorrhoeae** – Causes purulent inflammation.
     - Mycoplasma hominis & Ureaplasma urealyticum – Can cause chronic infection.
   - Post-Surgical & Postpartum Infections
     - D&C, C-section, IUD placement, or abortion.
   - Mumps Virus (Viral Oophoritis)
     - Occurs in post-pubertal females, can lead to ovarian atrophy.
   - Tuberculosis (TB Oophoritis)
     - Seen in **pelvic TB cases**, causes chronic inflammation and **ovarian fibrosis**.

2. **Non-Infectious Causes (Non-Organic)**
   - **Autoimmune Disorders** – Hashimoto's thyroiditis, Addison's disease.
   - **Endometriosis** – Ectopic endometrial tissue in the ovary causing inflammation.
   - **Chemical Irritants** – Reaction to contraceptive devices or medications.

Clinical Features of Ovaritis

1. **Acute Ovaritis**
   - Severe lower abdominal pain, worsened with movement.
   - Fever (>38°C or 100.4°F).
   - **Purulent vaginal discharge** (yellow, green, or foul-smelling).
   - Pain during intercourse (dyspareunia).
   - Nausea, vomiting, malaise (in severe infections).

2. **Chronic Ovaritis**
   - Intermittent, dull pelvic pain.
   - **Menstrual irregularities** (prolonged/heavy periods, spotting).
   - Infertility due to ovarian dysfunction.
   - Hormonal imbalances (low estrogen, high FSH in autoimmune cases).

Complications of Ovaritis

1. Ovarian Abscess – Can rupture, causing peritonitis.
2. Infertility – Chronic inflammation damages ovarian tissue.
3. Ovarian Cysts or Fibrosis – Due to chronic infection or autoimmune damage.
4. Hormonal Imbalance & Premature Ovarian Failure (POF).
5. Ectopic Pregnancy – Due to damage to ovarian and tubal structures.

Diagnosis of Ovaritis

1. Clinical Examination
- Pelvic Exam – Reveals tender ovaries, cervical motion tenderness.
- Speculum Exam – Purulent cervical discharge (if STI-related).

2. Laboratory Tests
- CBC (Complete Blood Count) – Elevated WBC count (suggests infection).
- Cervical & Vaginal Swabs – Tests for STIs (Chlamydia, Gonorrhea, Mycoplasma).
- Autoimmune Panel – If autoimmune oophoritis is suspected.
- Anti-Müllerian Hormone (AMH) & FSH Tests – Assess ovarian function.

3. Imaging Studies
- Transvaginal Ultrasound (TVUS) – Detects ovarian abscess, cysts, or fluid collection.
- MRI/CT Scan – Used in suspected cases of autoimmune or chronic oophoritis.
- Laparoscopy – Gold standard for definitive diagnosis, helps identify adhesions, abscesses, or fibrosis.

Allopathic Management of Ovaritis

1. Antibiotic Therapy (Based on Cause)
- Mild to Moderate Cases (Oral Therapy)
    - Doxycycline 100 mg BID x 14 days (for Chlamydia).
    - **Azithromycin 1g single dose** (alternative to doxycycline).
    - Metronidazole 500 mg BID x 14 days (for anaerobic bacteria).
- Severe Cases (IV Therapy & Hospitalization)
    - Ceftriaxone 1g IV + Doxycycline + Metronidazole.
    - **Gentamicin + Clindamycin IV** (for polymicrobial infections).

2. Autoimmune Oophoritis Management
- **Corticosteroids** – Prednisone to reduce inflammation.
- **Hormone Replacement Therapy (HRT)** – For premature ovarian insufficiency.

3. Surgical Management
- **Ovarian Drainage** – If abscess is present.

- **Oophorectomy (Ovary Removal)** – In severe, non-responsive cases.

Dosage & Potency Guidelines

Remedy	Potency	Dosage
Belladonna	30C–200C	3-4 times daily (acute)
Apis Mellifica	30C–200C	3 times daily (acute)
Arsenicum Album	30C	Every 4-6 hours
Sepia	200C	Once daily (chronic)
Pulsatilla	30C–200C	1-2 times daily
Lachesis	200C	Once daily (chronic)
Bryonia	30C–200C	3 times daily
Kali Carbonicum	200C	Weekly dose
Thuja	200C	Once daily (chronic)
Tuberculinum	1M	Once a month
Ignatia	30C	2-3 times daily
Staphysagria	30C	2-3 times daily

Pelvic Pains

Aetiology-

Endometriosis

In endometriosis, cells that normally line the inside of the uterus (the endometrium) grow inappropriately outside on organs such as the ovaries, bladder, or rectum.

Symptoms you may have:
- Pelvic pain or cramps before or during your period
- Pain during or after sex
- Pain when you ovulate
- Painful bowel movements
- Rectal bleeding during your period
- Pain when you urinate
- Lower back pain
- Infertility
- Spotting between periods
- Bloating in your abdomen

Adenomyosis

This condition is similar to endometriosis. Cells that normally line your uterus (the endometrium) invade the muscle tissue of the uterus wall (the myometrium). Many women with adenomyosis don't have any symptoms.

Symptoms you may have:
- Pain during your period
- Feeling of pressure on your bladder or rectum
- Heavy periods
- Periods that last longer than usual
- Spotting between periods

Interstitial Cystitis

Women with interstitial cystitis have an inflamed bladder. The inflammation is not caused by an infection. This condition tends to affect women in their 30s and 40s.

Symptoms you may have:
- You need to urinate very often
- Often feeling an urgent need to urinate
- Discomfort when you urinate
- Pain during sex

Urinary Tract Infection

Bacteria are usually the cause of urinary tract infections. Infections can involve any part of the urinary tract, including the kidneys, bladder, and urethra. Urinary tract infections are much more common in women than in men.

Symptoms you may have:
- Feeling pressure in your lower pelvis
- Pain or a burning sensation when you urinate
- Needing to urinate often
- Often feeling an urgent need to urinate
- Needing to get up at night to urinate
- Cloudy urine
- Blood in urine
- Urine has strong or bad smell
- Only a trickle of urine comes out
- Lower back pain

Pelvic Inflammatory Disease

This is an infection of the uterus, fallopian tubes, or ovaries that causes them to become inflamed and infected. Most often, it is a sexually transmitted bacterial infection, like gonorrhea or chlamydia. These bacteria enter the uterus through the vagina and leave the fallopian tubes to infect surrounding organs like the ovaries. Scars left by the infection may cause chronic pelvic pain; however, more commonly the pain is acute.

Symptoms you may have:
- Vaginal discharge having an unusual color, texture, or odor
- Abdominal or pelvic pain in a specific area or more widespread
- Pain during sex
- Irregular or missed periods
- Menstrual cramps that are worse than usual
- Frequent need to urinate
- Pain when you urinate
- Pain when you ovulate
- It hurts when you press on certain areas of your pelvis
- Lower back pain
- Fatigue
- Fever
- Nausea

Pelvic Congestion Syndrome

Pelvic congestion is just like the varicose veins that some women have in their legs, but it affects the veins of the pelvis. Blood backs up in the veins, making them become enlarged and engorged. Pelvic congestion causes chronic pelvic pain in some women.

Symptoms you may have:
- Pain starts 7-10 days before your period
- Pelvic pain is worse when you sit or stand
- Lying down relieves pelvic pain
- Lower back pain
- Aches in your legs
- Pain during sex

Irritable Bowel Syndrome

Chronic pelvic pain sometimes isn't only due to problems with reproductive organs or the urinary tract; other organs in the pelvic area, if "diseased," can present as pelvic pain. Irritable bowel syndrome, an intestinal condition that often causes pain, may be the cause.

Symptoms you may have:
- Diarrhea
- Constipation
- Incontinence
- Flatulence
- Bloating
- Pain relieved by a bowel movement

Uterine Fibroids

Fibroids are noncancerous tumors that grow in, and on, the wall of the uterus. Not all women who have them notice symptoms, but for some, fibroids can be painful.

Symptoms you may have:
- Heavy periods
- Feeling pressure or fullness in your abdomen
- Need to urinate frequently
- Pain or cramps during your period
- Constipation
- Hemorrhoids

Tubo ovarian mass
- Mostly one sided
- Always along with palpable mass on abdominal examination
- Associated pressure symptoms like frequent urination, retension of urine, bowel irritation, indigestion etc. present

- Bearing down sensation may be present in huge mass
- Senasation as if something live, moving thing in abdomen
- Sudden acute pain episodes may present with sudden twisting of tumours
- Ca 125 raises in chocolate cyst or Cancer of ovary
- If fluid containing is called cystic.

Levator Syndrome

Sometimes, spasms of a pelvic muscle called the "levator ani" cause pelvic pain.
Symptoms you may have:
- Pain is related to sitting
- Pain doesn't seem to be related to bowel movements
- You wake up at night in pain
- Pain usually lasts less than 20 minutes at a time

Pelvic Support Problems

Sometimes women have pelvic pain when the muscles and ligaments that hold organs in place weaken. This causes organs like the uterus, the bladder, or the rectum to move from their normal places and herniate into the vagina. The vagina may also change shape. Pregnancy and giving birth may cause these kinds of problems.
Symptoms you may have:
- Leaking urine
- Feeling like something is falling out of your vagina
- Difficulty with bowel movements
- Lower back pain
- Pain during sex
- Pelvic organs bulge into the vagina, or even stick out the vaginal opening, in severe cases

Vulvodynia

Vulvodynia is pain that affects the vulva for no apparent reason. The pain of vulvodynia may be constant or it may come and go.
Symptoms you may have:
- Burning or stinging sensations in the vulva
- Pain when something presses on the vulva, like during sex or when you straddle a seat
- Pain in your inner thighs

Pelvic Adhesions-
- In PID
- ENDOMETROISIS

- Retroverted uterus
- Tuberculosis
- Uterine cancer
- Post operative

Psychological Causes

For some women, the root of pelvic pain is psychological. That's not to say that the pain isn't real. There just isn't an identifiable physical cause. Some people have emotional problems that only show up as physical symptoms. Women who have suffered sexual abuse or assault often have chronic pelvic pain afterward.

Symptoms you may have:
- Depression
- Anxiety
- Substance abuse
- Stress

OTHER CAUSES –

Appendicitis, Diverticulitis, Gaseous distention, Renal colic.

Diagnosis

- **Pelvic exam.** This can reveal signs of infection, abnormal growths or tense pelvic floor muscles. Your doctor checks for areas of tenderness. Let your doctor know if you feel any discomfort during this exam, especially if the pain is similar to the pain you've been experiencing.
- **Lab tests.** During the pelvic exam, your doctor may order labs to check for infections, such as chlamydia or gonorrhea. Your doctor may also order bloodwork to check your blood cell counts and urinalysis to check for a urinary tract infection.
- **Ultrasound.** This test uses high-frequency sound waves to produce precise images of structures within your body. This procedure is especially useful for detecting masses or cysts in the ovaries, uterus or fallopian tubes.
- **Other imaging tests.** Your doctor may recommend abdominal X-rays, computerized tomography (CT) scans or magnetic resonance imaging (MRI) to help detect abnormal structures or growths.
- **Laparoscopy.** During this surgical procedure, your doctor makes a small incision in your abdomen and inserts a thin tube attached to a small camera (laparoscope). The laparoscope allows your doctor to view your pelvic organs and check for abnormal tissues or signs of infection. This procedure is especially useful in detecting endometriosis and chronic pelvic inflammatory disease.
- **Pap smear-** To rule out PID, cervical erosion, cancerous cause of pelvic pain

Management

Medications

- **Pain relievers.** Over-the-counter pain remedies, such as aspirin, ibuprofen (Advil, Motrin IB, others) or acetaminophen (Tylenol, others), may provide partial relief from your pelvic pain. Sometimes a prescription pain reliever may be necessary. Pain medication alone, however, rarely solves the problem of chronic pain.
- **Hormone treatments.** Some women find that the days when they have pelvic pain may coincide with a particular phase of their menstrual cycle and the hormonal changes that control ovulation and menstruation. When this is the case, birth control pills or other hormonal medications may help relieve pelvic pain.
- **Antibiotics.** If an infection is the source of your pain, your doctor may prescribe antibiotics.
- **Antidepressants.** Some types of antidepressants can be helpful for chronic pain. Tricyclic antidepressants, such as amitriptyline, nortriptyline (Pamelor) and others, seem to have pain-relieving as well as antidepressant effects. They may help improve chronic pelvic pain even in women who don't have depression.

Other therapies

for chronic pelvic pain

- **Physical therapy.** Stretching exercises, massage and other relaxation techniques may improve your chronic pelvic pain. A physical therapist can assist you with these therapies and help you develop coping strategies for the pain. Sometimes physical therapists target specific points of pain using a medical instrument called transcutaneous electrical nerve stimulation (TENS). TENS delivers electrical impulses to nearby nerve pathways. Physical therapists may also use a psychology technique called biofeedback, which helps you identify areas of tight muscles so that you can learn to relax those areas.
- **Neurostimulation (spinal cord stimulation).** This treatment involves implanting a device that blocks nerve pathways so that the pain signal can't reach the brain. It may be helpful, depending on the cause of your pelvic pain.
- **Trigger point injections.** If your doctor finds specific points where you feel pain, you may benefit from having a numbing medicine injected into those painful spots (trigger points). The medicine, usually a long-acting local anesthetic, can block pain and ease discomfort.
- **Psychotherapy.** If your pain could be intertwined with depression, sexual abuse, a personality disorder, a troubled marriage or a family crisis, you may find it helpful to talk with a psychologist or psychiatrist. There are different types of psychotherapy, such as cognitive behavioral therapy and biofeedback. Regardless of the underlying cause of your pain, psychotherapy can help you develop strategies for coping with the pain.

Surgery

- **Laparoscopic surgery.** If you have endometriosis, doctors can remove the adhesions or endometrial tissue using laparoscopic surgery. During laparoscopic surgery, your surgeon inserts a slender viewing instrument (laparoscope) through a small incision near your navel and inserts instruments to remove endometrial tissue through one or more additional small incisions.
- **Hysterectomy.** In rare complicated cases, your doctors may recommend removal of your uterus (hysterectomy), fallopian tubes (salpingectomy) or ovaries (oophorectomy). There are important health consequences to having this procedure. Your doctor will discuss the benefits and risks in detail before recommending this option.

Cause of Pelvic Pain	Key Symptoms	Homeopathic Remedies	Indications for Use
Dysmenorrhea (Menstrual Cramps)	Severe cramping, radiating pain, nausea, backache	Magnesia Phosphorica, Colocynthis, Cimicifuga	Spasmodic pain, better by warmth and pressure
Endometriosis	Chronic pelvic pain, dyspareunia, heavy bleeding	Sepia, Lachesis, Belladonna	Bearing-down pain, sensitivity to touch, heat intolerance
Pelvic Inflammatory Disease (PID)	Fever, tenderness, discharge, deep aching pain	Mercurius Solubilis, Hepar Sulph, Kali Bichromicum	Purulent discharge, burning pain, sensitivity
Ovarian Cysts	Sharp, unilateral pain, bloating, nausea	Apis Mellifica, Lycopodium, Pulsatilla	Stinging pain, right-sided pain, worse from pressure
Fibroids (Uterine Tumors)	Heavy bleeding, pressure, dull pain	Calcarea Carbonica, Thuja, Trillium Pendulum	Fibroids with excessive bleeding, weakness
Ectopic Pregnancy	Severe lower abdominal pain, dizziness, bleeding	Sabina, Viburnum Opulus, Arnica	Threatened miscarriage, sharp pain, bruised sensation
Pelvic Congestion Syndrome	Dull, aching pain, worse standing, varicosities	Pulsatilla, Hamamelis, Sepia	Dragging pain, worse in the evening

Interstitial Cystitis	Bladder pain, urinary urgency, burning sensation	Cantharis, Staphysagria, Equisetum	Painful urination, frequent urination, burning pain
Post-Surgical Pelvic Pain	Scarring, tenderness, pain post-operation	Staphysagria, Arnica, Calendula	Pain after incision, bruised feeling, slow healing
Psychosomatic Pelvic Pain	Vague pain, anxiety, emotional distress	Ignatia, Gelsemium, Natrum Muriaticum	Pain linked to emotions, grief, suppressed emotions

Puberity

Puberty in males and females involves a series of hormonal, physical, and psychological changes. These changes are regulated primarily by the hypothalamic-pituitary-gonadal (HPG) axis, leading to sexual maturity and the development of secondary sexual characteristics. Below is a detailed breakdown of the changes in both males and females during puberty.

Hormonal Changes

In Males:

1. **Gonadotropin Release**: Increase in luteinizing hormone (LH) and follicle-stimulating hormone (FSH).
2. **Testosterone Production**: Stimulates development of male secondary sexual characteristics and spermatogenesis.
3. **Growth Hormone Increase**: Promotes growth spurts.

In Females:

1. **Gonadotropin Release**: Increase in LH and FSH stimulates ovarian function.
2. **Estrogen Production**: Leads to breast development, uterine growth, and regulation of the menstrual cycle.
3. **Progesterone**: Supports menstrual regulation post-ovulation.

Physical Changes

In Males:

1. **Genital Growth**: Enlargement of the testes and penis.
2. **Spermatogenesis**: Onset of sperm production, marking fertility.
3. **Voice Deepening**: Thickening of vocal cords leads to a deeper voice.
4. **Facial and Body Hair**: Growth of hair on the face, chest, arms, and legs.
5. **Muscle Growth**: Increase in muscle mass and strength.
6. **Height Spurt**: Significant growth spurt, usually later than females.
7. **Acne and Body Odor**: Due to increased activity of sebaceous and sweat glands.

In Females:

1. **Breast Development**: Earliest visible sign, starting with breast buds (thelarche).
2. **Menarche**: Onset of menstruation, usually around age 12–13.
3. **Hip Widening**: Pelvic structure changes to prepare for childbirth.
4. **Pubic and Axillary Hair**: Hair growth in the pubic region and underarms.
5. **Height Spurt**: Occurs earlier than in boys but ends sooner.
6. **Acne and Body Odor**: Similar to males, due to hormonal changes.

Psychological and Emotional Changes

In Males:
1. **Aggression and Risk-Taking**: Often linked to surges in testosterone.
2. **Increased Libido**: Development of sexual interest and attraction.
3. **Mood Swings**: Changes in mood due to hormonal fluctuations.
4. **Independence**: Desire for autonomy and identity development.

In Females:
1. **Emotional Sensitivity**: Increased awareness of body image and self-esteem.
2. **Mood Swings**: Fluctuations often linked to the menstrual cycle.
3. **Increased Social Awareness**: More focus on relationships and peer interactions.
4. **Self-Consciousness**: Due to visible physical changes like breast development.

Timing and Duration of Puberty

Aspect	Males	Females
Onset	9–14 years	8–13 years
First Visible Sign	Testicular enlargement	Breast budding
Growth Spurt Timing	Later stages of puberty	Early to mid-puberty
Duration	3–5 years	2–4 years

Milestones Comparison

Change	Males	Females
Secondary Hair Growth	**Facial, chest, and pubic hair**	Pubic and axillary hair
Reproductive Maturity	**Sperm production (spermarche)**	Menarche (first menstruation)
Body Shape Changes	**Broadening shoulders, muscle mass**	Widening hips, fat deposition
Skin Changes	**Thicker skin, acne**	Softer skin, acne
Voice Changes	**Significant deepening**	Slight deepening

Precaucious And Delayed Puberity

Precocious Puberty vs. Delayed Puberty

Puberty is the phase of physical and sexual maturation triggered by hormonal changes. **Precocious puberty** refers to early onset, while **delayed puberty** refers to a delayed start of these developmental changes. Below is a detailed explanation of both conditions, followed by a 25-point comparative table.

Precocious Puberty

1. **Definition**: Onset of secondary sexual characteristics before age 8 in girls and before age 9 in boys.
2. **Types**:
   - **Central Precocious Puberty (CPP)**: Early activation of the hypothalamic-pituitary-gonadal (HPG) axis.
   - **Peripheral Precocious Puberty**: Hormone production independent of the HPG axis.
3. **Causes**:
   - Idiopathic (common in girls).
   - Brain tumors, infections, or trauma.
   - Hormone-secreting tumors (e.g., adrenal or ovarian).
   - Genetic syndromes (e.g., McCune-Albright syndrome).
4. **Symptoms:**
   - Early breast development in girls.
   - Early testicular and penile growth in boys.
   - Accelerated growth and bone age.
   - Pubic or axillary hair, acne, body odor.
5. **Consequences:**
   - Early growth spurt but premature closure of growth plates, leading to short adult stature.
   - Emotional or psychological stress.
6. **Management:**
   - GnRH analogs to delay further puberty.
   - Addressing underlying causes if peripheral.

Delayed Puberty

1. **Definition**: Absence of secondary sexual characteristics by age 13 in girls and by age 14 in boys.
2. **Types:**
   - **Constitutional Delay**: A temporary delay with eventual normal puberty (common).
   - **Pathological Causes**: Disorders affecting the HPG axis or gonads.

3. **Causes**:
   o Genetic predisposition.
   o Chronic illnesses (e.g., diabetes, celiac disease).
   o Hypogonadotropic hypogonadism (e.g., Kallmann syndrome).
   o Hypergonadotropic hypogonadism (e.g., Turner syndrome, Klinefelter syndrome).
4. **Symptoms**:
   o Lack of breast development in girls.
   o Lack of testicular enlargement in boys.
   o Delayed growth spurt.
   o Lack of pubic hair or other secondary characteristics.
5. **Consequences**:
   o Emotional stress due to being out of sync with peers.
   o Potential impact on fertility if untreated.
6. **Management**:
   o Treat underlying conditions.
   o Hormone therapy (e.g., testosterone or estrogen).

Comparative Table: Precocious vs. Delayed Puberty

Aspect	Precocious Puberty	Delayed Puberty
Definition	Early onset of puberty	Late onset of puberty
Age Threshold	<8 years in girls, <9 years in boys	>13 years in girls, >14 years in boys
Growth	Early growth spurt, shorter adult stature	Delayed growth spurt, normal adult height
Causes	Brain lesions, genetic syndromes, tumors	Chronic illnesses, genetic syndromes
Hormonal Activation	Early activation or independent production	Lack of activation or response
Bone Age	Advanced	Delayed
Psychological Effects	Emotional stress due to early maturation	Emotional stress due to delayed maturation

Types	Central, Peripheral	Constitutional, Pathological
Prevalence	More common in girls	More common in boys
Symptoms (Girls)	Breast development, menstruation	Absence of breast development
Symptoms (Boys)	Testicular enlargement, voice deepening	Lack of testicular enlargement
Secondary Characteristics	Early pubic hair, acne, body odor	Absence of secondary characteristics
Management Approach	GnRH analogs, treat underlying cause	Hormone therapy, treat underlying cause
Growth Velocity	Accelerated	Reduced before puberty onset
Impact on Adult Height	Reduced due to early epiphyseal closure	Typically normal
GnRH Levels	Elevated in central forms	Low in hypogonadotropic forms
Diagnosis	Bone age assessment, hormone levels	Bone age assessment, hormone levels
Associated Syndromes	McCune-Albright, hypothalamic hamartoma	Turner, Klinefelter, Kallmann
Familial Trends	May or may not have familial linkage	Often familial
Onset Speed	Rapid	Gradual
Treatment Duration	Until appropriate pubertal timing achieved	Until normal progression is established
Risk of Malignancy	Higher with hormone-secreting tumors	Low

Pubertal Hormones	High for age	Low for age
Reproductive Impact	Early fertility potential	Potential infertility if untreated
Psychological Counseling	Often required	Often required

Prevalence	Less common overall	More common overall
Family History	Less commonly linked to family history	Often linked to delayed parental puberty
Bone Density	Early increase but risk of osteoporosis later	Delayed accrual of bone density
Behavioral Changes	Premature mood swings or aggression	Lack of age-appropriate mood changes
Sexual Development Stage	Advanced for age	Immature for age
Fertility Issues	Early but normal fertility in some cases	Potential infertility, depending on cause
Obesity Link	Often associated with obesity in girls	Can delay puberty in both genders
Neurological Symptoms	Possible (e.g., headaches, vision changes)	Rare unless underlying CNS cause
Skin Changes	Acne, early oiliness	Dry skin or delayed skin maturation
Voice Changes (Boys)	Early deepening	Delayed deepening
Testicular Volume (Boys)	Increased early	Remains small for age
Breast Development (Girls)	Premature thelarche	Absent or delayed thelarche
Pubic Hair Onset	Early appearance	Delayed appearance
Underlying Endocrine Issues	Frequently linked (e.g., adrenal hyperplasia)	Rarely linked unless endocrine deficiency
CNS Imaging Need	Often required to rule out lesions	Rarely needed unless specific symptoms

Societal Perception	May cause social isolation due to early onset	May cause peer-related stress or teasing
Impact on School Performance	Can be distracted by early hormonal changes	Sometimes affected due to low confidence
Hormonal Markers	Elevated estradiol/testosterone for age	Suppressed estradiol/testosterone for age
Height Predictions	Short due to early epiphyseal closure	Normal or taller due to extended growth
Risk of Metabolic Disorders	Higher risk of metabolic syndrome later	Reduced or normal risk
Cognitive Development	Matches age but emotional maturity differs	Matches chronological age
Intervention Timing	Requires immediate intervention to prevent complications	Observation often sufficient for constitutional delay
Psychiatric Disorders	Increased risk of depression or anxiety	Increased risk of low self-esteem
Growth Hormone Role	May overlap with excess GH stimulation	May require GH for delayed growth
Pubertal Sequence	Disordered or advanced	Orderly but delayed
Nutritional Influence	Over-nutrition or obesity triggers earlier onset	Malnutrition can cause delayed onset

Precocious Puberty Remedies

1. Calcarea Carbonica

This remedy suits chubby, fair, and sluggish children with early menses and excessive sweating on the head. They are often slow to develop mentally but fast physically. They fear darkness, illness, and being alone. Sensitive to cold and easily fatigued. Delicate digestion and aversion to exertion are common.

2. Phosphorus

Best for tall, slender children who mature too quickly and have a tendency for bleeding. These children are affectionate, crave company, and are very sensitive to external impressions. Often exhibit early breast development or menstruation. They love cold drinks and dislike being alone. Easily exhausted and mentally active.

3. Lachesis

This is suited to girls with intense early sexual energy and strong emotional expressions. Left-sided symptoms are prominent, such as left ovarian pain. Worse after sleep and from tight clothing. Talkative, suspicious, and jealous. The remedy fits those who feel worse during or before menses.

4. Medorrhinum

Indicated for children who show premature sexuality, restlessness, and a desire for stimulation. Often used in cases with a family history of sycosis (gonorrhea miasm). They may be hyperactive, daring, and crave excitement. Sleep in the knee–chest position. Often better at the seaside and at night.

5. Sulphur

A great antipsoric, often prescribed for early development along with skin issues or itching of genitals. Suits untidy, intellectual children with a philosophical bent. They dislike bathing, are warm-blooded, and prone to offensive discharges. Crave sweets and are mentally curious but physically lazy.

Delayed Puberty Remedies

1. Pulsatilla

Gentle, emotional girls with delayed menses and changeable moods respond well to Pulsatilla. They tend to be chilly but feel better in the open air. Crave affection and sympathy, and often cry easily. Hormonal disturbances are common, and physical symptoms are mild and shifting.

2. Silicea

Children with delayed growth, late puberty, and weak immune systems benefit from Silicea. They are shy, chilly, and prone to infections. Often have sweaty, smelly feet and are mentally timid but determined once they decide. They may have difficulty assimilating nutrients, affecting development.

3. Baryta Carbonica

This is the remedy for dwarfish, immature children—both physically and mentally. Suited to extremely shy individuals with a fear of strangers and criticism. Often delayed in speech and puberty. They are chilly and sensitive to cold and prone to frequent throat infections.

4. Calcarea Phosphorica

Indicated for tall, thin, growing children who suffer from bone pains and slow maturation. They may be restless, dissatisfied, and always want to go somewhere else. Menses may be late and scanty. They are prone to anemia and poor assimilation of calcium and phosphate.

5. Sepia

Used in cases of hormonal imbalance leading to delayed or suppressed menses. Girls may be irritable, indifferent to loved ones, and fatigued. Pelvic organs are often weak or congested. Better with vigorous exercise and worse with cold or damp conditions. Has a strong affinity with female reproductive organs.

Puberity Menorrhagia

Definition
Puberty Menorrhagia is excessive or prolonged menstrual bleeding occurring in adolescent girls between **menarche (first period) and 19 years of age**. It is defined as:
- Blood loss > 80 ml per cycle
- Periods lasting more than 7 days
- Irregular or frequent heavy cycles

It is often due to **immature hypothalamic-pituitary-ovarian axis**, leading to anovulatory cycles and hormonal imbalances.

Types of Puberty Menorrhagia

1. **Anovulatory Puberty Menorrhagia (Common)**
    - Irregular cycles with excessive bleeding
    - Due to immature hormonal regulation

2. **Ovulatory Puberty Menorrhagia**
    - Heavy but regular cycles
    - Due to local uterine causes

Risk Factors
- **Hormonal Imbalance** (immature HPO axis)
- Polycystic Ovarian Syndrome (PCOS)
- Thyroid Disorders (Hypothyroidism, Hyperthyroidism)
- **Blood Disorders** (von Willebrand disease, thrombocytopenia)
- Obesity and Insulin Resistance
- Emotional Stress and Eating Disorders

Etiological Factors (Causes)

1. **Hormonal Imbalance**
    - Immature Hypothalamic-Pituitary-Ovarian (HPO) axis
    - Anovulatory cycles (no proper egg release)
    - Unopposed estrogen causing excessive endometrial growth

2. **Uterine Causes**
    - Endometrial hyperplasia
    - Fibroids, polyps

3. **Systemic Disorders**
   - Coagulation disorders (platelet dysfunction, hemophilia)
   - Hypothyroidism
   - Liver or kidney disease

4. **Lifestyle and Psychological Factors**
   - Obesity (excess estrogen production)
   - Stress, anxiety, eating disorders

Clinical Features
- Heavy bleeding (>80 ml per cycle)
- Periods lasting >7 days
- Irregular or frequent cycles
- Pallor, weakness, fatigue (due to anemia)
- Dizziness, shortness of breath
- Clots or flooding (sudden excessive bleeding)

Complications

Maternal (Adolescent) Complications
- **Anemia** (low hemoglobin, fatigue, weakness)
- Emotional distress, depression, anxiety
- Infertility (long-term anovulation in PCOS cases)
- Hypovolemic shock (extreme blood loss, rare but serious)

Fetal (Future Pregnancy) Complications
- Irregular ovulation leading to infertility issues later
- Increased risk of miscarriage due to endometrial instability

Diagnosis

1. **History & Clinical Examination**
   - Menstrual history (cycle length, flow, associated symptoms)
   - Family history of bleeding disorders
   - BMI, signs of PCOS or thyroid dysfunction

2. **Investigations**
   - CBC (Complete Blood Count) – To check anemia
   - Coagulation Profile (PT, APTT, INR) – To rule out bleeding disorders
   - **Hormonal Profile** (LH, FSH, Estradiol, Prolactin, TSH) – To assess endocrine causes
   - **Pelvic Ultrasound (USG)** – To rule out fibroids, polyps, PCOS
   - **Endometrial Biopsy** (if abnormal thickening is seen)

Modern Medicine Treatment

Treatment	Indications
Iron Supplements	Treats anemia and restores hemoglobin levels
Combined Oral Contraceptives (COCs)	Regulates menstrual cycle, reduces excessive bleeding
Progestins (Medroxyprogesterone, Norethisterone)	Stops excessive bleeding in anovulatory cycles
Tranexamic Acid (Antifibrinolytic)	Reduces heavy bleeding by preventing clot breakdown
NSAIDs (Mefenamic Acid, Ibuprofen)	Relieves pain and decreases blood flow
Thyroid Hormone Therapy	If menorrhagia is due to hypothyroidism
Desmopressin (DDAVP)	For bleeding disorders like von Willebrand disease
Dilatation & Curettage (D&C)	For excessive, life-threatening bleeding
Blood Transfusion	Severe anemia or hypovolemic shock

Homeopathic Management

Homeopathic Remedy	Indications for Use
Aconitum Napellus	Sudden onset of heavy bleeding with anxiety and fear
Belladonna	Bright red, profuse bleeding with heat and throbbing pain
Calcarea Carbonica	Heavy periods in overweight girls, profuse sweating
Chamomilla	Dark, clotted, painful menstruation with irritability
Cimicifuga (Actaea Racemosa)	Irregular, painful menses with emotional distress
Ferrum Metallicum	Pale, anemic girls with heavy, watery bleeding
Lachesis	Excessive dark bleeding, intolerance to tight clothing
Nux Vomica	Heavy periods with spasmodic pains, anger, irritability
Phosphorus	Sudden, bright red bleeding with weakness and thirst
Pulsatilla	Irregular, changeable flow with weepiness and mild temperament

Homeopathic Remedy	Indications for Use
Secale Cornutum	Thin, dark bleeding, excessive weakness
Sepia	Scanty, irregular menses with pelvic dragging sensation
Sulphur	Bright red, hot, offensive bleeding with itching
Thlaspi Bursa Pastoris	Profuse bleeding with large clots, frequent periods
Ustilago Maydis	Continuous dark bleeding with uterine cramps

Polycystic Overies

Definition

PCOD (Polycystic Ovarian Disease):

Polycystic Ovarian Disease (PCOD) is a common condition where the ovaries contain multiple small cysts (fluid-filled sacs) due to hormonal imbalances. It is characterized by irregular menstrual cycles, excessive androgen levels (like testosterone), and ovulation problems. PCOD primarily refers to a condition with cystic changes in the ovaries and hormonal disturbances, but it does not always lead to severe metabolic or long-term health complications.

PCOS (Polycystic Ovary Syndrome):

Polycystic Ovary Syndrome (PCOS) is a more complex and chronic hormonal disorder that not only affects the ovaries but also impacts metabolism, insulin sensitivity, and overall endocrine function. It includes irregular menstrual cycles, excess androgen production, ovulatory dysfunction, and multiple ovarian cysts. PCOS is associated with a higher risk of long-term complications like obesity, diabetes, infertility, and cardiovascular disease.

Comparison Between PCOD and PCOS

Point	PCOD (Polycystic Ovarian Disease)	PCOS (Polycystic Ovary Syndrome)
1. Definition	A condition with multiple ovarian cysts and hormonal imbalance, mainly affecting the ovaries.	A syndrome that includes multiple cysts, hormonal imbalance, ovulatory dysfunction, and metabolic issues.
2. Cysts	Presence of small cysts in ovaries, which are usually harmless.	Presence of cysts in ovaries, but these cysts are often larger and have a functional impact on the ovaries.
3. Hormonal Imbalance	Hormonal imbalance occurs but does not always lead to severe symptoms.	Hormonal imbalance is more severe, with higher androgen levels (male hormones), leading to significant symptoms.
4. Menstrual Irregularity	Irregular periods but not necessarily anovulation (absence of ovulation).	Irregular periods with a higher likelihood of anovulation, often leading to infertility.

Point	PCOD (Polycystic Ovarian Disease)	PCOS (Polycystic Ovary Syndrome)
5. Ovulation	Ovulation may occur but is irregular or delayed in some cases.	Ovulation is often absent or significantly delayed, leading to challenges in conceiving.
6. Symptoms	Mild symptoms like irregular periods, mild acne, or slight weight gain.	Severe symptoms like acne, male-pattern hair loss, excessive hair growth (hirsutism), and obesity.
7. Insulin Resistance	Insulin resistance is not always present.	Insulin resistance is common, and women with PCOS often have a higher risk of developing type 2 diabetes.
8. Fertility Issues	Fertility may be affected but is usually less severe.	Infertility is a common concern due to anovulation and hormonal disruptions.
9. Risk of Metabolic Disorders	Lesser risk of long-term metabolic disorders compared to PCOS.	Higher risk of developing obesity, diabetes, and cardiovascular diseases due to insulin resistance and metabolic disturbances.
10. Weight	Weight gain is not always associated with PCOD.	Weight gain and obesity are commonly associated with PCOS, and managing weight is often a key part of treatment.
11. Acne and Skin Problems	Mild acne may occur, but it is usually manageable.	Severe acne and other skin issues like oily skin, darkened skin patches (acanthosis nigricans), and excessive body hair (hirsutism) are more prominent.
12. Long-Term Health Risks	Generally, fewer long-term health risks, unless metabolic issues develop.	Increased risk of diabetes, endometrial cancer, cardiovascular diseases, and infertility.
13. Diagnosis	Diagnosed through ultrasound showing cysts and clinical signs, but not necessarily involving metabolic disturbances.	Diagnosis requires a more comprehensive approach, including ultrasound, blood tests (for hormone levels), and assessment of metabolic issues like insulin resistance.
14. Treatment Focus	Treatment primarily focuses on regulating the menstrual cycle and managing symptoms.	Treatment addresses hormonal imbalances, insulin resistance, fertility issues, and long-term metabolic risks.

Point	PCOD (Polycystic Ovarian Disease)	PCOS (Polycystic Ovary Syndrome)
15. Management Approach	Lifestyle changes, diet, and medication (e.g., birth control pills) to manage symptoms.	Combination of lifestyle changes, weight management, medication (e.g., metformin for insulin resistance), and possible fertility treatments.

Types of PCOD:

PCOD can manifest in various forms, but the most common classification involves the following types:

1. **Classic PCOD:**
   - The most common form, characterized by multiple cysts on the ovaries and irregular menstrual cycles.

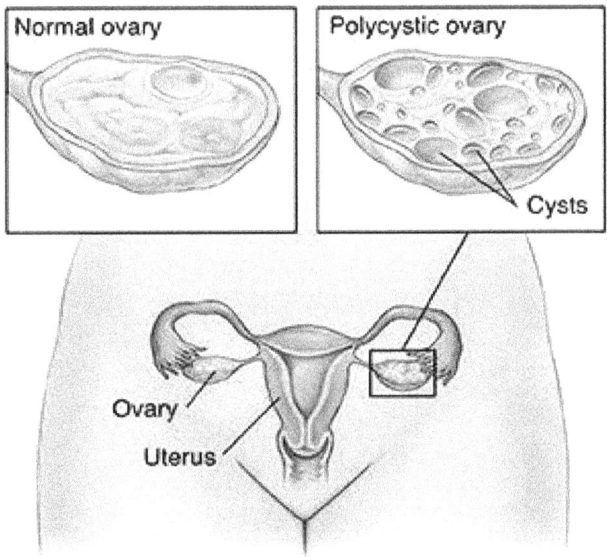

   - It is associated with hormonal imbalances, including elevated levels of androgens (male hormones), and may lead to infertility.

2. **Hyperandrogenic PCOD:**
   - This type is characterized by an excess of male hormones (androgens), leading to symptoms such as excessive hair growth (hirsutism), acne, and male-pattern baldness.

3. **Non-Hyperandrogenic PCOD:**
   - This form may not present with the typical signs of excess androgens (like hirsutism or acne) but still features cysts on the ovaries and irregular menstruation.

4. **Insulin-Resistant PCOD:**
    - This type is associated with insulin resistance, where the body's cells do not respond well to insulin. It can result in elevated insulin levels, leading to weight gain, metabolic issues, and an increased risk of type 2 diabetes.

Clinical Features of PCOD:

- **Irregular Menstrual Cycles**: Women with PCOD may have infrequent, irregular, or prolonged menstrual periods. Some may experience periods that occur only a few times a year.
- Excessive Androgen Symptoms:
    - **Hirsutism**: Excessive hair growth on the face, chest, back, or abdomen.
    - **Acne and Oily Skin**: Increased production of sebum (skin oil), leading to acne.
    - **Male-pattern Baldness**: Thinning hair or receding hairlines.
- **Polycystic Ovaries**: Multiple small cysts (usually 2–8mm in diameter) on one or both ovaries, detected via ultrasound.
- **Obesity or Weight Gain**: Many women with PCOD are overweight or obese, often due to insulin resistance.
- **Infertility**: Due to anovulation (lack of ovulation), many women with PCOD may struggle to conceive.
- **Depression or Anxiety**: Hormonal imbalances and the stress of dealing with symptoms can contribute to mental health issues.
- **Darkening of Skin**: Acanthosis nigricans, a condition causing dark, velvety patches of skin, usually found on the neck, armpits, and groin area.

Complications of PCOD:

- **Infertility**: Due to anovulation (failure of the ovaries to release an egg), women with PCOD may have difficulty getting pregnant.
- **Metabolic Syndrome**: PCOD increases the risk of developing obesity, insulin resistance, and type 2 diabetes.
- **Endometrial Cancer**: Irregular or infrequent periods can lead to the buildup of the uterine lining (endometrium), increasing the risk of endometrial cancer.
- **Cardiovascular Disease**: Women with PCOD have an increased risk of developing heart disease due to factors like obesity, insulin resistance, and high cholesterol.
- **Sleep Apnea**: PCOD, especially when associated with obesity, increases the risk of sleep apnea.
- **Psychological Impact**: The symptoms of PCOD, such as weight gain, acne, and hair growth, can lead to anxiety, depression, and low self-esteem.

Diagnostic Tests for PCOD:

1. **Clinical Evaluation**: A detailed medical history and physical examination to assess menstrual patterns, symptoms of androgen excess, and weight.
2. **Ultrasound**: Transvaginal ultrasound is typically performed to check for the presence of cysts on the ovaries. The presence of more than 12 follicles (2–9 mm in diameter) on one or both ovaries is a key diagnostic feature.

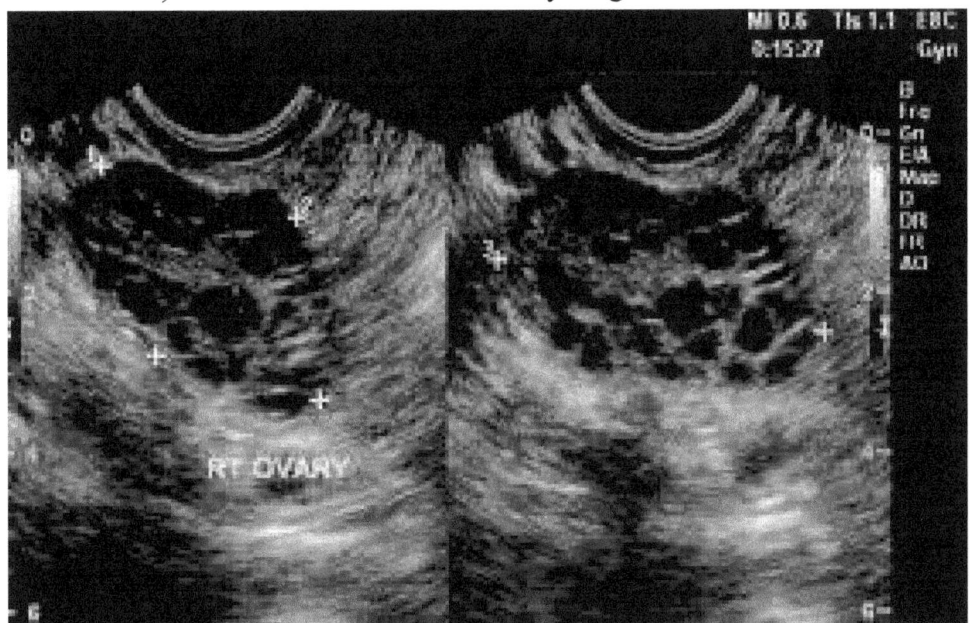

Honey Comb Like Appearance

1. Blood Tests:
   - **Hormone Levels**: Elevated levels of luteinizing hormone (LH), testosterone, and dehydroepiandrosterone sulfate (DHEAS) are common in PCOD.
   - **Thyroid Function Tests**: To rule out thyroid disorders, as symptoms may overlap with PCOD.
   - **Insulin Resistance**: Fasting insulin levels and glucose tolerance tests can help identify insulin resistance, a common issue in PCOD.
   - **Progesterone Level**: Low levels of progesterone may indicate a lack of ovulation.
   - **AMH level**- Raised
2. **Physical Examination**: A thorough examination for signs of hirsutism, acne, and obesity.

Medicinal Management:

1. **Hormonal Therapy**:
   - **Oral Contraceptives (Birth Control Pills)**: These help regulate menstrual cycles, reduce androgen levels, and control acne and hirsutism.
   - **Progestins**: Sometimes prescribed to regulate periods in women who cannot use oral contraceptives.

2. **Anti-Androgen Medications:**
   - **Spironolactone**: Often prescribed to reduce hirsutism and acne by blocking the effects of androgens.
   - **Finasteride**: Used to treat male-pattern baldness and excessive hair growth.
3. **Metformin:**
   - **Insulin Sensitizers**: Metformin is commonly prescribed in women with insulin resistance to improve ovulation and help with weight management. It can also reduce the risk of diabetes.
4. **Ovulation Induction:**
   - **Clomiphene Citrate (Clomid)**: A first-line medication for women who want to conceive. It induces ovulation.
   - **Gonadotropins**: If Clomid is ineffective, injectable gonadotropins may be used to stimulate the ovaries.
5. **Other Medications:**
   - **Dexamethasone**: A corticosteroid used to reduce elevated androgen levels.
   - **Glucocorticoids**: Sometimes prescribed in cases of severe hyperandrogenism.

Surgical Management:

1. **Ovarian Drilling (Laparoscopic Ovarian Diathermy):**
   - This is a surgical procedure where small holes are made in the ovaries using a laser or electrosurgical needle. It is performed in cases of severe PCOD where medical management is unsuccessful.
   - It can improve ovulation and fertility in some women.
2. **Laparoscopic Surgery:**
   - In cases where ovarian drilling is ineffective, laparoscopic surgery may be performed to remove the cysts.

Lifestyle Changes for PCOD:

1. **Weight Management**: Maintaining a healthy weight can help regulate menstrual cycles, reduce insulin resistance, and improve fertility. A balanced diet and regular exercise are key components.
2. **Exercise**: Regular physical activity (at least 30 minutes per day) can help control weight, reduce insulin resistance, and improve overall health.
3. **Diet**: A diet low in refined carbohydrates and sugars is beneficial for controlling insulin levels. Incorporating lean proteins, whole grains, healthy fats, and plenty of vegetables can help manage PCOD symptoms.
4. **Stress Management**: Stress can worsen hormonal imbalances, so practices such as yoga, meditation, and mindfulness are recommended.

5. **Sleep Hygiene**: Ensuring adequate and restful sleep is crucial for maintaining hormonal balance and overall well-being.

Homeopathic Remedies for PCOD:

Homeopathy offers several remedies based on individualized symptoms. Some common homeopathic remedies for PCOD include:

1. **Sepia:**
   - **Guiding Symptoms**: Women with PCOD who feel fatigued, irritable, and disconnected emotionally. They may experience irregular menstruation and a sensation of heaviness in the pelvic region.

2. **Lachesis:**
   - **Guiding Symptoms**: For women who experience irritability, excessive bleeding, and hot flashes. It is useful in cases where there is a history of hormonal imbalances or anger.

3. **Calcarea Carbonica:**
   - **Guiding Symptoms**: For women who have irregular periods, obesity, and a tendency to feel cold. This remedy is often prescribed for women who are overweight and struggle with PCOD-related weight gain.

4. **Natrum Mur:**
   - **Guiding Symptoms**: Women with PCOD who experience emotional distress, excessive thirst, and delayed or scanty periods. This remedy helps in restoring hormonal balance.

5. **Sulphur:**
   - **Guiding Symptoms**: For women with PCOD who have acne, oily skin, and a tendency toward hot flushes. It is also indicated when there is a feeling of weakness or tiredness.

6. **Pulsatilla:**
   - **Guiding Symptoms**: For women with emotional fluctuations, absent or delayed periods, and sensitivity to heat. This remedy is useful for women who experience changes in their cycle due to emotional stress.

7. **Agnus Castus:**
   - **Guiding Symptoms**: When menstrual irregularity is associated with hormonal imbalance and emotional instability.

8. **Berberis Vulgaris:**
   - **Guiding Symptoms**: For women with dark, oily skin, and acne. It helps in regulating the menstrual cycle and improving skin health.

9. **Thuja Occidentalis:**
   - **Guiding Symptoms**: Effective when cystic changes are present, particularly when ovarian cysts are present and affect menstrual regularity.
10. **Berberis Aquifolium:**
    - **Guiding Symptoms**: Used when there is a presence of skin problems like acne and oily skin associated with hormonal imbalances and PCOD.

Modern (allopathic) drugs and homeopathic remedies for the treatment of PCOD (Polycystic Ovarian Disease):

Aspect	Modern (Allopathic) Drugs	Homeopathic Remedies
Hormonal Regulation	**Oral Contraceptive Pills (OCPs)** – Regulates menstrual cycle by providing synthetic estrogen and progesterone. Examples: *Ethinyl estradiol + Drospirenone*	**Pulsatilla** – Helps regulate irregular cycles, particularly when periods are suppressed.
Ovulation Induction	**Clomiphene Citrate (Clomid)** – Stimulates ovulation by blocking estrogen receptors.	**Sepia** – Helps improve ovarian function and restore natural ovulation.
Insulin Resistance	**Metformin** – Improves insulin sensitivity, reducing androgen levels and aiding ovulation.	**Lachesis** – Useful in cases of insulin resistance with hormonal imbalance.
Androgen Reduction (Acne, Hirsutism)	**Spironolactone, Flutamide, Cyproterone Acetate** – Anti-androgens reduce acne and unwanted hair growth.	**Thuja Occidentalis** – Reduces excessive hair growth and balances hormones.
Weight Management	Metformin, Orlistat, GLP-1 agonists (e.g., Liraglutide) – Help in weight loss for obese PCOS patients.	**Calcarea Carbonica** – Used for weight gain due to hormonal imbalance and sluggish metabolism.
Emotional & Mental Health	**SSRIs (e.g., Fluoxetine, Sertraline)** – Prescribed for anxiety and depression in PCOS patients.	**Natrum Muriaticum** – Helps with mood swings, depression, and emotional imbalances related to PCOS.

Retroversion Of Uterus

Defination:-

Retrodisplacement of uterus where it tilted backwards on its transverse axis passing through the utero-vaginal junction.

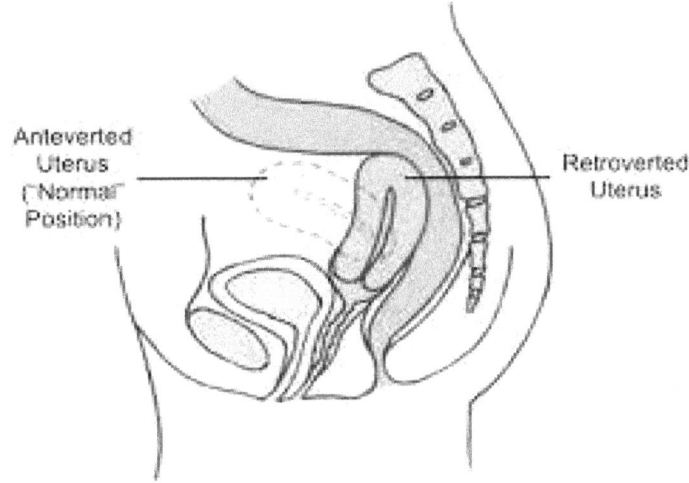

Degrees Of Retroversion :-

I st degree:- Fundus of uterus directed towards sacral promontory.

II nd degree :- Fundus of uterus lies in hallow of sacrum.

III rd degree :- Fundus of uterus lies over rectum,in pouch of duglus.

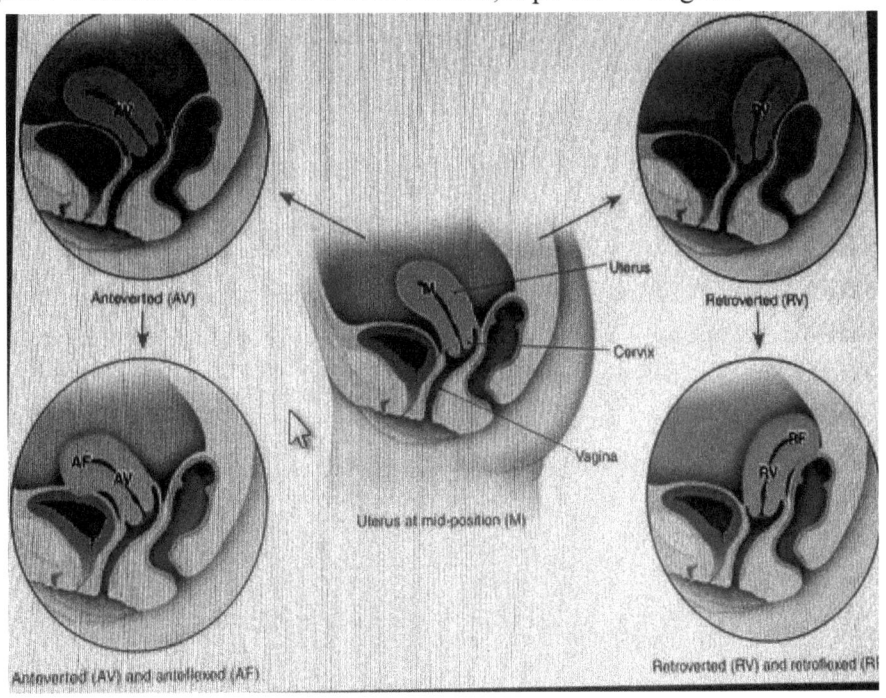

Incidence :-
-25 % occurance after 1st confinement.
-10% occurance in nulliparous.
AETIOLOGY :-

Congenital causes-
-developmental defect at puberity
-uterine hypoplasia
-shallow vagina
-short vaginal wall

Aquired causes-

-Puerpural retroversion:-due to increased weight of uteus due to hyperplasia in pregnancy and laxed vaginal and perineal supports,postdelivery retroversion of uterus is common.
-Uterine prolapse :-Prior to every prolapse there is retroversion.
-Adhesions or Endometroisis
-Fibroid,huge ovarian cyst in uterovascical pouch.

Types Of Retroversion:-
1. .Mobile or uncomplicated retroversion
2. Fixed or complicated retroversion

Clinical Features :-
Most of mobile types of retroversion cases doesn'nt produces any symptoms.

BACKACHE- Low,sacral bachache due to pressure of uterus over pelvic vessels leads to pelvic venous congestion.

MENSTRUAL DISORDERS – Menstrual irregularities like congestive dysmenorrheal,menorrhagea,leucorrhea

DYSPARENIA –Painfull sexual intercourse due to prolapsed ovaries in POD and congested uterus.

INFERTILITY – Due to changed direction of cervix in retroversion.

BEAR DOWN SENSATION- Continous bearing down sensation as if something is coming down from vagina or something moving inside the abdomen i.e, sense of womb displacement.This is due to laxed supports of uterus.

SIGNS-

P/V EXAM- Cervix directed downwards,forwards,towards pubic symphysis.

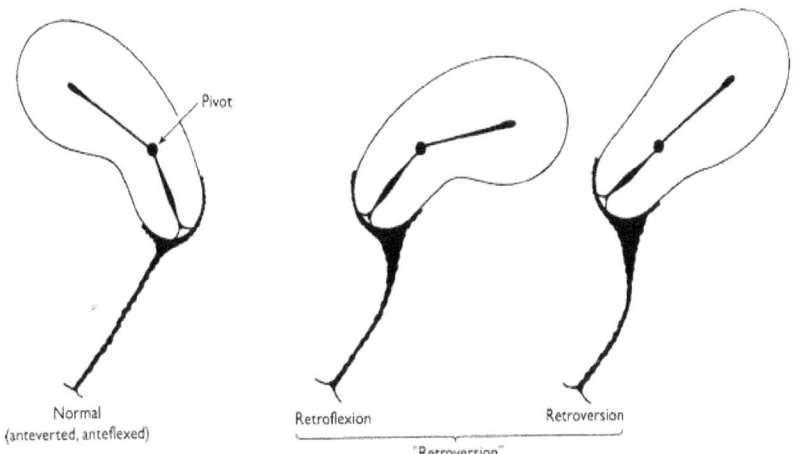

P/A EXAM- Non palpable uterine fundus as it tilted backwards.

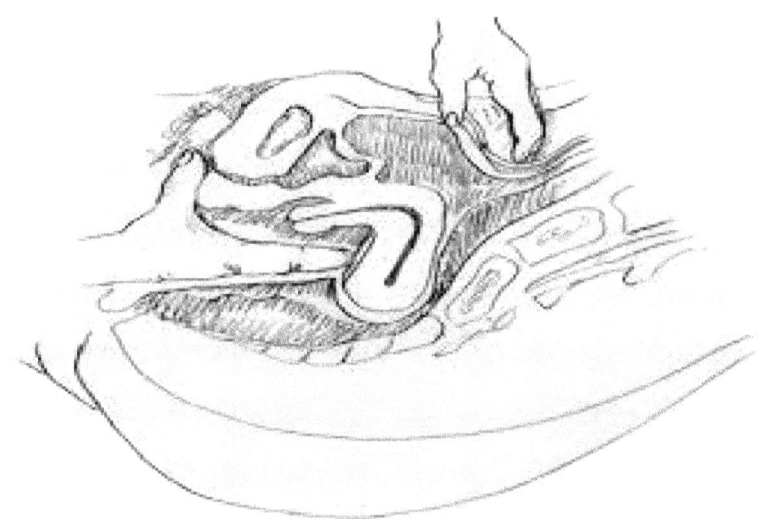

P/R EXAM- Palpable uterine fundus in POD.

Diagnosis :-

-USG
-P/V Exam
-P/A Exam
-P/R Exam

MANAGEMENT :-

Preventive Management -

-good puerperal management.
- abdominal and vaginal support
-avoid multiple MTP
-avoid multiple deliveries
-avoid forcible deliveries

-avoid excessive fundal pressure

-early detection of fibroid,cysts,adhesions and their management before retroversion become fixed.

Curative Management –

-no symptoms ,no management.

-Pessary treatment,applicable only in mobile type of retroversion,advicable even during pregnancy.

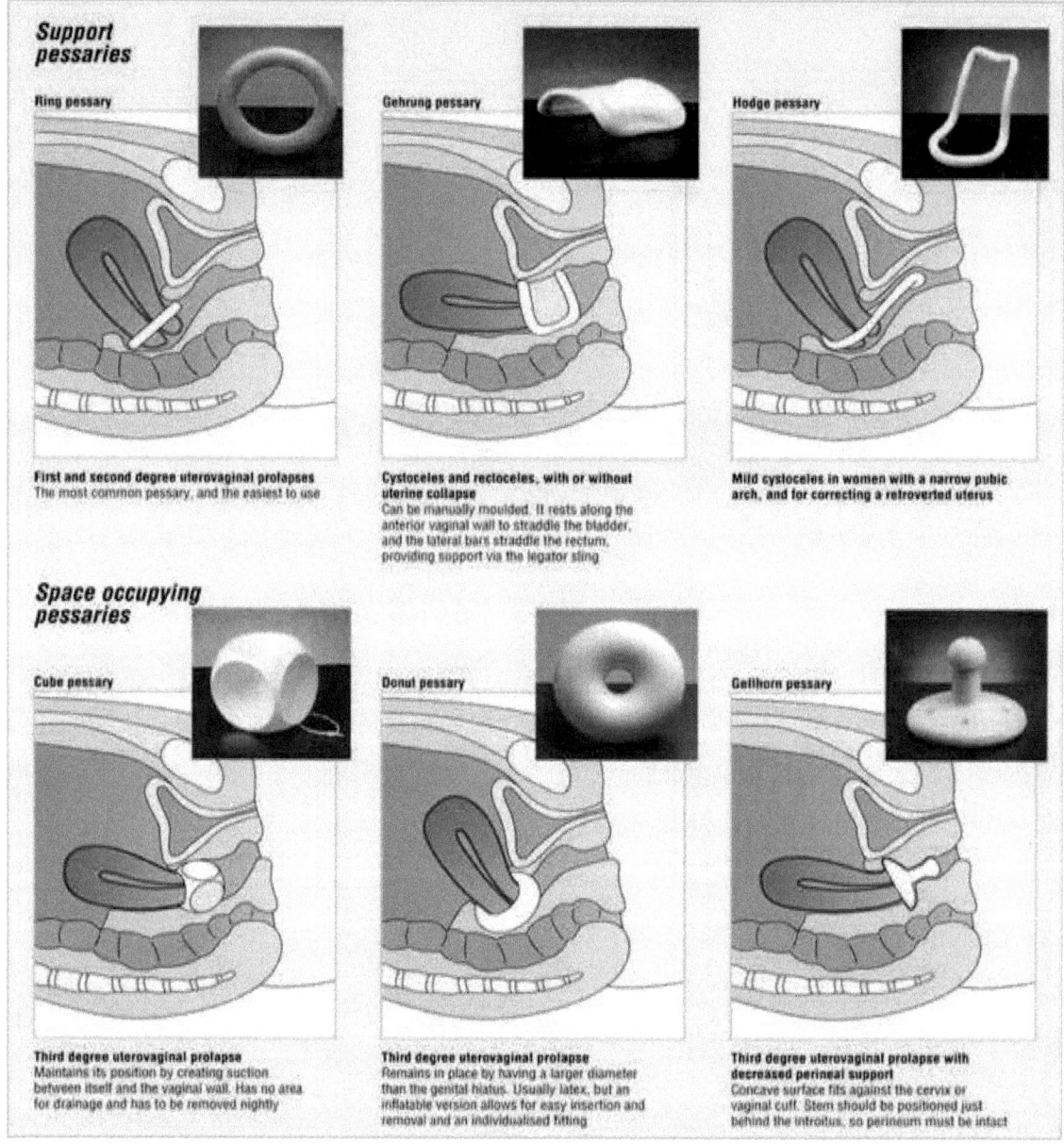

Pessary test positive-

It is said to be positive when all symptoms disappears after pessary introduction but reappears after removal of pessary.

Contraindications-
-Fixed retroversion
-PID,Pelvic inflammatory diseases.
-Laxed perineum.
Other indications of pessary management-
-Pregnancy with prolapse
-Puepural prolpase
-Pt .not want hysterectomy for prolapsed.
-Until hysterectomy done in prolapsed uterus.

Surgical Management-
-If pessary test positive
-In cases of infertility with h/o habitual abortion
-In complicated or fixed type of retroversion
-in fixed type with tubo-ovarian mass,pelvic adhesions.
HOMOEOPATHIC MANAGEMENT :-

Helonias-
Retroversion and prolapsed in women which exhausted due to mentle and physical hardwork,luxuiry and indolence,RECUURENT ABORTIONS AND DELIVERIES with complete tiredness of back and lower limbs.Dancing uterus,consciousness of constantly moving uterus in abdomen.Heavyness of abdomen.Fault finding nature of low spirited own with offensive ,profuse,brownish menorrhagea and foul leucorrhea. Pruritus vulva with ulcered cervix.Patient feels better when occupied.

Podophyllum-
Laxed perineum due to lifting heavy wt,during puerperal retroversion. Mobile type of retroversion causes irritation of rectum and hence diarrhea alternate with constipation.Uterus tilted over rt. Overy causes congestion and rt.sided menorrhagea.Severe dysparenia with intolerance of even light touch of undergarments. PREGNANCY WITH RETROVERSION, patient feels better by LYING ON ABDOMEN.

Sepia And Lil.Tig -

Sepia	Lilium tigrinum
1. Bearing down pressure, from back to abdomen.	1. Bearing down, everything forcing down, as if contents of the pelvis were being pushed down through a funnel, the out let being vagina.
2. Must cross legs to prevent protrusion of parts.	2. Must support vulva with hand or cross legs.
3. Here the patient feel cold more.	3. Here the patient feels heat more.
4. Mentally the patient is very much indifferent and apathetic.	4. Mentally the patient is always hurried and worried.
5. Complete absence of Sexual desire.	5. Sexual desire much more marked.

Study Methods to Rule Out Ovulation.

I. Clinical Methods to Assess Ovulation

1. **Menstrual History:**
   - Regular menstrual cycles (21–35 days) are often indicative of ovulation.
   - Irregular or anovulatory cycles suggest ovulatory dysfunction.

2. **Basal Body Temperature (BBT):**
   - Method:
     - The woman records her temperature every morning before getting out of bed.
     - A mid-cycle rise in basal temperature (0.3–0.6°C) due to progesterone confirms ovulation.
   - Limitations:
     - Can be affected by external factors such as illness, stress, or poor compliance.

3. **Cervical Mucus Changes:**
   - Method:
     - During ovulation, cervical mucus becomes clear, stretchy, and slippery ("egg-white consistency"), indicating high estrogen levels.
   - Limitations:
     - Subjective, requires patient education, and may be altered by infections or medications.

4. **Mittelschmerz (Ovulatory Pain):**
   - Some women experience mild pelvic pain around the time of ovulation, which may indicate follicular rupture.
   - Not a reliable or objective indicator.

II. Hormonal Assessments

1. **Serum Progesterone Levels:**
   - Method:
     - A blood sample is taken on day 21–23 of a 28-day cycle (luteal phase).
     - Serum progesterone >3 ng/mL indicates ovulation.
   - Benefits:
     - Gold standard for confirming ovulation retrospectively.
   - Limitations:
     - Requires precise timing based on the menstrual cycle.

2. **Luteinizing Hormone (LH) Surge Testing:**
   o Method:
     - Home ovulation prediction kits (OPKs) detect the LH surge in urine, which precedes ovulation by 24–36 hours.
   o Benefits:
     - Non-invasive and provides real-time prediction.
   o Limitations:
     - False positives can occur in conditions like PCOS.

3. **Follicle-Stimulating Hormone (FSH) and Estradiol Levels:**
   o Measured in the early follicular phase (day 2–5) to evaluate ovarian reserve and ovulatory function.

4. **Anti-Müllerian Hormone (AMH):**
   o Reflects ovarian reserve but does not directly assess ovulation.
   o Useful in evaluating conditions like PCOS or diminished ovarian reserve.

5. **Prolactin and Thyroid Function Tests:**
   o Hyperprolactinemia or thyroid dysfunction can cause anovulation.
   o Elevated prolactin or abnormal TSH levels may indicate underlying hormonal imbalances.

III. Imaging and Ultrasound Studies

1. **Transvaginal Ultrasound (TVUS):**
   o Follicular Monitoring:
     - Sequential ultrasounds track the growth and rupture of the dominant follicle.
     - Key Findings:
     - Pre-ovulatory follicle: 18–24 mm.
     - Follicular rupture and subsequent corpus luteum formation confirm ovulation.
   o Benefits:
     - Reliable, real-time assessment.
   o Limitations:
     - Requires multiple visits and skilled personnel.

2. **Ultrasound Indicators of Ovulation:**
   o Disappearance of the dominant follicle.
   o Free fluid in the pouch of Douglas post-ovulation.
   o Appearance of a corpus luteum.

IV. Endometrial and Cervical Evaluations

1. **Endometrial Biopsy:**
   - Method:
     - Performed in the late luteal phase (day 21–24 of a 28-day cycle).
     - Histological evaluation identifies secretory changes that confirm ovulation.
   - Limitations:
     - Invasive and not commonly used unless absolutely necessary.

2. **Cervical Smear or Ferning Test:**
   - During ovulation, cervical mucus dried on a glass slide exhibits a fern-like pattern due to high sodium chloride levels.
   - Simple but less reliable.

V. Specialized Tests

1. **Urinary Metabolites of Hormones:**
   - Tests measure metabolites of estrogen and progesterone (e.g., pregnanediol glucuronide).
   - Benefits:
     - Non-invasive.
   - Limitations:
     - Not widely available and lacks real-time accuracy.

2. **Serum Inhibin B Levels:**
   - Inhibin B is secreted by granulosa cells of developing follicles.
   - Low levels suggest poor follicular development or anovulation.

3. **Serum Estradiol Monitoring:**
   - Rising estradiol levels during the follicular phase reflect follicular development.
   - Peak estradiol levels occur just before ovulation.

VI. Advanced Techniques

1. **Laparoscopy with Chromopertubation:**
   - Direct visualization of ovulation through laparoscopic observation of the ovaries.
   - Chromopertubation assesses tubal patency simultaneously.
   - Reserved for cases where infertility is combined with suspected pelvic pathology.

2. **Ovarian Biopsy:**
   - Rarely performed due to its invasive nature.
   - Used in research or in cases of refractory ovulatory dysfunction.

VII. Imaging-Based Alternatives

1. **Magnetic Resonance Imaging (MRI):**
   - Occasionally used in complex cases to evaluate ovarian or pelvic abnormalities.
2. **Saline Infusion Sonography (SIS):**
   - Evaluates endometrial and ovarian changes during the menstrual cycle.

Common Conditions Leading to Anovulation

1. **Polycystic Ovary Syndrome (PCOS):**
   - Chronic anovulation with multiple small follicles.
   - Diagnosis is aided by hormonal tests, AMH, and ultrasound findings.
2. **Hypothalamic Amenorrhea:**
   - Low gonadotropins due to stress, excessive exercise, or eating disorders.
   - Diagnosed by low FSH, LH, and estradiol levels.
3. **Premature Ovarian Insufficiency (POI):**
   - Elevated FSH and low estradiol levels indicate poor ovarian function.
   - AMH levels are also significantly reduced.
4. **Thyroid Disorders and Hyperprolactinemia:**
   - Directly disrupt the hypothalamic-pituitary-ovarian axis.

USG IN OBS/GYN

USG in ANC:

1. **Confirmation of Pregnancy:**
   - Detection of an intrauterine pregnancy.
   - Exclusion of ectopic pregnancy or molar pregnancy.
2. **Dating of Pregnancy (Gestational Age Assessment):**
   - Accurate estimation of gestational age using crown-rump length (CRL) in the first trimester.
   - Reduces errors in calculating the expected date of delivery (EDD).
3. **Assessment of Fetal Viability:**
   - Identification of fetal cardiac activity.
   - Monitoring for early pregnancy complications like missed abortion.
4. **Screening for Fetal Abnormalities:**
   - Detection of structural anomalies (e.g., anencephaly, spina bifida).
   - Nuchal translucency measurement in the first trimester for chromosomal abnormalities (e.g., Down syndrome).

5. **Monitoring Fetal Growth and Development:**
   - Evaluation of fetal growth parameters (e.g., biparietal diameter, femur length, abdominal circumference).
   - Assessment of intrauterine growth restriction (IUGR) or macrosomia.
6. **Assessment of Amniotic Fluid:**
   - Measurement of amniotic fluid index (AFI) or single deepest pocket.
   - Diagnosis of oligohydramnios or polyhydramnios.
7. **Placental Localization and Function:**
   - Identification of placental location (e.g., low-lying placenta, placenta previa).
   - Detection of placental abnormalities like placenta accreta.
8. **Evaluation of Multiple Pregnancies:**
   - Determination of chorionicity and amnionicity.
   - Monitoring for complications like twin-twin transfusion syndrome (TTTS).
9. **Assessment of Fetal Position and Presentation:**
   - Detection of malpresentation (e.g., breech, transverse lie).
10. **Doppler Studies for Fetal Well-Being:**
    - Assessment of uteroplacental and fetal circulation (e.g., umbilical artery, middle cerebral artery Doppler).
    - Useful in cases of fetal growth restriction or preeclampsia.
11. **Guidance for Invasive Procedures:**
    - Real-time guidance for procedures like amniocentesis, chorionic villus sampling (CVS), and cordocentesis.
12. **Assessment of Cervical Length:**
    - Prediction of preterm labor using transvaginal ultrasound.
    - Monitoring in cases of cervical incompetence.
13. **Monitoring Maternal Conditions:**
    - Identification of uterine anomalies, fibroids, or adnexal masses.
    - Assessment of complications like uterine rupture or scar dehiscence.

Types of Ultrasound in ANC:

1. **Transabdominal Ultrasound (TAUS):**
   - Performed by placing the probe on the abdomen.
   - Used for routine assessments and third-trimester evaluations.
2. **Transvaginal Ultrasound (TVUS):**
   - Performed by inserting a probe into the vagina.

o Provides better resolution in early pregnancy and for assessing cervical length.

3. **3D and 4D Ultrasound:**
   o Provides detailed views of fetal anatomy.
   o 4D ultrasound adds real-time imaging for better visualization of fetal movements and expressions.

4. **Doppler Ultrasound:**
   o Evaluates blood flow in the umbilical artery, uterine arteries, and fetal vessels.
   o Used in high-risk pregnancies (e.g., preeclampsia, IUGR).

5. **Level II Ultrasound (Anomaly Scan):**
   o Detailed examination of fetal anatomy between 18–22 weeks.
   o Identifies structural anomalies and markers of chromosomal abnormalities.

6. **Biophysical Profile (BPP):**
   o Combines ultrasound with fetal heart rate monitoring.
   o Assesses fetal well-being by evaluating movements, tone, breathing, and amniotic fluid.

Timing of USG in ANC:

1. **First Trimester (6–13 weeks):**
   o Confirmation of pregnancy.
   o Dating scan.
   o Early anomaly screening (nuchal translucency).

2. **Second Trimester (18–22 weeks):**
   o Detailed anomaly scan.
   o Placental localization.
   o Growth assessment.

3. **Third Trimester (28–40 weeks):**
   o Monitoring fetal growth and well-being.
   o Doppler studies for high-risk cases.
   o Assessment of fetal presentation and amniotic fluid.

Role of USG in the Puerperal Period

The puerperal period, also known as the postpartum period, refers to the time following childbirth, lasting about 6 weeks, during which the body undergoes significant physiological changes. USG is commonly used to evaluate and manage complications during this period.

1. **Postpartum Hemorrhage (PPH)**
   - Role of USG:

- Identifies retained products of conception (RPOC) or clots in the uterine cavity.
- Detects uterine atony or subinvolution of the uterus.
- Assesses the size and shape of the uterus to detect abnormalities.

2. **Retained Products of Conception (RPOC)**
   - Role of USG:
     - Identifies echogenic material within the uterine cavity.
     - Differentiates between clots and placental tissue using Doppler imaging (vascularity assessment).

3. **Endometritis (Postpartum Infection)**
   - Role of USG:
     - Evaluates the endometrial thickness and detects retained products or infected tissue.
     - Identifies fluid collections or abscesses in the uterine cavity.

4. **Uterine Rupture or Scar Dehiscence**
   - Role of USG:
     - Assesses uterine integrity in women with a history of cesarean section or uterine surgery.
     - Identifies any defects, hematomas, or abnormal thinning at the scar site.

5. **Pelvic Abscess or Hematoma**
   - Role of USG:
     - Detects pelvic collections or hematomas in the broad ligament, pelvic cavity, or cesarean section incision site.
     - Differentiates between simple and complex fluid collections.

6. **Uterine Subinvolution**
   - Role of USG:
     - Monitors uterine size and involution postpartum.
     - Detects conditions like adenomyosis or fibroids that may hinder normal involution.

7. **Postpartum Ovarian or Adnexal Complications**
   - Role of USG:
     - Diagnoses ovarian cysts, torsion, or masses postpartum.
     - Detects adnexal pathology that may mimic postpartum complications.

8. **Postpartum Thrombosis**
   - Role of USG (Doppler Studies):
     - Evaluates blood flow in pelvic veins to identify deep vein thrombosis (DVT) or pelvic vein thrombosis.

- Helps in early diagnosis of life-threatening conditions like pulmonary embolism.

Role of USG During Operative Procedures in Obstetrics

Ultrasound provides real-time guidance for various operative procedures, ensuring precision, reducing complications, and improving outcomes. Below are the main applications:

1. **Cesarean Section**
   - Role of USG:
     - Assesses placental location and identifies conditions like placenta previa or placenta accreta spectrum disorders (PAS).
     - Guides surgical incision to avoid placental disruption.
     - Helps detect uterine anomalies or fibroids that may complicate the procedure.

2. **Manual Removal of Placenta**
   - Role of USG:
     - Confirms complete removal of the placenta and absence of retained fragments.
     - Identifies uterine abnormalities that could hinder complete placental expulsion.

3. **Uterine Artery Embolization (UAE)**
   - Role of USG:
     - Guides embolization procedures for controlling intractable postpartum hemorrhage.
     - Assesses blood flow and vascular supply to uterine arteries using Doppler imaging.

4. **Evacuation of Retained Products**
   - Role of USG:
     - Provides guidance for dilatation and curettage (D&C) or vacuum aspiration.
     - Ensures complete evacuation of RPOC while minimizing the risk of uterine perforation.

5. **Drainage of Postpartum Abscess or Hematoma**
   - Role of USG:
     - Guides percutaneous or transvaginal aspiration of pelvic abscesses or hematomas.
     - Assesses the resolution of the abscess post-drainage.

6. **Operative Management of Ectopic Pregnancy**
   - Role of USG:
     - Guides laparoscopic or transvaginal procedures for ectopic pregnancies.
     - Assists in the localization of ectopic gestational tissue.

7. **Uterine Tamponade or Balloon Placement**
   - Role of USG:
     - Guides the placement of intrauterine balloon catheters (e.g., Bakri balloon) for managing severe PPH.
     - Confirms correct positioning within the uterine cavity.

8. **Placenta Accreta Spectrum (PAS) Management**
   - Role of USG:
     - Preoperatively evaluates placental invasion into the uterine wall.
     - Guides hysterectomy or conservative surgical management in cases of placenta increta or percreta.

9. **Intraoperative Doppler Studies**
   - Role of USG:
     - Evaluates blood flow dynamics in the uterine and pelvic vessels during complex surgeries.
     - Helps avoid inadvertent damage to vital vascular structures.

10. **Scar Integrity Monitoring**
    - Role of USG:
      - Assesses cesarean scar integrity intraoperatively or postpartum.
      - Identifies dehiscence or defects that may require surgical repair.

Role of USG in Gynecological Diagnosis

1. **Anatomical Evaluation of the Pelvic Organs:**
   - Visualizes the uterus, ovaries, fallopian tubes (if abnormal), and surrounding structures.
   - Detects structural abnormalities and pathologies.

2. **Diagnosis of Uterine Disorders:**
   - Identifies fibroids, adenomyosis, and congenital uterine anomalies.
   - Evaluates endometrial thickness and abnormalities, including hyperplasia or polyps.

3. **Ovarian Assessment:**
   - Detects ovarian cysts, polycystic ovarian syndrome (PCOS), and tumors.
   - Monitors ovarian follicle development in infertility treatments.

4. **Evaluation of Abnormal Uterine Bleeding (AUB):**
   - Determines the cause of bleeding, such as endometrial polyps, submucosal fibroids, or thickened endometrium.

5. **Assessment of Pelvic Pain:**
   - Helps diagnose conditions like ovarian torsion, ectopic pregnancy, endometriosis, or pelvic inflammatory disease (PID).

6. **Diagnosis of Adnexal Masses:**
   - Differentiates between benign and malignant ovarian or adnexal masses.
   - Characterizes masses using Doppler to assess vascularity.

7. **Guidance for Interventional Procedures:**
   - Provides real-time imaging for procedures like follicular aspiration, hysterosonography (saline infusion sonography), intrauterine device (IUD) localization, and biopsy.

8. **Monitoring Post-Surgical or Post-Treatment Conditions:**
   - Evaluates the outcomes of surgeries like myomectomy or ovarian cystectomy.
   - Monitors the effects of medical therapies on endometrial thickness or ovarian function.

9. **Assessment of Infertility:**
   - Detects uterine or tubal factors contributing to infertility.
   - Monitors ovarian follicles during ovulation induction or assisted reproductive techniques.

10. **Diagnosis of Early Pregnancy Complications:**
    - Identifies ectopic pregnancy, retained products of conception, or gestational trophoblastic disease.

11. **Screening for Pelvic Malignancies:**
    - Detects early signs of ovarian or uterine cancers, including endometrial cancer.
    - Monitors for recurrence after treatment.

12. **Evaluation of Menopausal and Postmenopausal Changes:**
    - Assesses endometrial thickness for abnormal bleeding in postmenopausal women.
    - Detects atrophic changes or pathological lesions.

13. **Assessment of Congenital Anomalies:**
    - Identifies Müllerian anomalies, including uterine septum, bicornuate uterus, or unicornuate uterus.

Types of USG Used in Gynecological Diagnosis

1. **Transabdominal Ultrasound (TAUS):**
   - Conducted with a full bladder for optimal visualization of pelvic organs.
   - Provides an overview of large pelvic masses or uterine anomalies.

2. **Transvaginal Ultrasound (TVUS):**
   - Provides higher resolution imaging of the uterus, ovaries, and adnexa.
   - Preferred for evaluating early pregnancy, endometrial abnormalities, and ovarian cysts.

3. **Doppler Ultrasound:**
   - Assesses blood flow in pelvic masses, uterine arteries, and ovarian vessels.
   - Helps differentiate between benign and malignant tumors.

4. **3D Ultrasound:**
   - Reconstructs three-dimensional images of the uterus or adnexa.
   - Useful in diagnosing uterine anomalies and endometrial pathology.

5. **Saline Infusion Sonography (SIS):**
   - Involves the infusion of saline into the uterine cavity to visualize the endometrium.
   - Detects intrauterine adhesions, polyps, or submucosal fibroids.

Indications of USG in Gynecology

Uterine Disorders
- Abnormal uterine bleeding (AUB).
- Fibroids (leiomyomas).
- Adenomyosis.
- Endometrial hyperplasia or carcinoma.
- Congenital uterine anomalies.

Ovarian and Adnexal Disorders
- Ovarian cysts (functional, dermoid, endometriomas).
- Polycystic ovarian syndrome (PCOS).
- Ovarian torsion.
- Adnexal masses (benign or malignant).
- Tubo-ovarian abscesses (TOA).

Infertility and Reproductive Health
- Monitoring follicular development.
- Diagnosing polycystic ovarian syndrome.
- Assessing uterine or tubal factors contributing to infertility.

Pelvic Pain
- Evaluation of suspected ovarian torsion or rupture.
- Diagnosis of ectopic pregnancy.
- Detection of endometriosis or pelvic inflammatory disease (PID).

Postmenopausal Evaluation
- Assessment of endometrial thickness in abnormal bleeding.
- Identification of atrophic changes or malignancies.

Pelvic Masses
- Differentiation of cystic, solid, or complex masses.
- Evaluation of size, vascularity, and malignant potential.

Early Pregnancy and Related Complications
- Confirmation and location of pregnancy.
- Diagnosis of ectopic pregnancy.
- Detection of gestational trophoblastic disease or molar pregnancy.

Others
- Localization and evaluation of intrauterine devices (IUDs).
- Follow-up of gynecological surgeries or interventions.
- Screening for gynecological cancers in high-risk individuals.

USG In OBS/GYN

USG in ANC:

1. **Confirmation of Pregnancy:**
   - Detection of an intrauterine pregnancy.
   - Exclusion of ectopic pregnancy or molar pregnancy.

2. **Dating of Pregnancy (Gestational Age Assessment):**
   - Accurate estimation of gestational age using crown-rump length (CRL) in the first trimester.
   - Reduces errors in calculating the expected date of delivery (EDD).

3. **Assessment of Fetal Viability:**
   - Identification of fetal cardiac activity.
   - Monitoring for early pregnancy complications like missed abortion.

4. **Screening for Fetal Abnormalities:**
   - Detection of structural anomalies (e.g., anencephaly, spina bifida).
   - Nuchal translucency measurement in the first trimester for chromosomal abnormalities (e.g., Down syndrome).

5. **Monitoring Fetal Growth and Development:**
   - Evaluation of fetal growth parameters (e.g., biparietal diameter, femur length, abdominal circumference).
   - Assessment of intrauterine growth restriction (IUGR) or macrosomia.

6. **Assessment of Amniotic Fluid:**
   - Measurement of amniotic fluid index (AFI) or single deepest pocket.
   - Diagnosis of oligohydramnios or polyhydramnios.

7. **Placental Localization and Function:**
   - Identification of placental location (e.g., low-lying placenta, placenta previa).
   - Detection of placental abnormalities like placenta accreta.

8. **Evaluation of Multiple Pregnancies:**
   - Determination of chorionicity and amnionicity.
   - Monitoring for complications like twin-twin transfusion syndrome (TTTS).

9. **Assessment of Fetal Position and Presentation:**
   - Detection of malpresentation (e.g., breech, transverse lie).

10. **Doppler Studies for Fetal Well-Being:**
    - Assessment of uteroplacental and fetal circulation (e.g., umbilical artery, middle cerebral artery Doppler).
    - Useful in cases of fetal growth restriction or preeclampsia.
11. **Guidance for Invasive Procedures:**
    - Real-time guidance for procedures like amniocentesis, chorionic villus sampling (CVS), and cordocentesis.
12. **Assessment of Cervical Length:**
    - Prediction of preterm labor using transvaginal ultrasound.
    - Monitoring in cases of cervical incompetence.
13. **Monitoring Maternal Conditions:**
    - Identification of uterine anomalies, fibroids, or adnexal masses.
    - Assessment of complications like uterine rupture or scar dehiscence.

Types of Ultrasound in ANC:

1. **Transabdominal Ultrasound (TAUS):**
    - Performed by placing the probe on the abdomen.
    - Used for routine assessments and third-trimester evaluations.
2. **Transvaginal Ultrasound (TVUS):**
    - Performed by inserting a probe into the vagina.
    - Provides better resolution in early pregnancy and for assessing cervical length.
3. **3D and 4D Ultrasound:**
    - Provides detailed views of fetal anatomy.
    - 4D ultrasound adds real-time imaging for better visualization of fetal movements and expressions.
4. **Doppler Ultrasound:**
    - Evaluates blood flow in the umbilical artery, uterine arteries, and fetal vessels.
    - Used in high-risk pregnancies (e.g., preeclampsia, IUGR).
5. **Level II Ultrasound (Anomaly Scan):**
    - Detailed examination of fetal anatomy between 18–22 weeks.
    - Identifies structural anomalies and markers of chromosomal abnormalities.
6. **Biophysical Profile (BPP):**
    - Combines ultrasound with fetal heart rate monitoring.
    - Assesses fetal well-being by evaluating movements, tone, breathing, and amniotic fluid.

Timing of USG in ANC:

1. **First Trimester (6–13 weeks):**
    - Confirmation of pregnancy.
    - Dating scan.
    - Early anomaly screening (nuchal translucency).

2. **Second Trimester (18–22 weeks):**
    - Detailed anomaly scan.
    - Placental localization.
    - Growth assessment.

3. **Third Trimester (28–40 weeks):**
    - Monitoring fetal growth and well-being.
    - Doppler studies for high-risk cases.
    - Assessment of fetal presentation and amniotic fluid.

Role of USG in the Puerperal Period

The puerperal period, also known as the postpartum period, refers to the time following childbirth, lasting about 6 weeks, during which the body undergoes significant physiological changes. USG is commonly used to evaluate and manage complications during this period.

1. **Postpartum Hemorrhage (PPH)**
    - Role of USG:
        - Identifies retained products of conception (RPOC) or clots in the uterine cavity.
        - Detects uterine atony or subinvolution of the uterus.
        - Assesses the size and shape of the uterus to detect abnormalities.

2. **Retained Products of Conception (RPOC)**
    - Role of USG:
        - Identifies echogenic material within the uterine cavity.
        - Differentiates between clots and placental tissue using Doppler imaging (vascularity assessment).

3. **Endometritis (Postpartum Infection)**
    - Role of USG:
        - Evaluates the endometrial thickness and detects retained products or infected tissue.
        - Identifies fluid collections or abscesses in the uterine cavity.

4. **Uterine Rupture or Scar Dehiscence**
    - Role of USG:

- Assesses uterine integrity in women with a history of cesarean section or uterine surgery.
- Identifies any defects, hematomas, or abnormal thinning at the scar site.

5. **Pelvic Abscess or Hematoma**
   - Role of USG:
     - Detects pelvic collections or hematomas in the broad ligament, pelvic cavity, or cesarean section incision site.
     - Differentiates between simple and complex fluid collections.

6. **Uterine Subinvolution**
- Role of USG:
  - Monitors uterine size and involution postpartum.
  - Detects conditions like adenomyosis or fibroids that may hinder normal involution.

7. **Postpartum Ovarian or Adnexal Complications**
   - Role of USG:
     - Diagnoses ovarian cysts, torsion, or masses postpartum.
     - Detects adnexal pathology that may mimic postpartum complications.

8. **Postpartum Thrombosis**
   - Role of USG (Doppler Studies):
     - Evaluates blood flow in pelvic veins to identify deep vein thrombosis (DVT) or pelvic vein thrombosis.
     - Helps in early diagnosis of life-threatening conditions like pulmonary embolism.

Role of USG During Operative Procedures in Obstetrics

Ultrasound provides real-time guidance for various operative procedures, ensuring precision, reducing complications, and improving outcomes. Below are the main applications:

1. **Cesarean Section**
   - Role of USG:
     - Assesses placental location and identifies conditions like placenta previa or placenta accreta spectrum disorders (PAS).
     - Guides surgical incision to avoid placental disruption.
     - Helps detect uterine anomalies or fibroids that may complicate the procedure.

2. **Manual Removal of Placenta**
   - Role of USG:
     - Confirms complete removal of the placenta and absence of retained fragments.

- Identifies uterine abnormalities that could hinder complete placental expulsion.

3. **Uterine Artery Embolization (UAE)**
   - Role of USG:
     - Guides embolization procedures for controlling intractable postpartum hemorrhage.
     - Assesses blood flow and vascular supply to uterine arteries using Doppler imaging.

4. **Evacuation of Retained Products**
   - Role of USG:
     - Provides guidance for dilatation and curettage (D&C) or vacuum aspiration.
     - Ensures complete evacuation of RPOC while minimizing the risk of uterine perforation.

5. **Drainage of Postpartum Abscess or Hematoma**
   - Role of USG:
     - Guides percutaneous or transvaginal aspiration of pelvic abscesses or hematomas.
     - Assesses the resolution of the abscess post-drainage.

6. **Operative Management of Ectopic Pregnancy**
   - Role of USG:
     - Guides laparoscopic or transvaginal procedures for ectopic pregnancies.
     - Assists in the localization of ectopic gestational tissue.

7. **Uterine Tamponade or Balloon Placement**
   - Role of USG:
     - Guides the placement of intrauterine balloon catheters (e.g., Bakri balloon) for managing severe PPH.
     - Confirms correct positioning within the uterine cavity.

8. **Placenta Accreta Spectrum (PAS) Management**
   - Role of USG:
     - Preoperatively evaluates placental invasion into the uterine wall.
     - Guides hysterectomy or conservative surgical management in cases of placenta increta or percreta.

9. **Intraoperative Doppler Studies**
   - Role of USG:
     - Evaluates blood flow dynamics in the uterine and pelvic vessels during complex surgeries.
     - Helps avoid inadvertent damage to vital vascular structures.

10. Scar Integrity Monitoring
- Role of USG:
  - Assesses cesarean scar integrity intraoperatively or postpartum.
  - Identifies dehiscence or defects that may require surgical repair.

Role of USG in Gynecological Diagnosis

1. **Anatomical Evaluation of the Pelvic Organs:**
   - Visualizes the uterus, ovaries, fallopian tubes (if abnormal), and surrounding structures.
   - Detects structural abnormalities and pathologies.

2. **Diagnosis of Uterine Disorders:**
   - Identifies fibroids, adenomyosis, and congenital uterine anomalies.
   - Evaluates endometrial thickness and abnormalities, including hyperplasia or polyps.

3. **Ovarian Assessment:**
   - Detects ovarian cysts, polycystic ovarian syndrome (PCOS), and tumors.
   - Monitors ovarian follicle development in infertility treatments.

4. **Evaluation of Abnormal Uterine Bleeding (AUB):**
   - Determines the cause of bleeding, such as endometrial polyps, submucosal fibroids, or thickened endometrium.

5. **Assessment of Pelvic Pain:**
   - Helps diagnose conditions like ovarian torsion, ectopic pregnancy, endometriosis, or pelvic inflammatory disease (PID).

6. **Diagnosis of Adnexal Masses:**
   - Differentiates between benign and malignant ovarian or adnexal masses.
   - Characterizes masses using Doppler to assess vascularity.

7. **Guidance for Interventional Procedures:**
   - Provides real-time imaging for procedures like follicular aspiration, hysterosonography (saline infusion sonography), intrauterine device (IUD) localization, and biopsy.

8. **Monitoring Post-Surgical or Post-Treatment Conditions:**
   - Evaluates the outcomes of surgeries like myomectomy or ovarian cystectomy.
   - Monitors the effects of medical therapies on endometrial thickness or ovarian function.

9. **Assessment of Infertility:**
   - Detects uterine or tubal factors contributing to infertility.

- o Monitors ovarian follicles during ovulation induction or assisted reproductive techniques.

10. **Diagnosis of Early Pregnancy Complications:**
    - o Identifies ectopic pregnancy, retained products of conception, or gestational trophoblastic disease.

11. **Screening for Pelvic Malignancies:**
    - o Detects early signs of ovarian or uterine cancers, including endometrial cancer.
    - o Monitors for recurrence after treatment.

12. **Evaluation of Menopausal and Postmenopausal Changes:**
    - o Assesses endometrial thickness for abnormal bleeding in postmenopausal women.
    - o Detects atrophic changes or pathological lesions.

13. **Assessment of Congenital Anomalies:**
    - o Identifies Müllerian anomalies, including uterine septum, bicornuate uterus, or unicornuate uterus.

Types of USG Used in Gynecological Diagnosis

1. **Transabdominal Ultrasound (TAUS):**
   - o Conducted with a full bladder for optimal visualization of pelvic organs.
   - o Provides an overview of large pelvic masses or uterine anomalies.

2. **Transvaginal Ultrasound (TVUS):**
   - o Provides higher resolution imaging of the uterus, ovaries, and adnexa.
   - o Preferred for evaluating early pregnancy, endometrial abnormalities, and ovarian cysts.

3. **Doppler Ultrasound:**
   - o Assesses blood flow in pelvic masses, uterine arteries, and ovarian vessels.
   - o Helps differentiate between benign and malignant tumors.

4. **3D Ultrasound:**
   - o Reconstructs three-dimensional images of the uterus or adnexa.
   - o Useful in diagnosing uterine anomalies and endometrial pathology.

5. **Saline Infusion Sonography (SIS):**
   - o Involves the infusion of saline into the uterine cavity to visualize the endometrium.
   - o Detects intrauterine adhesions, polyps, or submucosal fibroids.

Indications of USG in Gynecology

Uterine Disorders
- Abnormal uterine bleeding (AUB).

- Fibroids (leiomyomas).
- Adenomyosis.
- Endometrial hyperplasia or carcinoma.
- Congenital uterine anomalies.

Ovarian and Adnexal Disorders
- Ovarian cysts (functional, dermoid, endometriomas).
- Polycystic ovarian syndrome (PCOS).
- Ovarian torsion.
- Adnexal masses (benign or malignant).
- Tubo-ovarian abscesses (TOA).

Infertility and Reproductive Health
- Monitoring follicular development.
- Diagnosing polycystic ovarian syndrome.
- Assessing uterine or tubal factors contributing to infertility.

Pelvic Pain
- Evaluation of suspected ovarian torsion or rupture.
- Diagnosis of ectopic pregnancy.
- Detection of endometriosis or pelvic inflammatory disease (PID).

Postmenopausal Evaluation
- Assessment of endometrial thickness in abnormal bleeding.
- Identification of atrophic changes or malignancies.

Pelvic Masses
- Differentiation of cystic, solid, or complex masses.
- Evaluation of size, vascularity, and malignant potential.

Early Pregnancy and Related Complications
- Confirmation and location of pregnancy.
- Diagnosis of ectopic pregnancy.
- Detection of gestational trophoblastic disease or molar pregnancy.

Others
- Localization and evaluation of intrauterine devices (IUDs).
- Follow-up of gynecological surgeries or interventions.
- Screening for gynecological cancers in high-risk individuals.

Vaginitis

Definition -
- Vaginitis refers to the **inflammation of the vaginal tissues**, which may result in abnormal discharge, itching, discomfort, and pain in the vaginal area

Types of Vaginitis

1. **Bacterial Vaginosis (BV)**
   o Caused by an imbalance of the normal bacteria in the vagina, particularly **Gardnerella vaginalis** and **Atopobium vaginae**.

2. **Candidiasis (Yeast Infection)**
   o Primarily caused by an overgrowth of **Candida albicans** or other Candida species.

3. **Trichomoniasis**
   o Caused by the protozoan parasite **Trichomonas vaginalis**.

4. **Atrophic Vaginitis**
   o Due to thinning and inflammation of the vaginal walls, often caused by **low estrogen levels** during menopause or post-menopause.

5. **Allergic Vaginitis**
   o Caused by allergies to **latex**, **spermicides**, **douches**, or certain soaps and detergents.

Etiology (Causes) of Vaginitis

1. **Bacterial Vaginosis:**
   o **Overgrowth of anaerobic bacteria** like **Gardnerella vaginalis**. This disrupts the natural balance of vaginal flora.
   o Risk factors include multiple sexual partners, douching, lack of condom use, and antibiotic use.

2. **Candidiasis:**
   o Caused by the overgrowth of Candida species, usually Candida albicans. Risk factors include antibiotic use, pregnancy, diabetes, immunocompromised states, and increased estrogen levels.

3. **Trichomoniasis:**
   o Caused by the parasite **Trichomonas vaginalis**, typically spread through **sexual contact**.

4. **Atrophic Vaginitis:**
    - Commonly seen in post-menopausal women, due to the reduction in estrogen levels, leading to thinning of the vaginal walls and loss of lubrication.

5. **Allergic Vaginitis:**
    - Due to an allergic reaction to products like **douches**, **spermicides**, **latex**, or fragrances in soaps and detergents.

Clinical Features of Vaginitis

1. **Bacterial Vaginosis**
    - **Discharge**: **Thin, grayish-white, fishy-smelling** discharge, often more noticeable after intercourse.
    - **Itching**: Occasional itching, but usually minimal.
    - **Odor**: **Strong fishy odor**, especially after intercourse.
    - **Pain**: Rare, but may experience mild vaginal discomfort.

2. **Candidiasis**
    - Discharge: Thick, white, cottage cheese-like discharge.
    - **Itching**: **Severe itching** and irritation in the vaginal area.
    - **Pain**: Pain or discomfort during urination or sexual intercourse.
    - **Redness and Swelling**: In the vaginal and vulvar areas.

3. **Trichomoniasis**
    - Discharge: Frothy, yellow-green, and may have a foul odor.
    - Itching and Burning: Severe itching, burning sensation during urination and intercourse.
    - **Pain**: Pelvic pain and discomfort.
    - **Urinary Symptoms**: Painful urination and frequent urination.

4. **Atrophic Vaginitis**
    - Discharge: Dryness, minimal discharge, or slight watery discharge.
    - **Itching**: Vaginal itching and irritation.
    - Pain: Painful intercourse (dyspareunia), vaginal dryness, and burning.
    - **Urinary Symptoms**: Urinary urgency and frequent infections.

5. **Allergic Vaginitis**
    - **Discharge**: May or may not have discharge, often clear or slightly watery.
    - Itching and Swelling: Severe itching and swelling of the vulva and vagina.
    - **Pain**: Vaginal pain or soreness, typically associated with irritation from allergens.
    - **Redness**: Local redness and inflammation due to irritation.

Complications of Vaginitis

1. **Pelvic Inflammatory Disease (PID):**
   - Untreated vaginitis can lead to **PID**, causing inflammation of the reproductive organs.

2. **Infertility:**
   - Bacterial infections, especially **gonorrhea** and **Chlamydia**, can lead to scarring of the fallopian tubes and increase the risk of infertility.

3. **Recurrent Infections:**
   - **Chronic candidiasis** or **BV** can cause recurrent infections and affect the quality of life.

4. **Pregnancy Complications:**
   - Vaginitis, particularly **BV**, can increase the risk of **preterm labor**, **low birth weight**, and **infections** during childbirth.

5. **Sexual Transmission:**
   - **Trichomoniasis** can be sexually transmitted and may increase susceptibility to other STIs.

Diagnosis of Vaginitis

1. **Microscopic Examination:**
   - Wet mount to detect Trichomonas, Candida, or bacterial overgrowth.

2. **Gram Stain:**
   - For **BV**, a **Gram stain** will show a **clue cell** (vaginal epithelial cell with bacteria adhering to its surface).

3. **Culture:**
   - Culture for **Candida**, **Trichomonas**, or **Gardnerella** can confirm the diagnosis.

4. **pH Testing:**
   - **Vaginal pH** test: BV and Trichomoniasis usually result in a pH above 4.5. **Candidiasis** typically does not change the pH significantly.

5. **Nucleic Acid Amplification Tests (NAAT):**
   - For Chlamydia, gonorrhea, and Trichomonas.

Allopathic Drug Management of Vaginitis

Type of Vaginitis	Treatment (Allopathic)
Bacterial Vaginosis (BV)	- **Metronidazole** (oral or vaginal gel)
	- **Clindamycin** (oral or vaginal cream)

Type of Vaginitis	Treatment (Allopathic)
Candidiasis (Yeast Infection)	- Fluconazole (oral)
	- **Clotrimazole**, **Miconazole** (vaginal creams or suppositories)
Trichomoniasis	- Metronidazole (oral)
Atrophic Vaginitis	- **Topical estrogen** (creams, tablets, or rings)
Allergic Vaginitis	- **Antihistamines** (oral or topical)
	- **Steroid creams** (hydrocortisone or stronger for allergic reactions)

Homeopathic Therapeutic InDications for Vaginitis

1. **Borax**
   - Indications:
     - For candida infections, where there is severe itching, painful urination, and a thick white discharge.
     - Burning sensation in the vagina.

2. **Sepia**
   - Indications:
     - For **vaginal dryness** and **irritation**, especially in **post-menopausal women** or those with hormonal imbalances.
     - Heavy, offensive discharge, often with pelvic congestion.

3. **Natrum Muriaticum**
   - Indications:
     - For **itching, burning**, and **dryness** in the vaginal area.
     - Vaginal discharge with a stale odor, often following emotional stress or grief.

4. **Kali Bichromicum**
   - Indications:
     - For stringy, thick discharge with a foul odor.
     - Burning sensations in the vagina with painful intercourse.

5. **Mercurius Solubilis**
   - Indications:
     - For foul-smelling yellow discharge associated with bacterial vaginitis.
     - Excessive salivation, sore throat, and night sweats with vaginal infection.

6. **Pulsatilla**
    - Indications:
        - For itching and burning in the vagina with changeable symptoms.
        - Discharge may be yellow or greenish, with emotionally sensitive states.

7. **Graphites**
    - Indications:
        - For **itching, cracking,** and bleeding in the vaginal area with a thick, yellowish discharge.
        - Painful intercourse and vaginal fissures.

8. **Sulphur**
    - Indications:
        - For **itching, burning,** and **inflamed skin** around the vaginal area, especially if the patient has a **tendency to skin eruptions**.
        - Offensive discharge with a foul odor and worse at night

Vaginismus

Definition

Vaginismus is a **psychosexual disorder** characterized by **involuntary spasm of the vaginal muscles**, leading to pain and difficulty in vaginal penetration, including intercourse, tampon insertion, or gynecological examination. It is classified as a **female sexual dysfunction** and is primarily psychological but may have some physical contributors.

Types of Vaginismus

Type	Characteristics
Primary Vaginismus	- Present since the first attempt at vaginal penetration (lifelong condition). - Often linked to psychological trauma or fear of pain.
Secondary Vaginismus	- Develops later in life after a period of normal function. - May be due to infections, trauma, menopause, or emotional distress.
Global Vaginismus	- Occurs in **all situations** where penetration is attempted.
Situational Vaginismus	- Occurs only in **specific situations**, such as with intercourse but not with tampons.

Causes and Risk Factors

Category	Causes
Psychological Factors	- **Fear of pain** (dyspareunia) - Sexual trauma or abuse - Anxiety or stress about intercourse - Negative cultural or religious beliefs about sex
Physical Factors	- Pelvic inflammatory disease (PID) - Endometriosis - Vaginal atrophy (menopause-related) - Urinary tract infections (UTIs)
Relationship Factors	- Marital conflict - Performance anxiety - Lack of trust in partner

Category	Causes
Neuromuscular Factors	- **Overactive pelvic floor muscles** leading to reflex contraction

Clinical Features

Category	Symptoms
Vaginal Symptoms	- Involuntary vaginal muscle contractions - Burning, stinging, or tightness during penetration - Difficulty inserting tampons or undergoing gynecological exams
Psychological Symptoms	- Severe anxiety or fear of penetration - Avoidance of sexual activity
Relationship Issues	- **Emotional distress** affecting intimacy - Strained partner relationships due to fear of intercourse

Complications

Complication	Effects
Sexual Dysfunction	- Inability to engage in intercourse (dyspareunia)
Infertility	- Difficulty conceiving due to inability to have penetrative sex
Emotional & Mental Health Issues	- Depression, anxiety, low self-esteem
Marital/Relationship Strain	- Frustration and stress in intimate relationships
Avoidance of Medical Care	- Fear of gynecological exams leading to undiagnosed reproductive health issues

Diagnosis

Investigation	Findings
Clinical History	-History of **pain or fear during penetration** - Psychological and sexual history evaluation
Pelvic Examination	- May be difficult due to muscle spasms - If tolerated, examination may **exclude organic causes**

Investigation	Findings
Cotton Swab Test	- Assesses sensitivity and muscle response to touch
Psychological Assessment	- Evaluates underlying fear, trauma, or relationship issues

Allopathic Drug Management

Category	Drugs and Dosage
Muscle Relaxants	- **Diazepam (2-5 mg PO at bedtime)** – Helps relax pelvic floor muscles
Topical Anesthetics	- **Lidocaine gel (2-5%) applied locally** – Reduces pain during penetration
Botox Injections	- OnabotulinumtoxinA (50-100 units injected into vaginal muscles) – Relaxes involuntary contractions
Hormonal Therapy	- Topical estrogen cream (0.5g intravaginally daily for 2 weeks, then twice weekly) – Used for postmenopausal atrophy
Antidepressants/Anxiolytics	- **SSRIs (Fluoxetine 20 mg/day PO)** – If associated with anxiety or depression

Non-Pharmacological Management

- **Pelvic floor physical therapy** (Kegel exercises, desensitization techniques)
- Cognitive-behavioral therapy (CBT) (addresses fear and anxiety)
- **Dilator therapy** (gradual vaginal insertion with increasing sizes)
- **Couples counseling** (if relationship issues contribute to vaginismus)

Homeopathic Remedies for Vaginismus

Remedy	Indications
Sepia	- Vaginal dryness, pain, **aversion to intercourse** - Women who feel emotionally distant from their partners
Platina	- Extreme vaginal tightness and pain - Hypersexual thoughts but fear of actual intercourse
Lachesis	- Painful spasm during intercourse, especially during menopause - Fear of penetration
Staphysagria	- History of sexual trauma or abuse

Remedy	Indications
Ignatia Amara	- Suppressed anger, deep emotional wounds - Emotional distress, grief, or anxiety leading to sexual dysfunction
Causticum	- **Pelvic muscle weakness**, fear of intercourse - Involuntary muscle spasms
Pulsatilla	- Timid, emotional women with fear of intimacy - Vaginal dryness, burning pain
Hypericum	- Nerve pain in the vaginal region following injury or surgery

Various Obstretric And Gynaecological Procedure

1. Cesarean Section (C-Section)

Definition
A surgical procedure where a baby is delivered through an incision made in the mother's abdomen and uterus.

Indications
- **Maternal Indications**: Prolonged labor, uterine rupture, maternal infection (e.g., herpes), obstructed labor, maternal exhaustion.
- **Fetal Indications**: Fetal distress, abnormal fetal presentation (e.g., breech or transverse), cord prolapse, multiple gestation.
- **Placental Indications**: Placenta previa, placental abruption.
- **Other**: Elective reasons or previous C-section.

Brief Procedure
1. Preoperative preparations include sterilization, catheterization, and anesthesia.
2. A horizontal (Pfannenstiel) or vertical incision is made in the abdomen.
3. The uterine wall is incised, and the baby is delivered.
4. The placenta is removed, and the uterus and abdominal layers are sutured.

Anesthesia Required
- Regional anesthesia (spinal or epidural) is most commonly used.
- General anesthesia may be required in emergencies.

Complications
- **Maternal**: Infection, excessive bleeding, injury to surrounding organs (bladder, bowel), blood clots, anesthetic complications.
- **Fetal**: Breathing difficulties, minor surgical injuries.

Pre-Procedure Care
- Ensure fasting for 6–8 hours before surgery.
- Consent form signed after explaining risks.
- Preoperative blood tests (CBC, blood group, cross-matching).
- Prophylactic antibiotics and IV line placement.

Post-Procedure Care
- Pain management with analgesics.
- Monitoring for bleeding, infection, and clot formation.
- Encourage breastfeeding and ambulation.
- Remove sutures or staples around a week post-surgery if non-dissolvable.

2. Episiotomy

Definition
A surgical incision made in the perineum to enlarge the vaginal opening during childbirth.

Indications
- To prevent severe perineal tearing during delivery.
- Expedite delivery in cases of fetal distress.
- Assisted vaginal deliveries (forceps or vacuum).
- Rigid perineum that hinders the baby's descent.

Brief Procedure
1. Performed during crowning when the baby's head stretches the vaginal opening.
2. The incision is made in the midline or mediolateral direction.
3. Sutures are placed after delivery to repair the incision.

Anesthesia Required
- Local infiltration with lignocaine if no epidural is in place.
- Epidural anesthesia if already administered.

Complications
- Infection.
- Bleeding or hematoma formation.
- Pain during intercourse (dyspareunia).

Pre-Procedure Care
- Educate the mother about the need and benefits.
- Ensure sterile instruments.

Post-Procedure Care
- Pain relief with analgesics or topical ointments.
- Use sitz baths to soothe the area and prevent infection.
- Encourage gentle pelvic floor exercises once healing begins.

3. Forceps Delivery

Definition
A procedure where forceps (specialized instruments) are used to assist in delivering the baby's head during the second stage of labor.

Indications
- Prolonged second stage of labor.
- Fetal distress.
- Maternal exhaustion or inability to push effectively.
- Abnormal fetal position (e.g., occiput posterior).

Brief Procedure
1. The forceps are gently placed around the baby's head.
2. Traction is applied in synchronization with maternal contractions.
3. The baby is delivered, and the forceps are removed.

Anesthesia Required
- Regional anesthesia (epidural or spinal).
- Pudendal nerve block for minimal discomfort.

Complications
- **Maternal**: Vaginal or perineal tears, bleeding, infection.
- **Fetal**: Scalp injuries, facial nerve palsy, skull fractures.

Pre-Procedure Care
- Empty the bladder with a catheter.
- Ensure full cervical dilation and proper fetal position.

Post-Procedure Care
- Monitor the mother for bleeding or vaginal tears.
- Observe the baby for injuries like scalp hematomas.

4. Vacuum-Assisted Delivery

Definition
A procedure using a vacuum device to assist in delivering the baby's head.

Indications
- Prolonged second stage of labor.
- Fetal distress during delivery.
- Maternal exhaustion.

Brief Procedure
1. A suction cup is attached to the baby's head.
2. A vacuum is created, and gentle traction is applied during maternal contractions.
3. The baby's head is delivered.

Anesthesia Required
- Regional anesthesia (epidural or spinal).
- Pudendal block may also suffice.

Complications
- **Maternal**: Vaginal or perineal tears, bleeding.
- **Fetal**: Scalp bruising, cephalohematoma, intracranial hemorrhage.

Pre-Procedure Care
- Ensure adequate cervical dilation and assess fetal head position.
- Sterilize equipment.

Post-Procedure Care
- Observe the baby for scalp or neurological injuries.
- Provide maternal pain relief and wound care if tears occur.

5. Amniocentesis

Definition
A diagnostic procedure where amniotic fluid is aspirated for prenatal testing or fetal health assessment.

Indications
- Genetic testing (e.g., Down syndrome, spina bifida).
- Assessing fetal lung maturity.
- Detecting fetal infections or anemia.

Brief Procedure
1. Ultrasound guides needle placement into the amniotic sac.
2. A sample of amniotic fluid is aspirated.

Anesthesia Required
- Local anesthesia or no anesthesia; the procedure is minimally painful.

Complications
- Miscarriage (<1% risk).
- Amniotic fluid leakage.
- Preterm labor.

Pre-Procedure Care
- Explain the procedure and associated risks.
- Perform ultrasound to locate the placenta and fetus.

Post-Procedure Care
- Monitor for contractions or vaginal fluid leakage.
- Avoid strenuous activities for 24–48 hours.

6. External Cephalic Version (ECV)

Definition
A manual procedure to turn a breech fetus into the cephalic position.

Indications
- Breech or transverse lie after 36–37 weeks gestation.

Brief Procedure
1. Ultrasound confirms fetal position and placental location.
2. Tocolytics are administered to relax the uterus.
3. Gentle external pressure is applied to rotate the fetus.

Anesthesia Required
- None; tocolytics minimize discomfort.

Complications
- Fetal distress.
- Premature rupture of membranes.
- Placental abruption.

Pre-Procedure Care
- Non-stress test to ensure fetal well-being.
- Informed consent about risks.

Post-Procedure Care
- Monitor fetal heart rate for distress.
- Educate the mother on signs of labor.

7. Cerclage

Definition
A surgical procedure where a stitch is placed around the cervix to prevent premature dilation and preterm birth.

Indications
- Cervical insufficiency or a history of recurrent second-trimester losses.

Brief Procedure
1. A suture is placed around the cervix through the vaginal route.
2. The stitch is removed around 36–37 weeks or earlier if labor starts.

Anesthesia Required
- Regional or general anesthesia.

Complications
- Infection.
- Premature rupture of membranes.
- Cervical injury.

Pre-Procedure Care
- Ultrasound to assess cervical length.
- Administer prophylactic antibiotics.

Post-Procedure Care
- Monitor for contractions or signs of infection.
- Advise reduced physical activity if indicated.

8. Dilation and Curettage (D&C)

Definition
A procedure to remove tissue from the inside of the uterus for diagnostic or therapeutic purposes.

Indications
- Heavy or abnormal uterine bleeding.
- Postmenopausal bleeding.
- Retained products of conception (after miscarriage or childbirth).
- Endometrial biopsy for diagnosing cancer or other conditions.
- Treatment of incomplete or missed abortion.

Brief Procedure
1. The cervix is dilated using dilators or medication.
2. A curette or suction device is used to remove uterine tissue.

Anesthesia Required
- General anesthesia or local anesthesia with sedation.

Complications
- Uterine perforation.
- Infection (endometritis).
- Hemorrhage.
- Adhesions (Asherman syndrome).

Pre-Procedure Care
- Obtain informed consent.
- Ensure fasting if general anesthesia is used.
- Ultrasound may be done to assess uterine contents.

Post-Procedure Care
- Monitor for excessive bleeding or infection.
- Avoid intercourse or tampon use until healed.
- Follow-up with the doctor for histopathology results if performed.

9. Laparoscopy

Definition
A minimally invasive surgical procedure where a camera and instruments are inserted into the abdomen to diagnose or treat gynecological conditions.

Indications
- Diagnosis of pelvic pain, infertility, or endometriosis.
- Treatment of ovarian cysts, fibroids, ectopic pregnancy, or adhesions.
- Tubal sterilization.

Brief Procedure
1. A small incision is made near the navel.
2. The abdomen is inflated with carbon dioxide gas for better visibility.
3. A laparoscope and surgical instruments are inserted for diagnosis or treatment.

Anesthesia Required
- General anesthesia.

Complications
- Injury to surrounding organs (bladder, bowel).
- Infection or bleeding.
- Gas-related shoulder pain post-surgery.

Pre-Procedure Care
- Fasting for at least 8 hours.

- Blood tests and imaging (ultrasound, MRI) for surgical planning.

Post-Procedure Care
- Pain management.
- Encourage mobilization to prevent blood clots.
- Watch for fever, severe abdominal pain, or abnormal discharge.

10. Hysteroscopy

Definition
A diagnostic or operative procedure using a hysteroscope to view or treat conditions inside the uterus.

Indications
- Evaluation of abnormal uterine bleeding.
- Diagnosis of uterine abnormalities (polyps, fibroids, septum).
- Removal of retained intrauterine devices (IUDs).
- Endometrial ablation.

Brief Procedure
1. A hysteroscope is inserted through the cervix into the uterus.
2. Saline or gas is used to distend the uterine cavity for better visualization.
3. Operative tools may be used if needed.

Anesthesia Required
- Local, regional, or general anesthesia, depending on the procedure.

Complications
- Uterine perforation.
- Infection.
- Fluid overload.

Pre-Procedure Care
- Abstain from eating and drinking if general anesthesia is used.
- Administer prophylactic antibiotics if indicated.

Post-Procedure Care
- Monitor for fever, pain, or heavy bleeding.
- Rest and avoid strenuous activities for a few days.

11. Hysterectomy

Definition

Surgical removal of the uterus. Can be total (removal of uterus and cervix) or subtotal (uterus only).

Indications

- Uterine fibroids causing symptoms.
- Endometrial or cervical cancer.
- Severe endometriosis or adenomyosis.
- Chronic pelvic pain unresponsive to other treatments.

Brief Procedure

1. Can be performed via abdominal, vaginal, or laparoscopic approach.
2. Uterus is detached from surrounding structures and removed.
3. In some cases, ovaries and fallopian tubes are also removed (salpingo-oophorectomy).

Anesthesia Required

- General anesthesia or regional anesthesia (spinal/epidural).

Complications

- Infection, bleeding, or injury to adjacent organs.
- Blood clots.
- Hormonal changes if ovaries are removed.

Pre-Procedure Care

- Blood tests and imaging.
- Counseling on hormonal changes if ovaries are removed.

Post-Procedure Care

- Pain management.
- Early ambulation to prevent clots.
- Avoid lifting heavy objects for 6–8 weeks.

12. Colposcopy

Definition

A diagnostic procedure to examine the cervix, vagina, and vulva using a colposcope for abnormal tissue.

Indications

- Abnormal Pap smear results.
- Suspicion of cervical or vaginal dysplasia.

Brief Procedure
1. A speculum is inserted into the vagina.
2. The cervix is visualized, and acetic acid is applied to highlight abnormal areas.
3. A biopsy may be taken if necessary.

Anesthesia Required
- None or local anesthesia for biopsy.

Complications
- Bleeding or infection after biopsy.
- Mild discomfort.

Pre-Procedure Care
- Schedule the procedure when not menstruating.
- Avoid vaginal medications or intercourse 24 hours prior.

Post-Procedure Care
- Mild cramping or spotting may occur.
- Avoid tampons or intercourse until healing from biopsy.

13. Tubal Ligation

Definition
A permanent sterilization procedure involving blocking or cutting the fallopian tubes.

Indications
- Permanent contraception.

Brief Procedure
1. Can be done laparoscopically or during a cesarean section.
2. The fallopian tubes are blocked by clipping, cutting, or cauterizing.

Anesthesia Required
- General or regional anesthesia.

Complications
- Bleeding, infection.
- Rarely, failure leading to pregnancy.

Pre-Procedure Care
- Counseling on permanent nature of the procedure.
- Preoperative blood work.

Post-Procedure Care
- Avoid heavy lifting for a few days.
- Watch for signs of infection (fever, severe pain).

14. Endometrial Ablation

Definition
A procedure to destroy the uterine lining to reduce or stop heavy menstrual bleeding.

Indications
- Heavy menstrual bleeding not responsive to medical treatment.

Brief Procedure
1. Methods include thermal balloon, radiofrequency, or cryotherapy.
2. The endometrial lining is ablated using heat, electricity, or cold.

Anesthesia Required
- General or local anesthesia.

Complications
- Uterine perforation.
- Infection.
- Persistent bleeding.

Pre-Procedure Care
- Perform imaging (ultrasound) to evaluate the uterus.
- Rule out uterine cancer or pregnancy.

Post-Procedure Care
- Mild cramping and discharge are common.
- Avoid tampons and intercourse for 1–2 weeks.

15. Myomectomy

Definition
A surgical procedure to remove uterine fibroids (leiomyomas) while preserving the uterus.

Indications
- Symptomatic fibroids (e.g., heavy menstrual bleeding, pelvic pain, infertility).
- Large or rapidly growing fibroids.
- Desire to preserve fertility or avoid hysterectomy.

Brief Procedure
1. Performed through abdominal (open), laparoscopic, or hysteroscopic approach.

2. Fibroids are located and excised.
3. The uterine wall is repaired.

Anesthesia Required
- General anesthesia.

Complications
- Bleeding.
- Adhesion formation.
- Infection.
- Risk of uterine rupture in future pregnancies.

Pre-Procedure Care
- Imaging (e.g., ultrasound, MRI) to locate fibroids.
- Blood tests to assess hemoglobin levels.

Post-Procedure Care
- Monitor for excessive bleeding or infection.
- Encourage light activity to prevent blood clots.
- Contraception is recommended for a few months before trying to conceive.

16. Bartholin's Cyst Surgery

Definition
A surgical procedure to treat Bartholin's gland cysts or abscesses by drainage or removal.

Indications
- Recurrent or large Bartholin's cysts.
- Infected cyst or abscess.

Brief Procedure
1. **Incision and Drainage**: A small incision is made, and the cyst is drained.
2. **Marsupialization**: Edges of the cyst wall are sutured to create a permanent drainage opening.
3. In severe cases, the gland may be excised.

Anesthesia Required
- Local anesthesia with or without sedation.
- General anesthesia for gland excision.

Complications
- Infection or recurrence of the cyst.
- Scarring or discomfort.

Pre-Procedure Care
- Explain the procedure to the patient.
- Administer antibiotics if an abscess is present.

Post-Procedure Care
- Sitz baths to promote healing.
- Pain management.
- Monitor for signs of recurrence or infection.

17. Oophorectomy

Definition
Surgical removal of one or both ovaries.

Indications
- Ovarian cysts or tumors.
- Endometriosis.
- Ovarian torsion.
- Risk reduction in BRCA mutation carriers.

Brief Procedure
1. Can be performed via laparoscopic or open approach.
2. The ovary is identified, ligated, and removed.

Anesthesia Required
- General anesthesia.

Complications
- Bleeding or infection.
- Hormonal imbalance (if both ovaries are removed).
- Adhesion formation.

Pre-Procedure Care
- Imaging studies (ultrasound, MRI).
- Blood tests and counseling on hormonal effects (for bilateral oophorectomy).

Post-Procedure Care
- Hormone replacement therapy (if both ovaries are removed).
- Monitor for signs of infection or complications.

18. Cone Biopsy (Conization)

Definition
A surgical procedure to remove a cone-shaped section of abnormal tissue from the cervix.

Indications
- Diagnosis or treatment of cervical dysplasia or carcinoma in situ.

Brief Procedure
1. Performed using a scalpel (cold knife), laser, or loop electrosurgical excision procedure (LEEP).
2. A cone-shaped section of the cervix is removed.

Anesthesia Required
- Local anesthesia, regional anesthesia, or general anesthesia.

Complications
- Bleeding or infection.
- Cervical stenosis or incompetence.

Pre-Procedure Care
- Pap smear and colposcopy to assess abnormal tissue.
- Avoid intercourse or vaginal products before the procedure.

Post-Procedure Care
- Avoid heavy lifting and sexual activity for 4–6 weeks.
- Monitor for excessive bleeding or discharge.

19. Tubal Reanastomosis

Definition
A surgical procedure to restore fertility by reconnecting the fallopian tubes after tubal ligation.

Indications
- Desire for pregnancy after prior sterilization.

Brief Procedure
1. Performed via laparoscopic or open surgery.
2. The blocked segments of the fallopian tubes are reconnected.

Anesthesia Required
- General anesthesia.

Complications
- Ectopic pregnancy.
- Adhesion formation.

Pre-Procedure Care
- Hysterosalpingography (HSG) to assess tubal condition.
- Blood tests and counseling.

Post-Procedure Care
- Avoid strenuous activities for a few weeks.
- Follow-up imaging to confirm tubal patency.

20. Pelvic Floor Repair (Colporrhaphy)

Definition
A surgical procedure to repair weakened pelvic floor muscles and treat prolapse.

Indications
- Uterine, vaginal, or bladder prolapse.
- Urinary incontinence.

Brief Procedure
1. Anterior colporrhaphy repairs cystocele.
2. Posterior colporrhaphy repairs rectocele.
3. Vaginal tissues are tightened with sutures.

Anesthesia Required
- Regional or general anesthesia.

Complications
- Infection or bleeding.
- Dyspareunia (painful intercourse).

Pre-Procedure Care
- Pelvic examination and imaging.
- Bowel preparation may be needed.

Post-Procedure Care
- Avoid heavy lifting or straining.
- Use stool softeners to prevent constipation.

21. Vulvectomy

Definition
A surgical procedure to remove part or all of the vulva, usually for treating vulvar cancer or precancerous lesions.

Indications
- Vulvar cancer or precancerous conditions (VIN).
- Recurrent vulvar infections or lichen sclerosus.

Brief Procedure
1. Depending on the extent, partial or total removal of vulvar tissue is performed.
2. May include lymph node dissection in cancer cases.

Anesthesia Required
- General or regional anesthesia.

Complications
- Infection, wound healing issues.
- Lymphedema (if lymph nodes are removed).
- Altered sexual function.

Pre-Procedure Care
- Biopsy to confirm diagnosis.
- Counseling on the extent of surgery.

Post-Procedure Care
- Pain management and wound care.
- Monitor for lymphedema or infection.

22. Cervical Cerclage

Definition
A procedure where the cervix is stitched to prevent premature dilation and preterm birth.

Indications
- History of recurrent second-trimester miscarriages.
- Short cervix identified on ultrasound.

Brief Procedure
1. Sutures are placed around the cervix via vaginal (most common) or abdominal route.
2. The sutures are removed near term or if labor starts.

Anesthesia Required
- Regional or general anesthesia.

Complications
- Infection.
- Premature rupture of membranes.
- Cervical trauma.

Pre-Procedure Care
- Ultrasound to assess cervical length.
- Prophylactic antibiotics may be administered.

Post-Procedure Care
- Monitor for contractions or signs of infection.
- Advise avoiding strenuous activities.

www.ingramcontent.com/pod-product-compliance
Lightning Source LLC
LaVergne TN
LVHW070529070526
838199LV00075B/6739